Hospice Approaches to Pediatric Care

Charles A. Corr, Ph.D., is Professor in the School of Humanities, Southern Illinois University at Edwardsville, and a member of the Board of Directors of Hospice of Madison County (Granite City, Illinois). Previous volumes he has coedited include *Helping Children Cope with Death: Guidelines and Resources* (second edition, 1984) and *Childhood and Death* (1984).

Donna M. Corr, R.N., B.S.N., is Assistant Professor in the Nursing Faculty, St. Louis Community College at Forest Park, St. Louis, Missouri. With her husband, she is coeditor of *Hospice Care: Principles and Practice* (Springer Publishing Company, 1983).

Hospice Approaches to Pediatric Care

Charles A. Corr, Ph.D.
Donna M. Corr, R.N., B.S.N.

Editors

Springer Publishing Company
New York

Springer Publishing Company, Inc.
536 Broadway
New York, New York 10012

85 86 87 88 89 / 10 9 8 7 6 5 4 3 2 1

Library of Congress Cataloging in Publication Data

Main entry under title:

Hospice approaches to pediatric care.
Includes bibliographies and index.
1. Terminally ill children. 2. Hospice care. 3. Terminally ill children—Family relationships. 4. Children and death. 5. Death—Psychological aspects. I. Corr, Charles A. II. Corr, Donna M. [DNLM: 1. Grief—in infancy & childhood. 2. Hospices. 3. Terminal Care—in infancy & childhood. WS 200 H828]
RJ249.H67 1985 362.1'75 84-26736
ISBN 0-8261-4600-7

Printed in the United States of America

For Eric and Jess Wilkes,
and for Marjory Cockburn.

With respect, gratitude, and affection.

Contents

Preface *ix*

Contributors *xiii*

Part I Caring for Dying Children: General Principles 1

1. Developing a Hospice Program for Children 5
Dottie C. Wilson

2. The Dying Child: At Home 31
Ida M. Martinson and Marian Enos

3. Improving Care for Hospitalized Terminally Ill Children: A Practicable Model 43
Patricia Riordan Wheeler and Nancy Foerster Lange in consultation with Salvatore J. Bertolone

Part II Caring for Dying Children: Specific Applications 61

4. Home Care for Terminally Ill Children and Their Families 65
Belinda Barry Martin

5. Respite Care and the Dying Child 87
Rosalind Crenshaw Cutchins and Barbara S. Mease

6. Helen House: A Hospice for Children 107
Mother Frances Dominica

7. A Hospice Approach to Neonatal Care 127
Roberta Siegel, Susan H. Rudd, Cindy Cleveland, Linda K. Powers, and Robert J. Harmon

Part III Symbolic Interactions with Dying and Bereaved Children 153

8. Expressive Therapy with Children in Crisis: A New Avenue of Communication 155
Barbara Bouton Schmitt and Molly Hardy Guzzino

9. Amanda the Panda 179
JoAnn Zimmerman

Part IV Caring for Bereaved Children, Family Members, and Staff 195

10. Children's Grief: Individual and Family Dynamics 197
Stephen J. Fleming

11. Parental Bereavement 219
Charles A. Corr, Ida M. Martinson, and Kay L. Dyer

12. Self-Help Groups: Grieving Parents and Community Resources 241
Dennis Klass

13. An Approach to Caring: Caregiver Concerns 261
Marcia E. Lattanzi

Index 281

Preface

In an earlier book, *Hospice Care: Principles and Practice,* we sought to identify the basic principles that define hospice care and to show how they can be put to work in everyday practice. Our concerns in that undertaking were threefold. First, we wished to insist that *hospice is a philosophy, not a facility*—an outlook on care or, better yet, an approach to the giving of care, rather than a place in which services are offered. That approach is a coherent and unified way of delivering palliative care for the management of distressing symptoms when cure is no longer a reasonable expectation. It stresses maximizing present quality of life and, in many ways, is at its best when it enables those who can and who wish to do so to remain in their own homes. Second, we wanted to show that *hospice principles can be applied in diverse ways.* They are not limited, for example, to programs or settings that bear the label "hospice." Further, while the hospice approach is most closely identified with care for dying persons and their families, we wished to point out that this mode of care has relevance for many kinds of persons. Thus, hospice principles are applicable not only to those with cancer, but also to individuals coping with other terminal conditions, with chronic illnesses, and with bereavement. Third, we sought to make these points through *contributions from experts in the field,* each of whom was invited to speak authoritatively to a particular area of expertise.

In the present volume, we bring the same concerns to care that involves or is related to children. These children may be terminally ill, chronically ill, or bereaved survivors. Our scope also includes family members who are grieving the illness or death of a child, and those who care for such children and families. It is particularly appropriate that hospice approaches to pediatric care should be seen as not confined merely to the children themselves,—much less, exclusively to those who are dying—for the central message of hospice is that care must be addressed to the needs of whole persons and to every concerned individual. Death and chronic illness are not just biological events that only involve defective organs or malfunctioning biochemical systems. Instead, they are multidimensional phenomena with physical, psychological, social, and spiritual aspects. It is the whole child who is stressed by illness or bereavement, as well as his or her family and friends, and others who are drawn into the crisis. For all of these people, we strongly support a careful and comprehensive assessment of needs, the involvement of whatever professional and personal skills are useful in meeting those needs, the development of new initiatives, and the coordination of care insisted upon throughout this book. Further, we are particularly concerned that grieving children and other bereaved persons not be left to struggle alone. In the end, we seek to demonstrate that hospice approaches are relevant to pediatric care (conceived in this broad fashion), and that they can help in many ways to support or to improve quality of life.

We undertook this book as a result of a realization that those within the hospice movement and members of the pediatric health care community had much to learn from each other. Hospice workers have devoted the bulk of their efforts to the care of adult patients and particularly the elderly. Inevitably, however, they have found themselves involved with children—the second and third generation family members of their primary patients—who may need support both before and after the death of a relative. Further, hospice programs with a strong home care component are increasingly being asked to give aid where no other resources are available to make it possible for families with ill children to keep them at home. For these and other reasons, hospice personnel need to learn more about care involving children and about ways to adapt their underlying principles to new populations and situations.

Similarly, members of the pediatric community can benefit from the wealth of expertise that has recently been developed concerning needs of the dying and the bereaved. Pediatric caregivers have long been aware of children as members of family systems, and they have been open to psychosocial dimensions of care. At the same time, they—like many others in our society—have found it extraordinarily difficult to "give up," as it is often said, on efforts to prolong a child's life. One outcome has been beneficial: new techniques and therapeutic interventions have been developed that have increased survival and reduced death rates for many childhood diseases. But death and incurable conditions are not to be eradicated from childhood any more than from any other stage of life. Where they are inevitable or where the individual child and family unit judge that additional cure-oriented interventions have become too burdensome, it is the responsibility of the society and its health system not to quit but to turn to new and more relevant modes of care. The witness of hospice is that these new modes are no less active or aggressive than former strategies and that palliative care can be a rewarding option in certain limited situations.

Bringing hospice approaches to bear on pediatric care is potentially beneficial for a wide audience. Professional caregivers, volunteer helpers, students, parents, and the lay public can all learn from an enhanced understanding of hospice principles and their application to situations involving children. This is true even though there are as yet few landmarks in this field. These are early days for our subjects. But important beginnings have already been made in specific areas. And new initiatives continue to be launched. It is time to draw these diverse strands together, to identify what they have in common, and to point the way for the future. That is the purpose and the hope of this book.

Charles A. Corr, Ph.D.
Donna M. Corr, R.N., B.S.N.

Contributors

Salvatore J. Bertolone, M.D., is Assistant Professor of Pediatrics and Director, Pediatric Hematology/Oncology, University of Louisville School of Medicine, Louisville, Kentucky.

Cindy Cleveland, R.N., B.S.N., is Family Care Coordinator, Newborn Center, The Children's Hospital, Denver, Colorado.

Rosalind Crenshaw Cutchins, M.S., is Family Services Supervisor of Edmarc, Inc., Suffolk, Virginia.

Kay L. Dyer, R.N., B.S.N., has worked as a pastoral counselor and is currently a volunteer with Belleville Hospice, Inc., Belleville, Illinois.

Marian Enos, R.N., M.S., is Director of the People, Incorporated Epilepsy Program, Minneapolis, Minnesota. She was formerly associated with the University of Minnesota School of Nursing.

Stephen J. Fleming, Ph.D., is Associate Professor, Department of Psychology, Atkinson College, York University, Downsview, Ontario, Canada.

Mother Frances Dominica, S.R.N., R.S.C.N., F.R.C.N., is Superior General of the Anglican Society of All Saints and founder of Helen House, Oxford, England.

Molly Hardy Guzzino, M.A.A.T., is currently an art therapist at the San Marcos Treatment Center of the Brown Schools, San Marcos, Texas. Her early work on Chapter 8 was completed while she was Director of the Child Life Department at Tulane Medical Center Hospital, New Orleans, Louisiana.

Robert J. Harmon, M.D., is Associate Professor of Psychiatry, Division of Child Psychiatry, and Director of the Infant Psychiatry Clinic at the University of Colorado School of Medicine, Denver, Colorado. He is supported by Research Scientist Development Award 5K01 MH00281 and Research Project Grant 5 R01 MH34005 from the National Institute of Mental Health.

Dennis Klass, Ph.D., is Professor and Chairman of the Department of Theology, Webster University, St. Louis, Missouri.

Nancy Foerster Lange, R.N., is Pediatric Hospice Nurse, Hospice of Louisville, Inc., Louisville, Kentucky.

Marcia E. Lattanzi, R.N., M.A., is Director of Education and Bereavement, Boulder County Hospice, Inc., Boulder, Colorado.

Belinda Barry Martin, R.N., M.S.N., P.N.P., is Home Care Coordinator, Childrens Hospital of Los Angeles, Los Angeles, California.

Ida M. Martinson, R.N., Ph.D., F.A.A.N., is Professor and Chairperson of the Department of Family Health Care Nursing, School of Nursing, University of California, San Francisco, California. At the time of the work described in Chapter 2, she was Professor in the School of Nursing at the University of Minnesota, Minneapolis, Minnesota.

Barbara S. Mease, R.N., M.Div., is Director of Professional Services of Edmarc, Inc., Suffolk, Virginia.

Linda K. Powers, R.N., is Head Nurse, Department Head, Newborn Center, The Children's Hospital, Denver, Colorado.

Susan H. Rudd, M.S.S.A., is Perinatal Social Worker, Newborn Center, The Children's Hospital, Denver, Colorado.

Barbara Bouton Schmitt, M.A.A.T., is Coordinator of Education and Volunteers, and Expressive Therapist, Hospice of Louisville, Inc., Louisville, Kentucky.

Roberta Siegel, M.S.W., is Chief Perinatal Social Worker, Newborn Center, The Children's Hospital, Denver, Colorado.

Patricia Riordan Wheeler, R.N., M.S.N., R.N.C., F.N.P., was Executive Director, Hospice of Louisville, Inc., Louisville, Kentucky, at the time of writing Chapter 3.

Dottie C. Wilson is Director, Palliative Care Center, St. Mary's Hospital for Children, Bayside, New York.

JoAnn Zimmerman works as Amanda the Panda throughout the state of Iowa.

I

Caring for Dying Children: General Principles

When hospice principles are applied to situations involving children, it is only natural that a number of questions will be raised. For example, are hospice approaches to pediatric care desirable or even feasible? In what ways are these approaches unique? Why are they needed? Do they apply only to terminally ill and dying children, or do they also include parents, siblings, and other family members both before and after a death? What are the general principles that define this philosophy of care? How broad is its scope? What are the ways in which it can be implemented? Such questions deserve at least a preliminary response—something more than is contained in our prefatory remarks, something less than might be discovered by reading through this book as a whole. The three chapters in Part I introduce the general principles of hospice approaches to pediatric care, and thereby provide a provisional reply to the questions set forth above. We are especially pleased that these chapters were written by contributors who are widely acquainted with both hospice and pediatric care.

From her work in adult hospice care and at St. Mary's Hospital for Children in Bayside, New York, Dottie Wilson offers a detailed survey in Chapter 1 of the many distinctive elements in hospice care for children, the various dimensions of care that can fall under this heading and the many ways in which services can be provided either at home or in a health care facility, and the issues to be faced at each stage of program planning. This is both a review of constituent elements which can be individually adopted and adapted to local situations and existing programs, and an anticipation of components that will be taken up singly at greater length in later chapters of this book. We are fully aware that few programs are so fortunate as to be able to offer all of the services described here under a single administrative umbrella. But many can extend present services along one or another of these lines. That is certainly better than doing nothing, and it may be all that is needed in a specific community. Perhaps the most important point stressed in this chapter is the necessity and the value of careful assessment of needs and resources before an attempt is made to implement new services that are directed to children and families in connection with the poignant realities of dying, death, and bereavement.

In Chapter 2, Ida Martinson—who is perhaps the single foremost pioneer in this field—and Marian Enos set forth conclusions that were demonstrated beyond dispute in the Home Care Project in Minneapolis: under the right conditions and with appropriate support, dying children can not only be "sent" home to die, they and their families can achieve a healthy and meaningful time in their last days of life. The key to this innovative research project, as it is for all hospice care for ill and dying children, is that professional caregivers worked through and gave support to parents and other family members. Professionals did not "take over" the child's care and contribute to additional alienation or estrangement within the family. Lack of coordination—so frequently experienced in health care—was minimized, family resources were confirmed and utilized, and caregivers were themselves provided with ongoing support for their own legitimate needs. Anticipation of and preparation for difficult times was essential. Coordination of care and availability of support created a sense of underlying security that was invaluable for safe passage through crises. A caring community was created in and around the home and institutionalization, or integration within the health care system, was achieved when the results of this sort of care were demonstrably favorable.

About the time of the institutionalization phase in Minneapolis, an adult hospice program in Louisville, Kentucky, received a pediatric referral for home care. Much of the work of Hospice of Louisville with children has in fact been in the form of home care, but their personnel have also been involved in helping to prepare staff in a pediatric medical center to give improved care for dying children and in coordinating transitions in care between home and hospital. It is these latter subjects that Patricia

Wheeler and Nancy Lange primarily address in Chapter 3. In one sense, hospice approaches to pediatric care depend on a return to basic medical and nursing assessment and management; in another sense, they involve new sensitivity to the specific issues faced by dying children and their families, and the development of new skills required for appropriate responses to these issues. The intertwining of these aspects is clearly shown in this chapter, as are the underlying goals of integrating services and interventions in accordance with a collaborative model and in the interest of achieving quality time in living for both child and family.

1

Developing a Hospice Program for Children

Dottie C. Wilson

> Nothing would be done at all if a man waited until he could do it so well that no one could find fault with it.
>
> —*Cardinal Newman*

Introduction

One experience that all adults have in common is that we were once children; each of us can remember something of what it was like. One thing terminally ill children have in common is that they will never be adults. To many people this situation seems so shattering that they want to avoid involvement. But we can do something. We can make a start to improve the comfort, quality, and meaning of the short lives of these children by investing our talents and our skills, by sharing our knowledge and our time, by listening and caring.

Pediatric hospice programs are medically-directed health care programs specifically designed for dying children and their families. Staff and volunteers in such programs provide direct support and coordinate assistance available from other sources in order to meet the total needs of this unique population.

The concept of pediatric hospice care is a simple extension of the hospice philosophy. It is based on the premise that dying children and

The author acknowledges with sincere thanks the contributions to this chapter of Celia Berdes, M.S.P.H., and Burton Grebin, M.D.

their families, like dying adults and their families, can benefit from palliative care designed to maximize present quality of life. Although hospice planners focused first on adults because of their larger numbers, they have directed attention more recently to the smaller but perhaps more vulnerable group, the children.

While it has been recognized that the unmet needs of dying children demand attention, there continues to be debate as to the most beneficial approach, level, and location of care. This chapter will not attempt to resolve or even enter into that debate. Rather, it will describe our research and experience at St. Mary's Hospital for Children, raise pertinent questions, identify some of the problems we have experienced in answering these questions, and propose some approaches or guidelines. The discussion is organized around three general topics: (1) distinctive elements of hospice care for children; (2) dimensions of care, services needed, and ways they can be provided; and (3) steps and issues in program planning and development. These remarks are based on the author's nine years experience in hospice work, which has included both adult and pediatric hospice research, program planning, and service development.

By way of preface, it is important to note that there is no one right way to develop a pediatric hospice program. Each local situation—its needs, its resources, and the commitment of its people—determines the existence, dimensions, and quality of its own pediatric hospice care. Thus, it seems only fair to describe briefly the local situation on which is based much of our experience and our studies in the pediatric field. It is a unique situation, unlikely to be replicated elsewhere; however, its experience will provide useful information for others.

St. Mary's Hospital for Children is located in Bayside, Queens, which is part of metropolitan New York City. It was founded in 1870 by the Sisters of St. Mary, a religious order of the Episcopal Church. It is New York's only special purpose skilled nursing facility designed to meet the comprehensive needs of children with special medical problems. At present, these problems involve pediatric medicine, rehabilitation, pediatric allergy, birth defects, and genetic disease. For the past four years, St. Mary's has been developing its Palliative Care Center, a full-scale hospice program for children up to the age of 16 years, which will include home care, inpatient care in a specially designed ten-bed unit, day care, and bereavement care, as well as major education and research programs. Later, the Center may include outpatient clinic care, night care, and expanded community services.

The Center has been developed through the successful blending of the author's background in adult hospice work, the expertise of the hospital's management and staff in children and their needs, and the knowledge of the state's and city's regulatory agency officials in licensure and reimbursement. Concurrently, the work of others, both in the literature and in the community, has contributed greatly.

Among the benefits of this cooperative effort has been the identification of a number of clear distinctions between adult and pediatric hospice care. These distinctive elements affect both program planning and ongoing care provision.

Distinctive Elements

Apart from the distinction of being new and relatively untried, hospice care for children differs from hospice care for adults in a number of aspects: the patients themselves, the families, the caregivers, the location of care, and the influence of regulatory agencies (Wilson, 1982).

Patients

Distinctions can be seen in the size of the patient pool, the ages and developmental levels of the children, their diagnoses, and their length of hospice stay.

The Patient Pool. Fortunately, medical advances in recent years have succeeded in significantly reducing mortality rates in childhood. As a result, however, those children who are dying are so small in number that the diversity of a program necessary to meet their needs is difficult to develop and to support, both financially and qualitatively.

Age and Developmental Level. What age is a child? Although in an adult hospice a 20-year-old and an 80-year-old patient may not have similar needs, the diversity of needs and care requirements of children from birth to adulthood can become overwhelming. A child is a product of his or her chronological age, developmental age, and medical condition. Furthermore, variations in size, handicap, level of cognition and communication, and social and activity interests also affect service provision, staffing, and facility design (Stillion & Wass, 1979; Bluebond-Langner, 1978, pp. 3 –14).

Diagnoses. Considering the small size of the patient population, specialization in one terminal disease such as cancer may be unrealistic. Yet, a diversity of terminal conditions in children increases the need for a variety of service modalities and expanded staff knowledge and skills. This diversity compounds previously mentioned variations in patient age and ability.

Length of Hospice Stay. In the opinion of a number of the pediatricians contacted by the author, as well as those cited in the literature (e.g.,

Calman, 1978, p. 42), it is more difficult to establish in children than in adults when a disease is terminal and when hospice referral is appropriate. Length of stay, therefore, may be considerably shorter or very much longer than is usual in adult hospice programs. As a result, consistency in staffing and service provision may be particularly difficult to maintain.

Our research has identified dying children who are appropriate for hospice care as a small group, widely scattered geographically, with more variation than adults in size, interests, understanding, communication abilities, handicaps, diagnoses, prognoses, and length of stay. How can their needs be met? Were it not for the small patient population size, the method of choice would be a separate program for each combination of variables.

Families

Among the families of dying children, there are distinctions in size, responsibility, role as caregivers, and needs.

Size. The families of young patients tend to be larger than those of older ones. Parents and grandparents usually are still living, siblings are often still in the home, and school and neighborhood friends are part of the affected family group. Both because of the size of the family and because most of its members have not faced a pediatric death before, the task of meeting family needs requires special attention, skill, and time.

Responsibility. Parents are said to "own" their children. Since children are minors, parents make decisions for them. Since parents sometimes see the child's needs quite differently from the way the child or the staff see them, care provision and communication are affected. In adult hospice programs the wishes of the patient are paramount; in hospice care for children it is sometimes more difficult to determine whose wishes should be followed. Obviously, the age and cognitive level of the child are important factors here.

Care Provision. Most parents expect to care for their dependent children. They would feel more deprived than would the families of adult patients if this were not permitted (Northrup, 1974). Therefore, program design must emphasize parental participation in care. This should occur to the extent that parents (and other family members) are capable of caring for their child and feel comfortable doing so. Programs must include staff teaching to supplement parental involvement and inpatient facilities set up for round-the-clock parent presence (Stillion & Wass, 1979).

Needs. As a rule, families suffer the death of a child more severely than the death of an adult (Fischoff & O'Brien, 1976). And, because of the size of the family group and the differences in age within it, there are often more conflicts within the family. The frequency of major problems between parents of a child who has died is well documented (Lascari, 1978; Weisensee, 1976). Bereavement care, as a result, must be a major program component, with family support provided more frequently, to a larger number of bereaved members, and for a longer time than in typical adult hospice programs. To be successful, bereavement care must be provided by highly sensitive and skilled personnel.

In summary, families of pediatric hospice patients are characteristically larger and more visible, participate more, and often have more insistent psychosocial and other problems than those of adult hospice patients. A higher level of staff skill and a greater amount of staff time should be provided in order to address their needs adequately.

Caregivers

Distinctive problems related to caregivers are in the areas of knowledge, approach to care, and recruitment.

Knowledge. A natural result of the past emphasis on adult hospice care is that there is little available research, experience, and knowledge concerning the details of care for pediatric hospice patients. This is particularly apparent in techniques for pain and symptom management (Chapman & Goodall, 1979). As a result, quality of care may be jeopardized. Adapting existing knowledge to the care of children and seeking new approaches to medical management problems should be major program goals.

Approach to Care. Historically, adults have tended to view children as immune to adult concerns, perhaps because children are reticent or less able to communicate their feelings. Reports indicate that adults believe children do not feel pain, that they "bounce back" from painful tests and treatments quickly and retain little memory of them, and that they do not comprehend or worry about their condition or its effects on others. More recent studies disprove these beliefs (e.g., Eland & Anderson, 1977; Swafford & Allen, 1968). Although it may be difficult to learn the real needs of dying children, hospice staff members should be trained and encouraged to listen, watch, and be open to these patients even more than for adult patients. They should also urge family members and the public to do the same. Further research in this aspect is indispensable.

Recruitment. Many adult caregivers, like other adults, feel so strongly that childhood death is "unnatural" that they prefer not to care for dying children. For this reason, recruitment of program staff and volunteers means seeking very special people from a very small pool of those who are interested—a difficult and time-consuming task (Mount, 1980). For the same reason, support systems for pediatric hospice staff aimed at preventing burnout are even more important than for those caring for adults (Beszterczey, 1977).

Pediatric hospice caregivers, then, tend to have more challenges and less knowledge for work that requires more knowledge, a broader range of skills, and more sensitivity than what is customary in adult hospice care.

Regulatory Agencies

Most current legislation and regulations concerning health care programs seem to be based on the assumption that all patients are adults. Frequently, there is no precedent for approval of requested program details related to children. For example, reimbursement for the time babies spend sleeping in a day care program is a foreign concept to regulatory agencies, as is reimbursement for highly skilled attendants for youngsters at home with tracheostomies. Pediatric hospice planners may find themselves repeatedly applying for special acknowledgements or exemptions for what they consider to be essential program elements, which are not included or envisioned in existing regulations.

However, most regulatory officials, like those in the New York State Department of Health, are interested in and supportive of improved care for dying children. They may suggest ways to formulate program design in order to qualify under existing legislative guidelines. The end result may not meet the original and total expectations of the planners but still may meet major program goals. It is essential for pediatric hospice planners going through this process to have an open approach to what is possible and a clear understanding of what is essential.

Recognizing that any program or portion thereof can be helpful, pediatric hospice planners have the opportunity to make choices as to the design of their programs. Some comments concerning program choices follow.

Dimensions of Care

All or some of various hospice care dimensions can improve the quality and meaning of life for both dying children and their families. The ideal would be to have a sort of "cafeteria selection" of care components so that patients and families could be offered choices in meeting their many and frequently dissimilar needs. The ability of a pediatric hospice program to have unlimited choices of components and services, however, can be little more than a long-range goal in today's health care system. (To define our terms, "components" are the major care categories: home care, inpatient care, etc. Components are differentiated from "services," which refer to the care provided by the different hospice disciplines, such as physicians, nurses, volunteers, etc.)

The modalities and resources for both care and support that may be needed include all the standard hospice components and more. Among them are:

Home care
Day/night care
Inpatient care
Outpatient clinic care
Bereavement care
Respite care
Satellite care centers
Home maintenance and modification
Family support and self-help groups
Religious supports
Preschool and school participation
Community activities and supports
Community sources for equipment and materials
Transportation

In addition, research, education, and advocacy are valid and important program functions.

These dimensions of care are considered here under three general headings: the child at home, the child in an institution, and the family after the child's death.

The Child at Home

Home is, of course, the place most children want to be. At home, children are in familiar surroundings with their parents and siblings, their friends, their possessions, and their pets. They feel more secure and less afraid than in institutions. Their parents feel less fragmented, less guilty, and more in control than if their child were in a hospital; their siblings usually respond positively (Martinson, 1979). As family members participate in the care, they can see the patient's gradual deterioration and can face the approaching death more realistically. They tend to move through grieving and mourning processes together, which may help them avoid interpersonal problems and family breakups later on.

The primary goals of pediatric hospice planners should be to enable the child to remain at home as much and as long as possible. Home care, day/night care, outpatient clinic care, respite care, and many community supports can be provided or coordinated to make this possible.

Whenever a mother, father, or other responsible person is in the home and is able and willing to care for the child there with some outside help and support, then a pediatric hospice home care program is feasible for that child. Home care personnel can provide assessment, treatment, education (teaching the family how to provide care), preparation (teaching them what to expect), psychological support, and help in resolving home problems.

If the responsible family members are not able to be in the home consistently, perhaps because they have full-time or part-time jobs outside the home, then a day care (or night care) program may provide both health care services and child care during those hours. When the distance between homes and these programs is great, satellite day/night care centers may be established. It should be emphasized, however, that when care is split in this way (part at home and part elsewhere), attention must be paid to maintaining continuity of care.

If the child can be cared for at home but needs regular health care review by hospice staff familiar with his or her situation, then outpatient clinic care may be appropriate.

In cases where family members are caring for the child at home but are becoming tired, overburdened, and stressed, then respite care for the child in an inpatient facility should be available. With periodic respite care, the family of a child with a long-term illness gains a much-needed period of rest and revitalization and is soon able to resume care, refreshed. Respite care may be needed under other circumstances as well—when, for example, a sibling or parent is ill, particularly if someone is ill with a contagious disease which could spread to the already debilitated terminally ill child.

If the home needs renovation or repair to make care easier or to accommodate a child newly handicapped, home maintenance and modification services may be provided. Under certain circumstances, these services are reimbursable; if not, volunteer help may be sought. Similarly, hospice staff may draw upon community resources to obtain equipment (beds, wheelchairs, walkers, commodes, etc.), materials and supplies for patient care or patient activities, interests, and education, and meals or other basic necessities that may not otherwise be available.

Likewise, if the child is unable to attend school but wishes to keep up with classmates, participation of preschool or school staff members may be provided in the home environment. And if family members demonstrate needs in such areas as mental health, peer support, activities, tutoring, education of the child's schoolteachers and classmates, or religious counseling, then—again—community resources or staff and volunteer participation can be arranged. Parent, sibling, or whole family self-help and support groups may be available in the local community. Some are structured according to the patient's diagnosis (such as cancer); some offer assistance both during the terminal illness and after the death.

Any or all of these services can be supplied by or through a pediatric hospice program. They help meet the family's needs for knowledge, support, and problem solving, and they help meet the child's needs for care, support, an adequate home, and a capable and comfortable family group. In this way, despite inevitable difficulties, the time of dying can become a period of growth, accomplishment, and satisfaction for all concerned.

When all this is said, however, no discussion of home care should fail to mention one problem that sometimes occurs: the suitability of the home may be viewed differently by the staff, the family, and the child. If the child was comfortable in the home before the terminal illness and wants to be there, the wishes of the child must supersede any doubts of the staff as to its adequacy. Even if major modifications were to be made, the standards of health care staff might not be met. In such cases, staff members may need to be reminded that their role is to accept patients "where they are" and not where staff think they should be (a basic tenet of hospice care), and that this approach is as true for physical surroundings as for emotional and spiritual care (Ajemian & Mount, 1980; Davidson, 1975, pp. 59–71).

The Child in a Health Care Facility

Although the home may be the preferred location for the child, there are circumstances when inpatient care is necessary. For exclusively home care hospice programs, planners should insure that appropriate inpatient care is available and that continuity of care is maintained. Families are greatly reassured by the knowledge that alternatives exist if they find themselves unable to care for the child at home. They are further reassured when no guilt is attached to their choice of inpatient care.

The proper inpatient location for terminally ill children is thought by many to be the acute care facility where curative treatment had been provided previously (e.g., Saunders, 1980). In the acute care setting, the location, the staff, and the routines are known to the child and the child is familiar to the staff. This location has been considered particularly appropriate for cancer patients.

For the child who cannot be cared for at home and is to be admitted for an extended period of time, a pediatric skilled nursing facility may be the location recommended, where care is less crisis-oriented and procedures are usually noninvasive, and where education, activities, and peer companionship can be enjoyed.

A third alternative is the designated hospice inpatient unit, designed and staffed specifically for these children and their families. There, families continue to participate in the care, are welcome to stay all day and overnight, and are supported throughout the child's inpatient stay. Siblings and close friends of any age are welcome to visit, as are pets. Expertise in the medical needs of dying children, activities and therapies attuned to their abilities and wishes, and a warm, open, supportive environment help meet the patients' physical, psychosocial, and spiritual needs.

Inpatient admissions may be short-term to resolve management of new or exacerbated pain or other symptoms, followed by discharge home again. Such admissions may occur more than once for the child. Alternatively, admission may be made when the child is near death and needs more care than the family can provide. Inpatient care is appropriate in a number of circumstances: if the child's disease or symptoms are out of control and need monitoring and expert attention over time; if the caregivers in the home are unable or unwilling to care for the child adequately; if the home is not and cannot be renovated to become adequate for the child's care and safety; or if there is no home.

The inpatient facility, particularly a pediatric hospice inpatient unit, may also serve as the location for respite care and day/night care. Such an arrangement facilitates continuity of care and provides that familiarity of place so reassuring to the child. However, a pediatric hospice inpatient unit is difficult to design, to staff, and to make financially viable, particularly considering the small patient population and the preference for care in the home.

An inpatient hospice unit should not be thought of as a "terminal ward." Rather, it is a place where problems are resolved, expert care is provided, and support, understanding, and reassurance are offered to patients and families. It is also a place where preparation is made, whenever possible, for discharge back to home.

The Family After the Child's Death

Support of the family both before and after the death of a child is important. For older family members, the death of a child before that of the grandparents or the parents may seem "unnatural" and "wrong." Parents feel they have lost not only the child but the future they saw in that child, including, perhaps, the continuation of the family name. Each parent may not grieve the death of the child in the same way or at the same time as the other parent; each may be so grief-stricken that support of the other, however badly needed, is impossible (Schiff, 1977, pp. 57–82). As a result, marital and other relationships often may be at risk.

Support of families during the grieving period can have a significant impact on preserving the marriage, shortening the bereavement period, and making the grieving less distressing (Weisensee, 1976). As stated previously, bereavement care is most helpful when supplied by particularly sensitive and skilled personnel through frequent contacts with a family group over a long period of time.

Pediatric hospice planners will find that bereavement care is not reimbursable, even though it can be shown to be an important mode of preventive health care. The best approach may be one that is frequently successful in adult hospice programs, that is, volunteer bereavement caregivers supervised and supported by professional staff.

Two other questions may be raised by hospice planners: (1) Should community self-help and/or support groups be utilized? (2) Should bereavement care be offered to those whose children died but not within the hospice program? A beginning pediatric hospice program may be wise to do no more than sponsor existing self-help and support groups and evaluate their effectiveness. As the program develops, a bereavement care component specific to the identified needs of the hospice program's families may be established to supplement (or replace) community groups. Later on, when the hospice program's full complement of planned components is operating smoothly, bereavement care may be extended to those in need whose child was not a hospice patient. Additional evaluative studies should be conducted to determine the needs of this added group, and the program should be modified if these needs prove to be different or more intense.

The dimensions of care in all three of the above groupings (home care, inpatient care, bereavement care) require that services be provided and that staff and volunteers be available to provide them. As we have noted previously, pediatric hospice planners or managers face the task of selecting staff to provide these services from a small applicant pool, from which they must choose those with the highest levels of knowledge, skill, and sensitivity.

Services to be Provided

A large number of disciplines must be represented in the provision of high quality pediatric hospice care. Members of each discipline must possess a variety of skills to address the differing needs of the patient/family population. Such professionals work best together if they are willing and able to function as part of an interdisciplinary team to prioritize needs, to blend care provision, to assign roles and responsibilities, and to support each other. In addition, they should utilize and support the program's volunteers and include them within the team. Finally, they must incorporate the family and the child into the team.

At the same time, care must be organized in such a way as to meet regulatory and reimbursement requirements. If, for example, a bath for a home care patient is reimbursable only if given by a home health aide but not by a nurse, then baths should be given by home health aides.

Services to be provided may include those of physicians and dentists, nurses and nursing assistants, social workers and counselors, therapists and recreationalists, nutritionists, pharmacists, chaplains, educators, home health aides, homemakers and housekeepers, volunteers, and suppliers of equipment, materials, and transportation.

Physician Services

Physician services to pediatric hospice patients may be provided by the hospice's medical director and physicians, the family practitioner, the child's pediatrician, and/or the pediatric subspecialist in a major medical center. A pediatric psychiatrist and a dentist may be needed as well.

Physicians other than the pediatric hospice's medical director may lack sufficient skill or interest in the care of the terminally ill child. The heterogeneous knowledge of the family practitioner or the research concerns of the medical center specialist, for example, may militate against their learning additional skills needed for hospice work. These additional skills include pain and symptom management techniques, polypharmacy abilities, and counseling skills. In effect, physicians who already are highly skilled are being asked to gain new competencies to care for a small number of patients for a few hours a week. While this problem is not exclusive to pediatric hospices, it is significant and obstacles to recruitment of physicians are obvious.

Since high quality medical care is essential to good hospice care, attention should be directed early in program planning to finding the most suitable physicians available.

Nursing Services

Nurses are the backbone of pediatric hospice programs. They provide assessment, care, teaching, advocacy, and coordination of other services. Indeed, some existing programs are primarily nursing programs.

It may be difficult to find qualified people. How many nurses are there with pediatric experience, home care experience, and specialized training in a variety of disease conditions? An ideal candidate would also have an interest in terminal care, no "hidden agenda", ability to work as a member of an interdisciplinary team, and personal qualities of sensitivity and caring. Such a person should also be mature and stable in order to cope with the continual care of dying infants and children. It may be necessary first to find a person with some of these attributes and then to train that person in whatever skills are missing—an expensive but sometimes valid approach.

In addition to the services of licensed registered nurses, there may be need for licensed practical nurses, nursing assistants, aides, child care technicians, home health aides, and personal care workers. There has been some indication that more aide services and less nursing services are needed in the home, while more nursing services and less aide services are required for inpatient care. It is important to utilize the correct level of nursing caregiver in all cases in order to meet both the needs of the patient and the regulations for reimbursement.

Social Work and Counseling Services

The social, financial, and interpersonal needs of pediatric hospice patients and families differ from those of adults. It is seldom the breadwinner who is dying and there are likely to be few problems concerning wills, insurance, and so on. In both adult and pediatric terminal illness, however, the family is disrupted. In pediatric terminal illness, the future of the family is at stake. In particular, siblings will be affected by the experience (negatively or positively) for the rest of their lives and the parents' relationship is at risk. The dying child's intense anxiety and fear, together with the parents' feelings of anger, anxiety, and guilt, may call for professional assistance and intervention.

Medical social workers and counselors can help children and families cope with their emotional, interpersonal, financial, and social problems. With a thorough knowledge of community services, they can recommend help in many other areas. In addition, a social worker, or sometimes a counselor, is often in charge of the bereavement care component. In that capacity, he or she trains, coordinates, and supports volunteer bereavement caregivers. Clearly, such social workers and counselors must be good listeners, and sensitive to the needs, beliefs, and standards of others. They must be knowledgeable about current community resources and child welfare legislation and regulations.

There may be little reimbursement for social workers and counselors. Nevertheless, their role is so important to pediatric hospice care and to the interdisciplinary team that, if necessary, additional funding should be sought to supplement third party reimbursement.

Therapy Services

Although physical therapy and other therapeutic modalities are sometimes provided by adult hospices, a much broader range of therapy services is needed for pediatric hospice programs. These services may include: physical therapy; occupational therapy; speech and language pathology and audiology; respiratory therapy; recreation and play therapy; and music, art, and drama therapy.

Music, art, and drama therapists are particularly important in pediatric hospice care because they can help children express and resolve their fears and concerns. Such therapists also contribute greatly to improving quality and enjoyment in children's lives (Fagen, 1982). This help can be provided to both patients and siblings.

Financing these therapists and their supplies and equipment may be a problem, as reimbursement is limited. It may be possible to utilize skilled volunteers, but then it is essential to integrate such volunteers as active participants in the interdisciplinary team.

Other Service Providers

To provide consistent and high quality care, it is necessary to find the right people in each category, help them understand the hospice concept, include them as team members when appropriate, and support them in this stressful and arduous yet rewarding work.

Children and families may be stressed if the number of service providers is too large. ("Too large" should be defined by the individual family.) This should be avoided, if possible. However, a consistent hospice approach by all providers, gained through high-quality training, experience, and supervision, helps to reduce this stress.

Services may be provided in a number of ways: directly by hospice staff—both paid and volunteer, full-time or part-time; by contract with individual professionals on a fee-for-service basis; by contract with other health care agencies or institutions to provide one or more services by individuals whom they employ; or by utilization of existing staff in an agency or institution who can and will redirect the care of their dying pediatric patients to a hospice team approach. How the services are provided must depend on how the program is planned and developed.

Program Planning and Development

In this emerging field of pediatric hospice care, whatever it is possible to do in each situation and locality to accomplish all or part of whatever needs to be done should be attempted. How to go about developing the right program for each community's needs requires creativity and dedication, as well as facts and methodology. The steps in program development which follow may help provide guidelines for proceeding, whatever the scope of each planned program.

Program planning is detailed decision making. It is a design process through which are answered the questions: why, what, when, where, exactly for whom, by whom, and particularly how the program should be structured. This planning process is described here in three phases: initial planning—feasibility; operational planning—formal organization; detailed planning—component development. These are chronological phases. The first addresses the questions *why, what,* and *for whom;* the second addresses the questions *when, where, how,* and *by whom;* and the third deals with the specific details of *how.*

Initial Planning: Feasibility

Initial planning in any organization begins when a problem or unmet need is identified and addressed, and a solution is proposed. Pediatric hospice planning follows the same process. The steps are:

1. Identify a problem.
2. Learn about available solutions.
3. Consider and prioritize these solutions as to their appropriateness in resolving the problem.
4. Propose a solution.
5. Find the people and finances needed to conduct an investigation to determine the feasibility of the solution.

The feasibility of the solution is studied analytically in order to confirm or deny its practicality. The feasibility study may be conducted by outside consultants who are experienced in the field or by the planning staff of the initiating group. At the Royal Victoria Hospital, the initiating group employed graduate students to gather information using a questionnaire the group had designed (Mount, Jones, & Patterson, 1974). At St. Mary's Hospital for Children, a consulting firm was engaged to assist the hospital's planning group (ELM, 1979).

The feasibility study might address the following questions:

1. Who are the potential patients?
2. How many of them are there?
3. Where would they come from?
4. What are their needs?
5. How are they cared for now, and is there a need for something more or something else?

6. Are other organizations meeting or planning to meet this need?
7. Is the initiating group's organization or institution suitable for operating such a program?
8. What would it cost and how could it be financed?

A number of sources can be tapped to obtain the information necessary to answer these questions: one might call upon the initiating group staff, community physicians, discharge planners, other local health care providers, and institutional representatives, as well as search out available statistical data. It is the responsibility of the initiating group to define the initial goals of the program and to make a number of basic programmatic decisions throughout the study. These decisions help refine the scope of the study. Conversely, the study itself helps to delimit further the scope of the program. The following three examples may help clarify this process.

First, the question, "Who are the potential patients?", requires decisions as to patient ages, diagnoses, and prognoses that will be regarded as acceptable for program admission. Since most adult hospice programs only accept patients over the age of 18, one might assume that children's programs would accept those 18 years of age and younger. However, some pediatric organizations maintain a maximum limit of age 14 or 16, on the basis that those over that age do not consider themselves "children" and are also harder for the staff to manage. This suggests that there may be a special place for adolescent or teenage hospice programs. The value of a hospice program for the very young (those under, say, two years of age) may also be questioned on the basis that the child is not sufficiently aware for a hospice approach to make any difference. Against this it could be argued that the infant may need skilled management of distressing symptoms and the family may need hospice support. In fact, "neonatal hospice programs" have already been established in the United States to address just such issues (see Chapter 7 in this volume).

If cancer is the exclusive admission diagnosis, program planning is simpler with respect to, for example, referral sources and staff training. However, for a feasible program, the number of such patients may be too small. If patients with other terminal illnesses are to be accepted, it will be necessary to determine which illnesses and at what stages. This task may require that staff review past pediatric deaths in the area and obtain advice from pediatricians as to which of the diagnoses causing those deaths would have been appropriate for hospice care. Then, for the acceptable diagnoses, the average length of stay should be estimated to rule out those that could not fit hospice guidelines (e.g., guidelines which might stipulate "six months or less life expectancy" or "months rather than years").

Physicians have stated that their prognoses for terminally ill children tend to be less accurate than for adults, for all diagnoses. The period of hospice appropriateness may thus be longer or shorter than predicted, and may be longer or shorter than for adults with similar diagnoses and prognoses. This makes length-of-stay predictions and patient load planning very haphazard. Planning becomes even more uncertain when it is remembered that physicians do not always refer patients when they might otherwise first become eligible for hospice care, and that parents do not always accept such a referral. During the initial planning phase, it is important to be clear about diagnosis, stage, and prognosis in order to collect statistical data only within this framework. Even though the formal criteria for admission might state simply "incurable progressive disease for which aggressive treatment is not appropriate and from which the patient will die within weeks or months rather than years," more exact information is needed for program planning.

Second, the question, "How many of them are there?", requires a definition of the catchment area to be served. The geographic area to be included for home care and that for inpatient care need not be the same. Home care is usually the more restricted. It may be specified as either a radius around an institutional location within which a staff member can visit the home conveniently, or as a municipal demarcation such as a county, or as an area between designated landmarks or throughways. Because of the small and widespread patient population of pediatric hospice programs, it may be that their catchment areas for home care should be larger than for most adult programs. A large area may help insure the satisfaction of referring physicians as well, particularly if the program is the only one of its kind in the community.

Third, the question, "Is the initiator group's organization or facility suitable for the program?", requires decisions as to the model of program desired and the number of hospice-eligible patients that can be served in each component of that model. The many different structures of hospice programs are termed "models" (Wilson & English, 1985). There are two basic groups of hospice models: independent and dependent. An independent hospice may be a volunteer program, a licensed hospice home health agency, or a coordinating organization. A dependent hospice is a program formed as part of a hospital, a skilled nursing facility, a home health agency, or a consortium of these. Models within both independent and dependent groups are differentiated partly by their legal structure or ownership but primarily by the components they offer (home care, inpatient care, bereavement care, etc.).

The initiating group needs to choose the model best suited to its particular situation. This may be determined in part by addressing the questions, "What do patients in this area need?" and "How are these needs now being met (or planned)?" If none of the important service components are being provided now, or if the quality of those provided is not adequate, then a choice could be made as to which, if not all, the initiator group could provide. Alternatively, the choice may be made in terms of which are most needed. As a general rule, priority should be given to home care, if only one component can be provided. If all components are needed and can be provided, every attempt should be made to do so.

The number of eligible patients in the area, calculated in the feasibility study, should be compared to the number the initiating group has the resources to handle. In our own situation, because of the very large population base in New York City, a full-scale program (with all major components) could be planned. It was decided that resources for home care—estimated at 50 patients per year—could be arranged without difficulty. However, as the existing inpatient facility was already fully occupied, it was necessary to add new space to house a ten-bed inpatient unit for the estimated 80 inpatients per year. The appropriateness of the hospital's location was considered satisfactory for several reasons: although it was some distance from the heart of the city, it was on a beautiful site where parking was not a problem, it had a fine reputation in the community for high-quality pediatric care, and it had been an acceptable inpatient location for children and families from a wide geographic area for many years.

Based on a rigorous and positive feasibility study, the implementation decision must be made by the initiating group and the board of the sponsoring organization. Only then can operational planning begin.

Operational Planning: Formal Organization

In the operational planning phase, a series of discrete steps must be addressed carefully. The recommendations of the feasibility study staff may provide helpful guidelines. The operational planning steps are:

1. Obtain start-up funding from private sources.
2. Establish a formal organization and recruit a program director and medical director.
3. Develop a referral base.
4. Plan program components, services to be provided, and staffing required for the anticipated patient load.
5. Explore reimbursement and other ongoing funding.
6. If required, prepare Certificate of Need application(s).

The beginning of operational planning is usually years in advance of the provision of reimbursed care. Ordinarily, therefore, private funds must be sought to finance program development over this period. The feasibility study report can be a major factor in supporting foundation grant applications once an updated estimated budget and funding plan are added. Thus, it is only as a result of the continuing support of the New York Community Trust, through years that saw continually escalating costs, that the St. Mary's project has been able to continue.

Establishing a formal organization for an independent hospice program means deciding whether to be licensed or privately funded. For a dependent program, it may be a matter of deciding where in the parent organizational hierarchy the hospice program should fit, and obtaining the necessary authorizations. As soon as possible thereafter, the program director (or executive director, or administrator) should be employed to help in the remaining program development steps. The medical director should be identified also, and become involved in the planning at as early a stage as possible. Before filling these positions, of course, job descriptions and funds for salaries are needed.

The initiating group, the program director, and particularly the medical director, while proceeding with planning, should be making every effort to develop a solid, supportive referral base. Ongoing contacts with local pediatricians, medical societies, hospital caregivers, and discharge planners are needed to assure appropriate patient referrals later on.

Each of the planned program components should be thought through carefully, utilizing and expanding on the statistical data in the feasibility study concerning patients and services. This effort will enable the planners to determine for each component the staffing needed to supply the planned services to the anticipated patients for their expected length of stay. The results of this part of the study for the home care component at St. Mary's (see Table 1.1) may be a useful example.

The next step is to allocate costs to staffing and all other cost items in order to produce an operating expense total. Then the total reimbursement that would be available for, say, the number of patient days (inpatient care) or the number of visits (home care) must be determined. Finally, this total is compared with the total estimated operating costs. This exercise may be a rather sobering one, sending the planners back to the drawing board! If the two totals do not match, it may be decided to abandon or modify the program plan or to seek ongoing additional funding. If a Certificate of Need application is required, the findings in all of the previous steps can contribute to its preparation.

Detailed Planning: Component Development

Now that the Certificate of Need has been issued and/or the other planning steps have been completed, can the program begin? Probably not,

Table 1.1. Long Term Home Health Care Program. Personnel Required to Provide Annual Volume of Services for Palliative Care Patients within the Hospital's Catchment Area (N = 12.5)[1]

Discipline	Visits/Month (Calculated)	Total Visits/Year	*Provided By* Contract	*Provided By* Direct	Hours Direct Per Visits[2]	Total Hrs./Yr. Direct	Direct FTE's @2080 Hrs./Yr.
Home Health Aide	113	1356	676	680	5	3400	2.0[3]
Homemaker	54	648	648	—	—	—	—
Medical Social Worker	14	168	55	113	3	339	0.2
Nursing	106	1272	400	872	3	2616	1.4[3]
Nutrition	5	60	—	60	2	120	0.06
Occupational Therapy	5	60	30	30	2	60	0.03
Physical Therapy	16	192	60	132	2	264	0.13
Recreation	26	312	—	312	2	624	0.3
							4.12

1. 50 patients per year, with an average length of stay of three months equals 12.5 patients at any one time.
2. Figures include travel and ancillary time. They are based on a four-hour stay per visit for a home health aide and homemaker, and a half to one-hour stay for other professionals. Transportation time is estimated at 1½ hours per visit. Ancillary tasks are considered minor for the home health aide and homemaker, and of varying amounts for other professions.
3. FTE's (full-time equivalents) adjusted for minimum relief factor.

until all the details of how and when each component is to operate are in place. The steps in this phase of planning include the following *for each component*, although some parts of these steps may have been completed already:

1. Employ a director or coordinator for each component.
2. Plan carefully how each component will work.
3. Establish an overall chart or other scheduling device.
4. Finalize formal organization and internal reporting systems.
5. Fulfill remaining requirements of regulatory and reimbursement organizations.
6. Design physical layout of the space to be used, and arrange for renovation/construction and decoration.
7. Determine the materials and equipment needed and begin to obtain them.
8. Write a policy and procedure manual, which should include admission and discharge policies and procedures and death procedures.
9. Design forms for patient care, evaluation, and reports.
10. Plan staffing (if not already done).
11. Plan volunteer involvement.
12. Prepare job descriptions for planned personnel (both paid and volunteer) and select initial staff and volunteers.
13. Prepare orientation and training program for planned personnel, and train initial staff and volunteers.
14. Determine any other individuals, agencies, or community resources to be involved, and sign contracts with them.
15. Continue developing referral base, and sign transfer agreements with referring institutions, where applicable.
16. Set up advisory committees and hold at least one meeting of each before care begins.
17. Communicate frequently with other individuals and groups, both internal and external, to insure their continuing interest, involvement, and cooperation.

Because of the volume of work involved in completing these steps for each component, it is wise not to begin care in more than one component at a time. Even with a staggered overall plan, many different activities tend to take place at the same time in this phase. Also, along with the care components, it is necessary to develop the education and evaluation/research components of the program as well.

There are multitudes of questions to be answered in developing a pediatric hospice program. Probably the best guideline we have found for this work is the experimental approach: make the best decisions possible based on available information, record the reasons those decisions were made, carry them out, and then evaluate the results. In this way, something is done and much is learned.

It may be useful to consider examples of some of the questions that we encountered. In developing only one step in one component at St. Mary's, the interior design for the inpatient unit, the questions we faced included the following:

1. *Given a ten-bed unit and a patient age range from birth to 16 years, how many of each age group may there be at any one time?* Our response: there could be any mix. However, we are buying six or seven each of cribs and beds, and will see if that proves to be sufficient.

2. *Do children prefer single rooms or double, triple, or four-bedded rooms? Which do families prefer for their children and themselves?* We picked three two-bedded, one three-bedded, and one one-bedded rooms, largely because of the age/sex/interests mix.

3. *Do children prefer the view from their bedroom windows to be quiet (boats on the bay) or more active (playground, houses, cars)? Or which for what age group?* We chose both: two rooms on one side, three on the other. We are guessing that older patients may prefer the quieter view, younger ones the more active outlook.

4. *Should the bedrooms be large and activity areas small, or vice versa?* Our pediatricians advise that children will be out of their bedrooms and in activity areas if they possibly can. Therefore, we have relatively small bedrooms—but still large enough for a family member to sleep overnight with each child—and fairly large activity areas.

5. *What activities would dying children like to have? How can we provide activities for all age groups, interests, and handicaps?* We chose a number of activities: a quiet activity area for conversation, quiet games, story telling, and dramatic play; a noisier activity area for group games and television-watching; a crafts room; a laundry (for older patients and family members); a planting and greenhouse area; water play table; bean (not sand) box; a soundproof room for electronic games, computers, and music for the older ones; music therapy room; a pantry with refrigerator, freezer, microwave, coffee maker, and so on, from which meals prepared in the hospital kitchen are served and which is stocked with snacks and food from home; a dining and day room which can be used also for entertainments, films, and religious services (although the hospital's chapel is nearby); a quiet room with books for private conversations and reading; and a private room in which one can be alone. There is carpeting throughout for sitting and reclining. There are five small terraces or balconies for fresh air and sunshine. There is an elevator which permits private access. And, of course, those who are able may use the hospital's playground, swimming pool, and other activity areas.

6. *At what height should the bathroom fixtures be set? For a young child, an older one, or for a wheelchair-bound person?* We decided early in the planning that the space would be as comfortable and noninstitutional as possible, more like a home. We therefore chose colored bathroom fixtures at home heights, as well as door knobs at regular heights.

7. *What can we plan for the handicapped child?* We have done as much as we felt we could: wide doorways for beds and wheelchairs, grab bars and raised seat units in bathrooms, wheelchair access showers, lowered water fountain, wheelchair access sink in crafts room, special wheelchair bathroom which is intended for day care children, wheelchair access to parts of the pantry and to water play, two sets of handrails in hallways at different heights.

8. *What about television and telephones?* We plan to have television in the activity areas but not regularly in the bedrooms. However, if a weak, bedridden child too sick to enjoy other activities wants to watch TV, a small one attached to or close to the bed is available. Each child has a telephone available at the bedside. We plan to perform cost/benefit studies on these special items.

9. *What, in addition, do families need?* Based on our belief that family members would need a place to get away from time to time, we have a separate family lounge away from the unit, with bathroom, phone, and comfortable furniture. Also, when the death occurs they will need a place to be with the body for a while, and so there is a viewing room with anteroom in the unit, near the elevator.

There are many other questions: colors, textures, and materials; lighting; air circulation, and heating and cooling; window sizes and shapes; nurses' station design; nurse call system; bathing facilities for all ages and handicaps; storage for everything from nursing supplies to toys to parents' overnight bedding; and safety measures—terrace railings, for example.

There are many things to decide and little in the way of hard facts on which to base these decisions. Evaluation and research in this and other areas of decision making will give better answers in the future. Education and communication of evaluation results among all pediatric hospice programs over time should help future planners as well as the hospices themselves.

Conclusion

This chapter has offered a comprehensive picture of distinctions between pediatric and adult hospice care, dimensions of the care of dying children and their families, and guidelines for program planning. If each of these aspects is taken into consideration in planning the provision of terminal care for children, success in the development of a pediatric hospice program is possible.

Hard choices must be made; no one program can provide everything needed. Program planners and staff must capitalize on their own strengths and recognize their limitations, not only individually but also organizationally. They must work to establish a team of multitalented people to contribute to the effort.

As has been shown, pediatric hospice programs cannot be developed through a cookbook approach. Faced with a special population needing special services and considering the resources currently available, each community, it is hoped, will be able to develop its own equally valid solution to the challenge of providing pediatric hospice care. Only when these programs pool their cumulative experience and their knowledge gained through research will there be a clearer definition of valid, successful pediatric hospice care.

References

Ajemian, I., & Mount, B. M., "Cultural Considerations in Palliative Care," in I. Ajemian & B. M. Mount (Eds.), *The R. V. H. Manual on Palliative/Hospice Care.* New York: Arno Press, 1980, pp. 47–60.

Beszterczey, A., "Staff Stress on a Newly Developed Palliative Care Service: The Psychiatrist's Role," *Canadian Journal of Psychiatry,* 1977, *22,* 347–353.

Bluebond-Langner, M., *The Private Worlds of Dying Children.* Princeton, NJ: Princeton University Press, 1978.

Calman, K. C., "Physical Aspects," in C. Saunders (Ed.), *The Management of Terminal Disease.* London: Edward Arnold, 1978, pp. 33–43.

Chapman, J. A., & Goodall, J., "Dying Children Need Help Too," *British Medical Journal,* 1979, *1,* 593–594.

Davidson, G. W., *Living with Dying.* Minneapolis: Augsburg Publishing House, 1975.

Eland, J. M., & Anderson, J. E., "The Experience of Pain in Children," in A. K. Jacox (Ed.), *Pain: A Source Book for Nurses and Other Health Professionals.* Boston: Little, Brown & Company, 1977, pp. 453–473.

ELM Services, Inc., *Pediatric Hospice Feasibility Study: Final Report.* Washington, DC, 1979 (unpublished).

Fagen, T. S., "Music Therapy in the Treatment of Anxiety and Fear in Terminal Pediatric Patients," *Music Therapy: Journal of the American Association for Music Therapy,* 1982, *2,* 13–23.

Fischoff, J., & O'Brien, N., "After the Child Dies," *Journal of Pediatrics,* 1976, *88,* 140–146.

Lascari, A. D., "The Dying Child and the Family," *The Journal of Family Practice,* 1978, *6,* 1279–1286.

Martinson, I. M., "Caring for the Dying Child," *Nursing Clinics of North America,* 1979, *14,* 467–474.

Mount, B. M., "Personnel Selection: Applying the McMurray Principles to Palliative Care," in I. Ajemian & B. M. Mount (Eds.), *The R. V. H. Manual on Palliative/Hospice Care.* New York: Arno Press, 1980, pp. 431–448.

Mount, B. M., Jones, A., & Patterson, A., "Death and Dying: Attitudes in a Teaching Hospital," *Urology,* 1974, *4,* 741–747.

Northrup, F. C., "The Dying Child," *American Journal of Nursing,* 1974, *74,* 1066–1068.

Saunders, C., personal communications, October 1979 and October 1980.

Schiff, H. S., *The Bereaved Parent.* New York: Crown Publishers, 1977.

Stillion, J., & Wass, H., "Children and Death," in H. Wass (Ed.), *Dying: Facing the Facts.* Washington, DC: Hemisphere Publishing Corp., 1979, pp. 208–235.

Swafford, L. I., & Allen, D., "Pain Relief in the Pediatric Patient," *Medical Clinics of North America,* 1968, *52,* 131–136.

Weisensee, M., "A Myriad of Relationships," in I. M. Martinson (Ed.), *Home Care for the Dying Child: Professional and Family Perspectives.* New York: Appleton-Century-Crofts, 1976, pp. 71–85.

Wilson, D. C., "The Viability of Pediatric Hospices: A Case Study," *Death Education,* 1982, *6,* 205–212.

Wilson, D. C., & English, D. J., "Issues in Hospice Administration," in G. W. Davidson (Ed.), *Hospice: Development and Administration* (2nd ed.). Washington, DC: Hemisphere Publishing Corp., 1985, pp. 33–133.

2

The Dying Child: At Home

Ida M. Martinson and Marian Enos

Introduction

Since 1972—for more than ten years—we have been involved in research to identify and evaluate the nursing care required for the family of a child who is dying from cancer at home. Our study, "Home Care for the Child with Cancer," examined the feasibility and desirability of a home care alternative to hospitalization for children with cancer for whom cancer control treatment was no longer effective, that is, children who were dying. Within this alternative, the parents as primary providers of the child's care were assisted by nurses who provided professional nursing services via telephone and home visits. The child's physician served as a consultant to the family and to the nurse, and prescribed needed medication. In the first two years of the study, 37 boys and 21 girls died from cancer while participating in home care. Of those 58 participants, 46 died

The study discussed in this chapter was funded in part by Department of Health, Education, and Welfare, National Cancer Institute, Grant CA 19490. Appreciation is expressed to numerous staff members who aided in the Project. We also wish to thank Bill Henry and Gay Moldow who stepped in and carried on to the end of this research effort. They were aided by Emily Kulenkamp, Susan Nixon, Marion Simacek, Patti Carlson, and Nancy Olson. Finally, thanks are extended to Lois Anderson for her coordination role in all of this.

at home, 11 reentered and died in the hospital, and one died in an ambulance en route to the hospital. For the 46 children who died at home, the average length of involvement from initial nurse contact to time of death was 38.9 days. The average number of home visits was 13.4, with an average of 2.2 hours each in duration.

We identified six conditions as necessary prerequisites for the effectiveness of the home care alternative. Because we dealt with children, these conditions are child-oriented. But principles related to home care of a child with cancer are not limited to children or to cancer, and we suggest that they are equally valid for adults who can also be given the opportunity to die at home. The six conditions are: (1) cure-oriented treatment has been discontinued, so that the emphasis is now on care and adding quality to life; (2) the child wants to be at home; (3) the parents desire to have the child at home; (4) the parents, other children in the family, and/or significant others recognize their own ability to care for the ill child; (5) an available nurse is willing to be on call 24 hours a day for professional consultation and support; and (6) the physician agrees with the plan and is willing to be on call as consultant to the nurse and to the family.

In our project, after a child was referred by his or her physician, a nurse from the Home Care Project staff contacted the child's parents. This person explained the project to the parents and secured their informed consent. The family was then assigned and introduced to a primary care nurse who assumed immediate responsibility for providing the needed nursing services to the child at home. At the same time, a back-up nurse was also assigned to provide services when the primary care nurse was not available.

It is important to note that this Home Care Project differed from most adult hospice care programs in that the primary professional provider was acknowledged to be the nurse. The Project was also directed by a nurse. Physicians and other health team members, including clergy, maintained their traditional roles, but were particularly seen as consultants to nurses.

Results of The Study

The findings of our study suggest both that it is feasible to care for dying children at home and that in most cases it is also desirable to do so. Probably the most important statistic in support of this finding is that 46 out of 58 deaths that occurred in the study took place at home. Although parents were free to move their children to the hospital at any time, 80 percent of them made decisions to care for their children at home until the time of their death.

Comments from parents in the Home Care Project illustrate their perceptions of the desirability of caring for their children at home: "We were able to take our child camping over Labor Day weekend"; "She was able to be with her father, who is a mechanic, during the hours that she was feeling good"; and "I was able to take her grocery shopping. She can't talk any more, but she can nod her head at foods she wants me to buy."

Two issues were central to many of the findings in our study: the necessity of having primary care nurses support the parents in the care of their child, and the necessity of a nurse network to insure continuity of care for these patients. If home care and hospice care are to be offered in the future as alternatives for children and families in this situation, then the system of health care delivery will have to change, since home care nurses and networks of nurses will be required.

Parents and the Primary Care Nurse

One key advantage to *parental control* is that it clarifies the role and relationship of the nurse in the individual situation. That is, parents are encouraged to assume as much control as possible, while the nurse provides the needed supervision, guidance, and support. Whereas, at the outset, necessity led to the need for more parental control (the nurse was not there 24 hours a day unless requested), it was soon noted that parents were not only able but eager to assume the role of caregiver once the child was at home.

How much direct, professional nurse involvement is required for this sort of care? For the 46 children who died at home in the initial 24 months of the project, the number of home visits per family was an average of 12. The total hours per family were an average of 10, with a range from 1 to 306 hours. Telephone calls numbered an average of 20. The total hours involved for telephone calls were an average of four. The total professional nurse-involvement was an average of 24 hours. However, a nurse was at all times on call and available by telephone for a home visit if necessary.

What are some of the important *functions of the home care nurse?* In working with the family, the nurse attempts to teach the parents whatever is needed in order for them to be knowledgeable about the child's care and feel in control. In doing this, the nurse explains to parents what care is needed, what nursing procedures must be done, and what method is used; the nurse also discusses the physiological aspects of how the child may die and the feelings that can go along with that. Essentially, each nurse must sift through his or her individual experiences and educational background to find the best method of teaching the parents to assume effective control of the situation and to take over as much of their child's care as they wish, using the help of the nurse and that of others as they see fit. The home care nurse also provides verbal support and feedback to the family concerning the care they are giving to their child.

As death draws near, the child's medical needs often progressively lessen while other nursing needs increase. Relations within the family can be very complex at this time. The nurse may need to suggest resources to help the family maintain maximum functioning without undue fatigue. Without professional help from the nurse, parental control may not be possible.

Home care nurses perform a variety of other tasks as well. They instruct parents in any special techniques which they can master, such as administering oxygen. Services that the parents cannot do for their child, such as urinary catheterization, are done by nurses on visits to the home. The nurse goes to the home whenever and as often as the family requests, without questioning the necessity of the visit. No unnecessary home visits were requested. In addition, the nurse provides or arranges for any equipment and supplies that are needed, and serves as an intermediary between the family and the physician in securing medication.

At the death of the child, the nurse assists the family members and facilitates the removal of the child's body and the securing of a death certificate. Nurses also maintain contact with the family after the death of the child. They usually attend the funeral and visit or telephone the parents for a period of several weeks after the child's death. In all contacts with the family, the nurse spends much time providing emotional support to the child and parents in addition to providing technical nursing services and teaching.

Parents may find that the first days—and particularly the very first day—at home with the sick child are almost overwhelming. This is the time when they feel most helpless and in need of assistance. During this crucial period ready access to the nurse is most important. The nurse's role is to facilitate the care, guarantee that quality care is being provided, and offer reassurance to the family that this is in fact so. The nurse must study the family, assess their situation, and act accordingly. In so doing, the nurse needs to pose the following questions: How tired are the parents? Do they need additional short-term help such as a home health aide, a relative coming in to sleep one night, or possibly even the nurse staying overnight? The nurse will also need to look into resources for equipment and supplies, know where oxygen can be obtained if that may be necessary, know how to get drugs, and make sure that at night and on weekends adequate medications will be available. Resources such as equipment rental agencies, ambulance services, homemaker services, and perhaps financial agencies should be identified.

During maintenance periods when the child's condition is stable, families may only need a weekly visit from the home care nurse to attend to matters of nutrition, constipation, pain control, skin care, mouth care, medications, teaching of procedures, record keeping, and preparation for possible developments or for death itself. It is essential that the caregiver and the nurse, in their interactions, establish a daily ritual in home care, one that is determined by the unique objectives of the child and family.

Nurses doing this kind of primary professional nursing practice are effectively addressing certain inadequacies which are often associated with traditional health care delivery. Those difficulties include the avoidance and neglect by health care professionals which may occur in cases where there is no hope for cure. Also, the inconsistency and lack of communication among persons and organizations serving people who are at the end stage of life (and their families) often make coordination seem impossible. Financial problems may be an additional source of stress, especially lack of medical insurance coverage. The nurse who helps parents take charge of home care does much to counteract these and other types of stress.

Nursing Networks

Home care nurses who provide direct care in family situations involving a dying child will be most effective if there is *an active network of nurses* to work with them in an organized way. Other network members will be hospital nurses and/or hospice nurses, community nurses, community agency nurses, nurse consultants, and back-up nurses who can fill in from time to time. It is especially important that the primary care nurse have a back-up consultant in nursing upon whom to call for advice and assistance. If it is to be adequate at all, the home care alternative must draw upon the very best professional nurses on the scene. The nursing network serves such individuals as a support and guarantor for continuity of care.

For each of the families served by our Home Care Project, we needed to locate a home care nurse who would be available and close enough to make a home visit whenever the family requested. This was particularly difficult for that half of the children in our study who lived outside the Minneapolis-St. Paul metropolitan area, some of them in distant rural areas and in neighboring states. Nevertheless, while much time was often required to locate a nurse in such areas, a suitable nurse was always found.

For ten families whose child died during the first year of our study, the length of home care involvement was less than one week. This points to the necessity of moving quickly. If a decision is made to send a child home from the hospital on Friday, a nurse must be contacted immediately—not after the weekend—to help the family. Only a preestablished network will make such dispatch workable.

A nursing network is also essential to provide ongoing support for the home care nurse. Since such a nurse is practicing in a role of greatly increased responsibility, and since the family is often located at some distance from the referral institutions, less support and less equipment are available than in most traditional settings. Our experience has been that a series of telephone calls and a well-kept file in some network headquarters can be significant aids to the home care nurse.

A Case Study

In the network which gradually developed within the Home Care Project at the University of Minnesota, a project staff nurse would make initial contact with a family a few days before their child was to be discharged from the hospital. A case study will illustrate how this worked.

This particular patient was to return to the hospital weekly for three weeks to receive a new drug as an outpatient. Staff members in the Home Care Project spent a full afternoon telephoning nursing agencies near the family's home in order to locate a home care nurse. Finally, a public health nurse who lived 30 minutes from the family's home, agreed to serve as their home care nurse, and the local county public health agency agreed to provide a back-up nurse. The fundamental issues pertinent to the case were explained to the primary home care nurse. This was her first such case. After the telephone conversation, written materials concerning home care, medications which were to be given, and characteristics of the particular cancer diagnosed were mailed to her. While this was not an optimal way to recruit and inform the nurse, the rural character of Minnesota gave us no other practicable alternative.

This particular nurse proved to be quite resourceful; she sought out and read books on death and dying, and when she was unsure of the best approach to a specific problem, she contacted other nurses whom she knew or members of the Home Care Project staff. She was able to deal with some of the problems encountered by this family over the telephone. Once, for example, the child's mother called to say that she was having difficulty getting the child to take her pain medication since swallowing was difficult. Another time the mother phoned to say that the child was vomiting and experiencing increased pain. The nurse recommended administration of the antiemetic that was already in the home and called the project staff for a recommendation concerning pain. Following consultation with the physician, the project staff nurse recommended an increase in dosage to the home care nurse who relayed this to the mother. It should be noted that one or another of the project staff nurses was available for consultation with the home care nurse 24 hours a day. In other cases, the home care nurse contacted the child's physician directly or used her own judgment within ranges which were established by the physician. Another example of project staff involvement in this case was the recommendation that the child's primary nurse from the hospital telephone the home care nurse. She did so, and they discussed the child's past nursing care and current care. Contact between the hospital nurse and the primary home care nurse was a source of helpful information and support.

In this case, the home care nurse also called the minister to introduce herself and to update him on the patient's condition and prognosis. In addition, she contacted the local physician. She was thus part of a coordinated, caring health team, one which she helped to create and sustain.

Later, when the child died, the home care nurse informed the other members of the team and the nurse network. Four days later this nurse attended a memorial service for her patient.

Institutionalization

In the Home Care Project the network of involved institutions included physicians serving eight hospitals. Fifty-six percent of the physician referrals came from the University of Minnesota Hospitals, while the rest came from outside that source. Eventually, other physicians heard of the project and made contact with us. We learned from this that reforms would be necessary, both within such institutions and in their interactions, if home care programs for dying children and their families are to be successful. Reform occurred during the Home Care Project in Minnesota because we gave early attention to particular aspects of *institutionalization* of home care concepts.

For example, we are convinced that institutions wishing to offer home care services in the future—whether they are hospitals or hospice programs—will need to designate persons to be *coordinators* of that effort. Such a position would require 24-hour coverage. The coordinator's duties would include: obtaining and orienting home care nurses from the primary institutions, from other similar institutions, from public health agencies and visiting nurse associations, or from the community; providing consultation and support to such nurses; serving as primary home care nurse to selected local families when necessary; maintaining contact with nurses and physicians in hospital situations, clinics, and hospice programs; and linking home care services to other professional resources, including physicians, teachers, school nurses, social workers, clergy, and morticians.

In the Home Care Project, *parents* in the families who were included in the study were greatly involved during both the service and the institutionalization phases as consultants and as advocates for home care. As they spoke out in the community, these parents provided support for the concept of children dying at home rather than in the hospital. Their influence was also felt as they requested services and insisted that they be made available.

It is also necessary in the institutionalization of concepts that we address the *system resistances,* which are very strong factors. Resistances are based on values (e.g., the belief that the best available care should be in the hospital), traditions, past experiences, attitudes, professional entrenchment, reluctance toward change, expectations, timing, and inertia. All of these factors inhibit people from accepting a new concept and implementating change within the system. As the effectiveness of a research model project is demonstrated, resistance—whether potential or real—is natural. We must give our full attention to this resistance in an organized way.

In order to break down potential and real resistances, we must utilize administrative, educational, legislative, and media avenues. Each of these avenues was used in the Home Care Project during the institutionalization phase of our work.

We took several measures early to provide *a foundation for administrative support* of the Home Care Project. Shortly after the first case of providing direct home care services and before the funded project began, the principal investigator worked to aid a local hospital to develop a permanent home care program. Later, a children's hospital, a clinic, and public health care agencies were also involved.

Additional efforts to promote administrative support resulted in the establishment of two advisory committees. The first, a community advisory committee, consisted of nurse representatives from local public health nursing agencies, nurse clinical directors, directors of nursing from local hospitals, and representatives from the Minnesota State Department of Health. The second committee was composed of nurse clinicians who worked with children who had cancer within the hospital with which the project was affiliated, the University of Minnesota Hospitals.

Health professionals thus were involved with the project from the moment of its inception. Possibly they developed a proprietary feeling toward the project so that they wished to continue the services they felt were needed and desired by the community. Thus, in this way we generated some acceptance of the concept by using an administrative avenue. Eventually, through the advisory committee members, the project staff arranged to present the results of the research to staff members, administrators, and boards of directors of various institutions.

Another avenue of influence was *education*. Lectures, workshops, meetings, and personal communication between the Project staff and health professionals in local, state, and national agencies helped to teach the health community about home care and the progress of this project. It was no longer possible for a hospital, physician, or nurse to say "that can't be done" because these health providers had learned that home care for dying children was feasible.

The staff became active and working members on committees in the community—for example, an American Cancer Society educational committee on childhood cancer, a hospital home health services advisory committee, and a volunteer committee concerned with the care of families confronting death through terminal illness.

We prepared written materials and made them readily available to the medical community (see Bibliography). We shared general information about the research project and the results of the project, as well as the specific nursing care knowledge that we gained while providing this highly specialized home care. Thus, the publications became valuable in their own right to those who received them.

Manuals have also been prepared for both home care nurses and family caregivers to be used in caring for the dying child. The circulation of these manuals contributes to the desired changes in the overall system.

We have given informative presentations to classes in schools of nursing, as well as to various classes at the university. Members of our staff have made a number of appearances to organizations of nurses, physicians, chaplains, and other professionals.

In addition to using administrative and educational measures during the institutionalization phase, the Project staff also pursued both *legislative and media avenues*. Representatives of the Project made appearances before the Minnesota State Legislature Health Subcommittee on two different occasions, and Project staff conferred with then-Vice President Mondale and leading insurance agencies. We utilized mass media to a great extent. A documentary film, "Time to Come Home," was prepared and is being circulated to cancer societies, medical centers, professional organizations, and others. In addition, television and radio interviews have been aired. Over 60 articles and book chapters have been published in the literature of numerous disciplines, including medicine, psychology, sociology, and nursing (see Bibliography for representative examples).

Conclusions

As a result of extensive exploration and use of all four of these avenues of influence, we reduced system resistances and established the institutionalization of the home care concepts. It was important to include the institutionalization phase in the original research design. This was a continuing concern of the principal investigator who devoted much of her time and energy to laying the groundwork for this phase.

Three local institutions in Minneapolis-St. Paul have established a permanent home care program for children who have reached the end-stage of life, one that will enable them to die at home as requested by parents. They are the large, 700-bed university hospital that serves as a cancer referral center for six states; a small 100-bed pediatric hospital; and a large, private clinic. Each of these programs has followed the policy guidelines for the provision of home care services for dying children that were developed and utilized by the research project. In addition, there has been an acceptance of home care for dying children in communities outside our local area.

The Home Care Project concepts have been accepted and implemented in the overall system. The nursing research which was done played an important part in the positive response of the health care delivery system to societal needs. We were successful at least in part because we took advantage of the local response to the Project and because our staff was diligent in their attempts to counteract system resistances.

Another factor that facilitated the success of the Project was the general climate of the period. This included an ever-increasing interest in the topics of death and dying, an awareness in the lay and professional communities of rapidly increasing hospital and health care costs, a desire to find ways to reduce or contain costs, a movement for patients to stay out of health care facilities as much as possible, and finally an increase in consumerism as citizens made more demands on their health care system. Minnesota was, for instance, the first state to pass into law a Patient's Bill of Rights which is posted in every hospital. Perhaps the Home Care Project began at the right place at the right time.

Our questions now are broader than those questions asked at the beginning of the Project about feasibility and desirability of home care. These were answered in the affirmative. Now we are asking the following: Can we as a society have flexibility in our health care system? Can we develop the community services necessary to make such ventures work? Are we willing to let the consumer assume the major caregiving role? How can the health care system be responsive to the needs of society and be flexible in meeting those needs? Will nursing services be available?

In summary, if the general public is to be offered three alternatives of care—hospital, hospice, and home—then nursing research must play a dominant part in bringing about needed changes. Model research projects in hospice care designed and directed by nurses must now be carried out.

Nurses doing primary professional practice must be supported by nurse networks. Institutionalization of services must be a part of each project. Beneficiaries from the projects and nurses must become allies and pursue change through administrative, educational, legislative, and media avenues.

Bibliography

Carlson, P., Simacek, M., Henry W. F., Martinson, I. M., Montgomery, J., & Montgomery, K., "Helping Parents Cope: A Model Home Care Program for the Dying Child," in H. Wass & C. A. Corr (eds.), *Childhood and Death*. New York: Hemisphere, 1984, pp. 113–127.

Gronseth, E. C., Martinson, I. M., Kersey, J. H., & Nesbit, M. E., "Support System of Health Professionals as Observed in the Project of Home Care for the Child with Cancer," *Death Education*, 1981, *5*, 37–50.

Martinson, I. M., "Alternative Environments for Care of the Dying Child: Hospice, Hospital, or Home," in O. J. Sahler (ed.), *The Child and Death*. St. Louis: C. V. Mosby, 1978, pp. 83–91.

Martinson, I. M., "Care of the Dying Child—1," *Nursing Times*, 1983, *79*, 56–57.

Martinson, I. M., "Caring for the Dying Child," *Nursing Clinics of North America*, 1979, *14*, 467–474.

Martinson, I. M., "Dying Children at Home," *Nursing Times*, 1980, *76*, 129–132.

Martinson, I. M. (ed.), *Home Care: A Manual for Implementation of Home Care for Children Dying of Cancer*. Minneapolis, MN: University of Minnesota, School of Nursing, 1978 (offset).

Martinson, I. M. (ed.), *Home Care for the Dying Child: Professional and Family Perspectives*. New York: Appleton-Century-Crofts, 1976.

Martinson, I. M., Armstrong, G. D., Geis, D. P., Anglim, M. A., Gronseth, E. C., MacInnis, H., Kersey, J. H., & Nesbit, M. E., "Home Care for Children Dying of Cancer," *Pediatrics*, 1978, *62*, 106–113.

Martinson, I. M., Armstrong, G. D., Geis, D. P., Anglim, M. A., Gronseth, E. C., Macinnis, H., Nesbit, M. E., & Kersey, J. H., "Facilitating Home Care for Children Dying of Cancer," *Cancer Nursing*, 1978, *1*, 41–45.

Martinson, I. M., Geis, D. P., Anglim, M. A., Peterson, E., Nesbit, M. E., & Kersey, J. H., "When the Patient is Dying: Home Care for the Child," *American Journal of Nursing*, 1977, *77*, 1815–1817.

Martinson, I. M., & Henry, W. F., "Home Care for Dying Children: Costs and Consequences for the Family," *The Hastings Center Report*, 1980, *10* (2), 5–7.

Martinson, I. M., Nixon, S., Geis, D. P., YaDeau, R., Nesbit, M. E., & Kersey, J. H., "Nursing Care in Childhood Cancer: Methadone," *American Journal of Nursing,* 1982, *82,* 432–435.

Moldow, D. G., Armstrong, G. D., Henry, W. F., & Martinson, I. M., "The Cost of Home Care for Dying Children," *Medical Care,* 1982, *20,* 1154–1160.

Moldow, D. G., & Martinson, I. M., "From Research to Reality—Home Care for the Dying Child," *MCN: The American Journal of Maternal Child Nursing,* 1980, *51,* 159–166.

Moldow, D. G., & Martinson, I. M., *Home Care: A Manual for Parents.* Minneapolis, MN: University of Minnesota, School of Nursing, 1979 (offset).

"Time to Come Home," a documentary film; color, 24 minutes. Produced by Kenneth Greer with Ida M. Martinson. Minneapolis, MN: University of Minnesota, School of Nursing, 1979.

3

Improving Care for Hospitalized Terminally Ill Children: A Practicable Model

Patricia Riordan Wheeler and Nancy Foerster Lange
in consultation with Salvatore J. Bertolone

Introduction

Problems in Caring for Terminally Ill Children

A recent article in the American Psychological Association *Monitor* described the status of hospice care for children in the United States in the following way:"Today there are more than 800 [hospices]. But only about 20 of them have served dying children, and most of these have served one or two" (Cunningham, 1983, p. 9).

Our review of the professional literature reveals a similar imbalance. Compared to the hundreds of articles written regarding hospice care for adults, those addressing the needs of dying children are strikingly few. Though the professional community is beginning to recognize the tremendous need in this area, actual development and implementation of programs of palliative care for dying children fall far short of meeting the need. In addition, it is almost exclusively home care programs that address this area. Families who receive care in acute care settings are often deprived of this special dimension of care.

It is our belief that there are two major reasons for the overall lack of palliative care programs specifically designed for dying children. The first reason is that the death of a child from any cause is viewed as unnatural by family members and caregivers alike. Children are not supposed to die. They are supposed to live, nurtured and protected by adults, to maturity in the fullness of time. This deeply ingrained expectation makes the recognition of terminality in a child extremely difficult. Not only has nature failed if a child dies, but so have we, since we are the protectors of children. Add to this the emphasis on cure characteristic of the medical model in our society, and the forces against which we must struggle to be able to accept terminal or life-threatening illness in a child become even more formidable. With such an orientation, it is not surprising that caregivers—family members and others—are unwilling to embrace a concept that to many signifies death.

The second major reason for the relative nonexistence of hospice care for children stems from the first. Because of the tremendous emotional impact associated with a child's dying, professional caregivers often feel inadequate to meet the needs of patients and families, afraid of failing them again and afraid of the pain they, the caregivers, will feel as a result of their involvement. It is therefore easier to ignore the needs or to hope that someone else will meet them.

In terms of care based on hospice principles for hospitalized children, there are several additional influencing factors: no "in-house" hospice beds; no personnel trained in comprehensive terminal care; no community-based hospice program able to make hospital visits because of reimbursement and other problems; no free-standing hospice in the community; no pediatric component in the existing area hospice. These deterrents often exist even in communities where there is an awareness of the need for and value of hospice-type palliative care.

An Approach to Improved Care

In the summer of 1979, Hospice of Louisville, Inc., received its first pediatric referral. One of our volunteer nurses with a background in pediatrics began working with the child and family. Over the next several months, three more referrals came in. As the nurses and volunteers worked with these families and their special needs, they became more and more convinced of the need for a program designed specifically for children. These experiences were the major motivating factors in the development of what was to become one of the first formal pediatric hospice programs in the United States. From its inception to mid-August 1984, the program has served 79 children and families. During this time we have worked with children and families in the home, in the hospital, and in long-term care facilities.

Several problems have been identified in terms of maintaining a viable and effective program:

1. Variable levels of understanding of the nature of hospice care.
2. Hesitancy of health professionals to refer.
3. Reluctance of caregivers to become involved in palliative care for dying children.
4. Absence of coordination of caregivers' efforts.
5. Lack of continuity of care.

A tremendous amount of education was and is needed for professional and lay persons alike regarding the real purpose of hospice care, which is to affirm life and promote as much quality time as possible for the child and family who face a life-threatening illness. A true understanding of this goal not only eases caregivers' acceptance of the hospice philosophy, but helps them recommend and explain it to families in terms that are hopeful rather than hopeless. Anyone facing a life-threatening illness experiences profound responses and needs simply because the illness is there and is a *threat* to life. This does not say that death is directly imminent nor does it discount the possibility of remissions or stable periods. It simply recognizes the need for help when a life is threatened by disease.

No one person or even one agency is able to meet all of the needs of children and families facing terminal illness. This is especially true with terminally ill children who are in and out of acute care hospitals many times during an illness. A child's needs during hospitalization are singular and separate from other identifiable needs during the illness. The complex needs of the child are also inextricably intertwined with those of parents, siblings, and other family members. For these reasons, ongoing *coordination* of the family's care must be achieved in order to provide continuity of care from one caregiver to another, one agency to another, and one setting to another.

Our recognition of how these problems affect delivery of care for terminally ill children led us to identify means to overcome the problems. Since care of children in the home has been extensively addressed by others (e.g., Martinson et al., 1978; see also Chapters 2 and 4 in this volume), our concern here is especially for terminally ill children while they are in the hospital and as they move between hospital and home. What are their special needs? What are the needs of their families? What about the staff caring for them? How can hospice principles be applied in the acute care setting to meet those needs?

We must understand the principles of good terminal care as identified by the International Work Group in Death, Dying and Bereavement (1979) in order to answer these questions. In summary, these principles—originally divided into four categories (general, patient-oriented, family-oriented, and staff-oriented)—state that: the patient and family comprise the unit of care; the approach to care must be interdisciplinary; a major focus of care is symptom control—physical, psychological, social, and spiritual; care must be available 24 hours a day, with bereavement care offered to survivors; and caregivers, as well as the patient/family, must receive support and education.

If we keep these principles in mind while exploring the reactions and needs of hospitalized terminally ill children and their families, we will facilitate our understanding of how they can direct caregivers in meeting those needs.

The Hospital Setting and Terminally Ill Children

Hospitalizations for terminally ill children occur at different points along the continuum of remission-relapse and at varying frequencies. In the vast majority of terminal and other illnesses that are appropriate for hospice-type care, parents seem to prefer to have their children at home in familiar surroundings as much of the time as possible (Zimmerman, 1979). When hospitalization is necessary for these children, it is usually due to uncontrolled symptoms, particularly pain; other physical problems; parental exhaustion and fear; and the parents' desire to avoid an at-home death. Some families prefer the security of the hospital setting and support of the medical team (Kent, 1981). The hospital or pediatric medical center can be a safe and friendly place, where relationships may have been established early in the illness. Whatever the situation, there are specific needs associated with the hospitalization.

Needs of Children and Families

When a disease no longer responds to curative therapy, treatment and emphasis shift to palliative care and management of symptoms. As an illness progresses, staff must identify and address problems specific to each stage, while always remembering the child and family as a unit (Plant, 1977). It is important to the family that the child remain as alert and comfortable as possible until the end. Not all symptoms can be relieved by drug therapy. Some can only be helped by the caring personal contact and communication of the staff. Many symptoms will be eased by the presence and involvement of the child's parents or other significant people. This joint concern and involvement of family, friends, and the health care team can greatly influence the child's and family's emotional and spiritual well-being, and will give added support to the child (Chapman & Goodall, 1980).

The death of a child is extremely traumatic and presents special problems for the entire family (Farrow, 1981). Terminal illness does not automatically confer strength and a pulling together. The response of family members to terminal illness and impending death will be affected by their perception of their child's illness, the duration of the illness, previous experience with illness, preexisting family integration, available resources, and religious beliefs. Family reactions in dealing with stress induced by the terminal illness of a child are varied and intense. While some are easy for staff to understand and cope with, others are not. Families usually have no models as to how to behave. They move at their own pace. The most common family reactions or behaviors are denial, guilt, fear, depression, anger, and grief. Some of these reactions are rooted in feelings of helplessness and hopelessness. Staff must strive to give the family and child a sense of worth and a measure of control. Perhaps in our ambition and desire to do everything, we sometimes immobilize our patients and render them more helpless and depressed than they need be (Earnshaw-Smith, 1981).

If we are to understand family needs, we must talk unhurriedly with children and family members, and build trusting relationships. Our failure to develop these relationships will leave families bewildered and insatiably demanding. Families need information about the illness and they must know what to expect. Their feelings must be accepted without criticism, and the child and family must be helped to accept all feelings as normal. Families need help in setting realistic, short-term goals. Families should be educated in the care of their ill children, and allowed and encouraged to be with them. Neither the child nor the family should be so separated by treatment and routines that they are forced to terminate their relationships prematurely. Family strengths and effective coping mechanisms need to be identified and reinforced. Appropriate referrals should be made to supportive community resources and practical assistance should also be provided. Most importantly, families need staff presence and honest, open communication (Dobihal, 1974).

In order to assess the effect a fatal illness will have on both the sick child and on the siblings in the family, it is essential to have an understanding of how children perceive death, and to realize that a child's understanding is based on both his or her developmental level and chronological age, individual personality, past experiences with death and loss, and the family's religious beliefs (Sahler & Friedman, 1981).

Dying children often blame themselves and thus experience guilt for the disruption they see in their families, and the sadness and suffering they see in their parents. They need a clear and honest explanation of what is happening. They often need reassurance of what will happen to their parents following their death, and that they will one day be together again. It is not death itself that is so difficult for children to accept, but rather separation from parents. This fear is obviously intensified in the hospital setting (Earnshaw-Smith, 1981).

Even children who are not aware of their diagnosis and prognosis sense anxiety in those around them and respond to it. Children need and deserve direct, honest answers to their questions. Withholding information can increase tensions, and disturbing fantasies may flood the child's mind. Children need a safe, private environment to decrease feelings of loss of control. Reassurance, coupled with the presence of loved ones and supportive staff, can offer a child much-needed security. Play and/or expressive therapy can be beneficial, nonthreatening supports for hospitalized children dealing with a terminal illness (see Chapters 8 and 9).

Needs of Siblings

Siblings frequently feel abandoned by parents during the hospitalization of a terminally ill brother or sister. They become jealous of the difference in attention, which they may perceive as a difference in love. They may even wish their sister or brother would die; then, after the death, they may experience survivor guilt thinking they caused the death. During this particularly intense period of parental stress, siblings often lack much-needed parental support. Therefore, they need an alternate support system.

With the consent of the sick child, staff and parents should encourage and allow siblings to visit as often as they wish, and to be as involved in the care of their brother or sister as they choose. Siblings frequently exhibit fear of personally becoming ill or dying. They should be encouraged to express or act out feelings, that is, with puppets, clay, or drawing. Their questions should be addressed honestly, simply, and concretely, and according to the family's value system (Sahler & Friedman, 1981). It is better to deal with questions and emotions prior to the death in order to lessen pathological behavior problems after the death (Martinson et al., 1978).

Needs of Staff Members

Staff members frequently exhibit emotional responses similar to those of the family. Families may be on an emotional roller coaster, and staff may find themselves in the same predicament. And yet, the family's outlook will be greatly influenced by the personality and reactions of staff (Verwoerdt, 1965). This is why dealing with terminal illness and death in children requires a special degree of caring and maturity (Farrow, 1981). Staff members must be in touch with their own feelings before they can offer support to children and families.

Many people show little awareness of the psychological impact caused by working with terminally ill children and their families, or the stress it creates. Caring behavior is as much a part of the helping process as drugs and treatments, but such behavior puts the staff person in a very vulnerable position. Despite the best intentions, not all health care professionals perform well in caring for the terminally ill. The strain caused by daily involvement with dying children and their families may affect the ability of some to deal with such children and families in a sensitive and professional manner (Potter, 1980).

The interdisciplinary team approach is paramount as a support system for individual caregivers. It is necessary in terminal illness to develop supportive attitudes and to set realistic personal and professional goals and expectations. Staff must be aware of their own emotional limitations and time constraints. Staff, as well as children and their families, must recognize and utilize available emotional and psychological services and/or supports, either within the immediate setting or outside its boundaries (Hackley, 1977; see also Chapter 13).

Improving Care for Hospitalized Terminally Ill Children

An analysis of the needs of dying children, their family members, and their caregivers within the hospital setting reveals them to be well suited to an application of hospice principles of care. Nevertheless, we recognized early in our own work that this application frequently does not occur. It was this knowledge, in addition to our contacts with children and families, and our experiences of trying to deal with the problems of delivering effective care to terminally ill children, that led us to the development of a model for implementing improved care for dying children in acute care settings.

Delivery of this care will involve the concentrated efforts of many people: nurses, physicians, social workers, nutritionists, clergy, therapists, family members, friends, and so on. Not only must these people contribute their professional expertise and human presence to the care, but, to ensure its quality, they must do so as an interdisciplinary team. This is not always easily accomplished, and it requires true commitment to the common goal of maximizing quality of life for the child and family. "Members must resolve to break down interprofessional rivalries and set aside defensive attitudes. Communication is essential and requires both time and effort" (Abdellah et al., 1982, p. 12).

Success also requires that the team accept similar principles and standards of terminal care. The current recognition and acceptance by our society of the value of hospice principles and standards of care make their dissemination to caregivers easier. Education of these caregivers and coordination of their efforts in terminal care must be accomplished. As Abdellah and colleagues have stated (1982), "not all . . . health professionals have the necessary training to be effective in working with dying patients and their families" (p. 13).

When possible, use of hospice personnel already educated and experienced in terminal care to expand this care into acute care settings is a logical progression of the hospice movement. In other cases, there are often caregivers available who are educated and experienced in this area and interested in educating others. Though we can anticipate problems that may arise in implementing any plan to enhance a specific approach to care, let us explore a model which offers a vehicle through which this can be accomplished.

The Collaboration Model

Assumptions and Values

Hazzard (1971) defined a model as "a symbolic depiction in logical terms of an idealized relatively simple situation showing the structure of the original system" (p. 392). Note that this definition covers models of "situations" as well as those of concrete realities.

The value of a model is its ability to demonstrate not only that a situation exists, but *how* it exists or, prescriptively, how it *can* or *ought* to exist. Models may describe and functionalize already defined theory, or they may help conceptualize and build theory that has not yet been defined.

Systems theory has been well defined and used as a basis for practice models (Chin, 1969; Bertalanffy, 1968). Along with developmental theory, it offers a strong framework for the model we propose.

Assumptions. The assumptions underlying the development of the collaboration model for care of terminally ill persons were adopted from the assumptions listed by the International Work Group in Death, Dying and Bereavement (1979). Since we are focusing the model on hospitalized terminally ill children, we will list those assumptions most germane to that population and setting.

1. The care of the dying is a process involving needs of the patient, family, and caregivers.
2. The problems of the patient/family facing terminal illness include a wide variety of issues: psychological, legal, social, spiritual, economic, and interpersonal.
3. Health care services customarily lack coordination.

4. Patients' needs may change over time.
5. The varied problems and anxieties associated with terminal illness can occur at any time of day or night.
6. The growing body of knowledge in symptom control, patient/family-centered care, and other aspects of the care of the terminally ill is now readily available.
7. Good terminal care presupposes emotional investment on the part of the staff.

In terms of caring for dying children, let us add the following assumptions:

8. The death of a child is considered "unnatural," no matter what its cause.
9. Families and caregivers of dying children may experience more acute needs for consistent psychological and emotional support than families and caregivers of dying adults.
10. No one discipline can meet all of the needs of dying children and their families.

There are two final assumptions necessary to the existence of the model:

11. The human being is an open system interacting with an environment, which is both internal and external.
12. Interaction between humans and environment can produce positive or negative consequences.

Values. The values implied by a model are necessary to illustrate that the goal of the model is worth attaining.

1. The uniqueness of the hospice philosophy lies in its strict focus on the terminally ill person and on his or her family. This focus produces specialized approaches to terminal care that benefit those experiencing and coping with dying.
2. Application of specialized knowledge to the delivery of care to dying children and their families is important for the welfare of those persons.
3. The concern of health care personnel for terminally ill children and their families is to provide the family group with the means to attain quality time during the terminal illness.
4. Collaboration among caregivers and between caregivers and those they serve, promotes quality care for the child and his or her family with a minimum of expenditure of energy. This pre-

serves patient and family energy for the participation in quality time available to them.

5. Qualified hospice personnel have the obligation to promote collaboration through dissemination of specialized knowledge and coordination of ongoing application of hospice principles to care of terminally ill children in any setting.

Goals and Recipients

Goals. The *primary or ultimate goal* of this model is quality care for hospitalized terminally ill children and their families (see Table 3.1). Quality care is defined as care based on the principles set forth by the International Work Group in Death, Dying and Bereavement which underlie standards for terminal care. Since these principles are the foundation of the hospice approach to terminal care, it is logical that experienced hospice personnel be instrumental in facilitating the delivery of this care if they are available. In the absence of such hospice workers, another caregiver educated and experienced in this area must assume this role. In this model, facilitation takes the form of educating hospital personnel and others involved, who may be unfamiliar with these principles and stan-

Table 3.1 Major Components of the Collaboration Model

Goals
Initial: Education of caregivers and coordination of care
Primary: Quality care for hospitalized terminally ill children and their families

Patients or Recipients
Initial: Health-care personnel and other caregivers
Primary: Terminally ill children and their families

Intervention

Framework
Initial: Situations related to education of caregivers or coordination of care
Primary: Situations for caring occurring in hospital or associated with transfer between hospital and home

Procedure
Initial: Dissemination of information
Primary: Delivery of quality care to hospitalized terminally ill children and their families

Agent
Initial: Health-care personnel
Primary: All caregivers, including family

dards. It also leads to coordinating aspects of care from several different sources. Hence, the education of caregivers and the coordination of care become our *initial or proximate goals.*

The criteria for measuring the accomplishment of the primary goal will be those standards of care developed by the National Hospice Organization that are pertinent to an acute care setting (National Hospice Organization, 1982). These criteria must be applied to each individual situation.

Recipients. As described in the previous section, there are actually two levels at which activity occurs within the model, and so *two different recipients* for our actions. Activity directed toward accomplishing the initial goal—facilitation through education and coordination—is aimed at *health-care personnel and others* who are involved in the care of the child and family while they are in the hospital. These persons may have little or no expertise in the area; they may be quite knowledgeable and experienced; or they may fall anywhere in between. Because they are usually identified with a specific department in their institution with specified prescribed duties, they are unable to act as coordinators of total care.

Activity related to the primary goal—delivery of quality care by the hospice and the hospital personnel—is then received by *the child and family.* The child may be in the early or the late stages of terminal illness. Family and child may be experiencing the stresses associated with the illness anywhere along the continuum of distress from minor to overwhelming. They may be very familiar with the hospital setting or totally new to it. Whatever the situation, the goal remains quality care.

Intervention

The three major aspects of the intervention component of the model are *framework, procedure,* and *agent.* Each may be viewed in relation to the initial and primary goals discussed earlier.

Framework—Initial Goal. Any time, place, or situation contributing to coordination of care and/or the education of: (1) caregivers by those familiar with principles of terminal care; or (2) members of the care team by each other of specifics related to cases.

Framework—Primary Goal. Any situation occurring at any time during a dying child's stay in an acute care hospital setting.

Obviously we are focusing here on dying children in the hospital. We must keep in mind, though, that children often are in and out of the hospital several times during a terminal illness. Therefore, while we focus on the hospital setting, we must remember that quality care by its very nature must include continuity of care. When the hospitalized child goes home, our framework must expand; part of the activity which the child and family received in the hospital, along with part of the team, must go home with them.

Procedure—Initial Goal. Educate caregivers and coordinate care. There are several effective and efficient ways to educate personnel involved with hospitalized children as regards the components of quality care for terminally ill children.

1. Hospital staff educated and experienced in therapeutic terminal care may informally share this knowledge with other caregivers within or outside of the hospital.
2. Appropriately trained and experienced personnel may conduct inservice education classes for various departments within the hospital that are frequently involved in terminal care, for example, nursing, pharmacy, dietary, and so on.
3. Informal meetings between local hospice workers and specific inpatient staff will acquaint these staff members with the hospice concept and philosophy. This may engender further interest and desire for knowledge.
4. Hospital pediatric staff may educate hospice workers about pediatric care in general if the hospice staff do not have experience in working with children.
5. Staff conferences about a dying child should include all persons involved in the care, including those from outside clinics or agencies. Such conferences offer excellent opportunities for sharing knowledge.
6. A hospice volunteer training course conducted in the hospital itself offers knowledge to a large number of inpatient staff which will beneficially influence care they give to their terminally ill patients.
7. Identification of an interested and committed pediatrician to serve as medical consultant to the interdisciplinary team is essential. This role should include formal and informal education of other physicians in the area of hospice care for terminally ill children.
8. Presentation of the hospice philosophy and principles of care at grand rounds held for hospital and community pediatricians, and at local meetings of the pediatric society, will acquaint physicians with the workings and availability of the hospice concept for terminally ill children both at home and in the hospital.
9. Hospice personnel should address the staffs of other agencies that are involved in caring for the child and family to explain the

process of delivering care based on hospice principles and to emphasize the importance of continuity in that care.
10. The family and, as appropriate, the child, should receive ongoing education regarding the care plan of which they will be part.

If possible, the major responsibility for the educational components of the model related to hospice-type care should fall to hospice personnel. They are specially trained in the area, are experienced in delivering this care, and are not hampered by the time constraints placed on others in terms of additional job commitments. Care of the terminally ill and coordination of that care *is* their job.

Coordination of hospice care in the hospital is accomplished through the following actions of the designated coordinator or worker assigned to each case:

1. Know who is involved in the care of the child and family.
2. Attend all staff conferences regarding the child and encourage other involved persons to attend.
3. If the child is a patient of a local hospice program, invite hospital personnel to hospice team meetings when the case is presented to the hospice interdisciplinary team.
4. Encourage open discussion of all aspects of care by team members.
5. Follow up meetings by sending written summaries of information and plans to those who attended as well as to those who did not.
6. Avoid duplication of services to the family by supporting hospital personnel in the expert care they give and supplementing in areas of hospice expertise.
7. Encourage continued contact through phone calls, mail, or visits between closely involved hospital personnel and the child and family during time periods when the child is out of the hospital.
8. Stay informed of what happens to the child and family while they are in the hospital, and keep hospital staff informed of what happens to them while they are home.

Procedure—Primary Goal. Deliver quality care to hospitalized terminally ill children and their families. Delivery of care based on hospice principles must be consistent to assure ongoing quality care. To accomplish this, all major caregivers must incorporate these principles into their assessment, planning, implementation, and evaluation of the care they give. Care must be given as a team with agreement as to components of care, and continuity assured by methods discussed earlier. Family members and children when appropriate must be active members of the team, involved in all four steps of the delivery of care. As care is evaluated and outcomes noted, modifications must be made as necessary to assure the desired outcome of quality time for children and families as they experience terminal illness.

Agent—Initial Goal. Health care personnel, involved caregivers, patient, and family members. As discussed earlier, hospice personnel are well-equipped to educate caregivers about hospice principles and standards and to coordinate team efforts. Other caregivers will share knowledge related to care in their areas of expertise.

Agent—Primary Goal. All caregivers, including family. Obviously, hospital and hospice personnel will be directly involved in delivering care. The child and family, as members of the care team, can also be viewed as agents. They certainly have input into the development of the care plan; families are often involved in direct physical care of the child and are always influential in emotional, psychological, and spiritual care. With proper education and guidance, the family will become an agent of quality care for itself.

Applying the Model

Application of the collaboration model to the delivery of care to dying children and their families requires several conditions: (1) acceptance of its goals by caregivers and families; (2) understanding of which parties are intended to benefit from the particular goals and interventions; and (3) determination of who will participate in the implementation of the intervention procedures designed to achieve those goals (see Figure 3.1). Use of the model with pediatric patients at Hospice of Louisville has been possible because of the presence in some measure of each of these conditions. The philosophy of the hospice program to go wherever the patient is, as well as the interest and participation of the pediatric health care community, have made implementation a reality. The goals are accepted by all as valuable and worthy of ongoing effort, while the recipients are also generally accepted.

Most of the activity envisioned by the model occurs within the intervention component. We have attempted essentially all of the steps outlined in that component with varying levels of success. Several factors have led to positive results in our community. First, when a child is referred to our hospice program, he or she has nearly always been in the hospital before, and has therefore developed relations with hospital staff.

Figure 3.1 A Collaboration Model for Improving Care for Hospitalized Terminally Ill Children

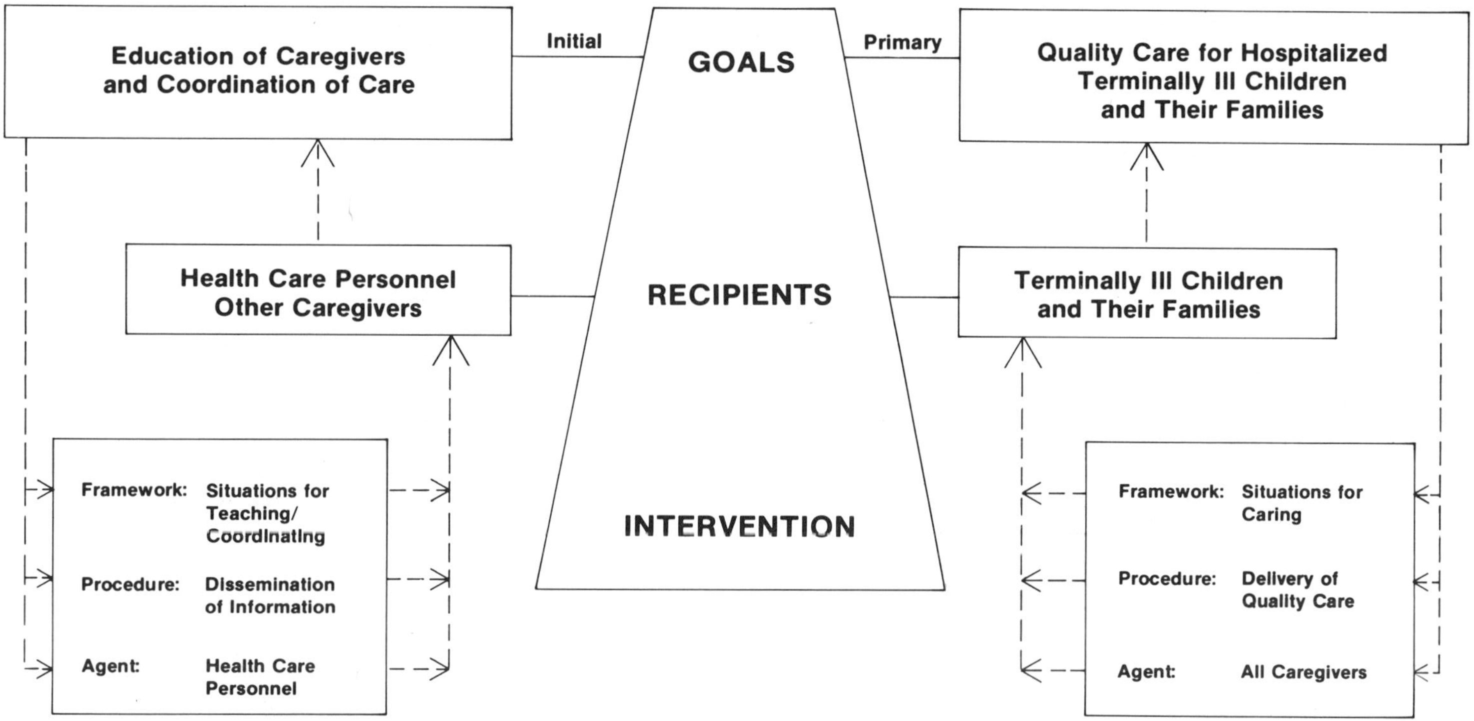

Second, physicians, clinic staff, and hospital staff in our area are generally supportive of hospice involvement, and are certainly cognizant of the principles of hospice care. Third, the clinic and hospital nurses who work with terminally ill children and their families are tremendously experienced, compassionate, and knowledgeable. The relationships between these nurses and their patients and families are strong and supportive. Furthermore, relationships between these nurses and the hospice nurses are characterized by mutual respect and support. All are committed to the best care possible for each child and family, and they regularly exchange knowledge and information through formal and informal channels. Finally, the freedom of the hospice nurse to act as coordinator, and to follow the child from hospital to home and back, allows ongoing communication and continuity of care.

Problems we have encountered are similar to those described by others. Professional jealousies, misunderstanding of the true focus of hospice care, confusion over roles, and lack of communication have all become apparent at one time or another. We are aware that these are problems that will come and go. We also recognize that such problems must be dealt with openly and early if they are to be prevented from interrupting the attainment of the model's goals. Areas of the model that need continuing work are education of caregivers, communication, and support of caregivers. If these are ongoing, we have found that the patient and family-centered activities in the model are much more effectively accomplished.

Conclusion

The last several years have shown a marked growth in the area of pediatric hospital care. Recognition of the unique needs of children and the inclusion of families in giving and receiving care have added significantly to its quality. What, then, is different or distinctive about hospice care for dying children in hospitals? These children are dying in a society which rejects death in general, one that views the death of a child as particularly unnatural and unfair. A special understanding of the effects of these views on the needs, reactions, and coping mechanisms of hospitalized terminally ill children and their families is essential in order to be able to give these family groups the care and support they need. A second important factor is that while a child with an episodic illness goes home from the hospital well, a child with a life-threatening illness will move between hospital and home several times during the course of his or her disease. This fact, in conjunction with the wide range of needs the child and family experience, makes ongoing coordination and continuity of care essential to meeting these needs. Interdisciplinary team members from all agencies, along with family members, must work together and communicate regularly to avoid loss of caring and support during periods of change or less intense contact with health professionals.

It is not necessary to have a formal pediatric hospice program to give care based on hospice principles to terminally ill hospitalized children. But it is essential to have an understanding of the unique needs and problems faced by these children and their families, and to aggressively seek out or develop the resources and methods necessary to assist these families as they struggle to maintain their integrity, to care for their members, and to experience the fullness of their lives.

References

Abdellah, F. S., Harper, B. C., & Lanceford, J. L., *Report of Hospice Care in the United States.* Washington, DC: U.S. Department of Health and Human Services, Health Care Financing Administration, 1982.

Bertalanffy, L. V., *General Systems Theory.* New York: Braziller, 1968.

Chapman, J. A., & Goodall, J., "Helping a Child to Live Whilst Dying," *Lancet,* 1980, *1,* 753–756.

Chin, R., "The Utility of Systems Models and Developmental Models for Practitioners," in W. G. Bennis, et al. (eds.), *Planning of Change.* New York: Holt, 1969.

Cunningham, S., "Hospices Find Place for Family," *APA Monitor,* April 1983, 9–10.

Dobihal, E. F., "Talk or Terminal Care?", *Connecticut Medicine,* 1974, 38, 364–367.

Earnshaw-Smith, E., "Dealing with Dying Patients and Their Relatives," *British Medical Journal,* 1981, *282,* 1779.

Farrow, G., "Helen House: Our First Hospice for Children." *Nursing Times,* 1981, *77,* 1433–1434. (See also Chapter 6, this volume.)

Hackley, J. A., "Full Service Hospice Offers Home, Day and Inpatient Care," *Hospitals,* 1977, *51,* 84–87.

Hazzard, M. E., "An Overview of System Theory," *Nursing Clinics of North America,* 1971, *6,* 385–393.

International Work Group in Death, Dying and Bereavement, "Assumptions and Principles Underlying Standards for Terminal Care," *American Journal of Nursing,* 1979, *79,* 296–297.

Kent, J., "Life Before Death," *Nursing Times,* 1981, *77,* 1435.

Martinson, I., Armstrong, G. D., Geis, D. P., Anglim, M. A., Gronseth, E. C., MacInnis, H., Kersey, J. H., & Nesbit, M. E., "Home Care for Children Dying of Cancer," *Pediatrics,* 1978, *62,* 106–113. (See also Chapter 2 above.)

National Hospice Organization, *Standards of a Hospice Program of Care,* 1982.

Plant, J., "Finding a Home for Hospice Care in the U.S.," *Hospitals,* 1977, *51,* 53–61.

Potter, J. F., "A Challenge for the Hospice Movement," *New England Journal of Medicine*, 1980, *302*, 53–55.
Sahler, O. J. Z., & Friedman, S., "The Dying Child," *Pediatrics in Review*, 1981, *3*, 159–164.
Verwoerdt, A., "Communication with the Fatally Ill," *CA: A Cancer Journal for Clinicians*, 1965, *15*, 105–111.
Zimmerman, J. M., "Experience with a Hospice Care Program for the Terminally Ill," *Annals of Surgery*, 1979, *189*, 683–690.

Bibliography

Dickoff, J., & James, P., "A Theory of Theories: A Position Paper," *Nursing Research*, 1968, *17*, 197–203.
Fomufod, A. K., "Chronically Ill Institutionalized Children: Psychosocial Effects of Prolonged Hospitalization of the Terminally Sick Child," *Social Science and Medicine, Part A: Medical Psychology and Medical Sociology*, 1980, *14A*, 239–242.
Martinson, I., *Home Care: A Manual for Implementation of Home Care for Children Dying of Cancer*. Minneapolis: University of Minnesota, 1978.
Riehl, J. P., & Roy, C., *Conceptual Models for Nursing Practice*. New York: Appleton-Century-Crofts, 1974.
Whitfield, J. M., Siegel, R. E., Glicken, A. D., Harmon, R. J., Powers, L. K., & Goldson, E. J., "The Application of Hospice Concepts to Neonatal Care," *American Journal of Diseases of Children*, 1982, *136*, 421–424. (See also Chapter 7 below.)

II

Caring for Dying Children: Specific Applications

The four chapters that comprise Part II all draw upon the general principles set forth in Part I and apply them in specific and distinctive ways for implementing hospice approaches to pediatric care. Each of these chapters explores the full range of needs experienced by a selected population of terminally ill or chronically ill children and their families. In each case, a variety of distressing diseases or conditions is envisioned, and each chapter addresses the provision of services at multiple levels from the physical to the psychosocial and the spiritual. The settings and the ways in which such services are offered differ greatly. What binds the whole together is a shared concern for maximizing quality of life even when cure is no longer a reasonable expectation and death may be close. Readers may best respond to this concern and reward our contributors not by slavishly duplicating their programs, but by learning from their insights and extrapolating to local contexts. A firm grasp of basic goals, keen sensitivity to actual needs, and hard work in providing services must be the guiding rules.

In Chapter 4, Belinda Martin sets forth a thorough description of a home care program with hospital-based coordination that relies heavily upon service providers from the community. We stress home care in this way because the home, in our judgment, is the primary health care setting for children and families. The hospital may well be the primary center for medical and cure-oriented care, but health and quality of life are originally and extensively promoted in the home. Thus, hospice care for children and families is perhaps best rendered in their homes—at least for those who wish to be at home and who are able to do so with appropriate support. Note, however, that home care is perceived here only as one option to be offered to children and their families, that the possibility of rehospitalization is always kept open, and that the goal is to normalize daily living and to improve quality of life—not necessarily to have the death occur at home.

Hospice approaches are, of course, not confined either to full-time home care or to traditional inpatient care, for it is the philosophy of care, not the setting, that defines these approaches. One especially interesting kind of hospice service is respite care. This is so because the main problems for families with terminally ill children may not be pain or technical issues of symptom management, but simply the physical and emotional burden of caring for a severely disabled child. Parents may only need a short break of a few hours or days to attend to other matters or to refresh themselves in order to be able to continue their own care for the child. Respite care is a particularly important way of supporting parents and families because it reinforces their own sense of autonomy and competence.

Respite care can be offered as an independent, community-based service or in a free-standing, purpose-built facility. Characteristics of the former are outlined in Chapter 5 by Rosalind Cutchins and Barbara Mease. They include the alternatives of in-home or center-based respite care, the value of mainstreamed care including healthy, disabled, chronically ill, and terminally ill children in a single program, and the encouragement of mothers and fathers in their rightful roles as parents. Similarly, in Chapter 6 Mother Frances Dominica reports the genesis of the idea for Helen House in Oxford, its construction, and the operation of its combined program of respite and terminal care. What stands out in this account is a basic trust and friendship. The point is not so much dying, but the way in which an institution of this sort can contribute to continuity of care and normality of living in the present moment.

The final chapter here, by Roberta Siegel, Susan Rudd, Cindy Cleveland, Linda Powers, and Robert Harmon, carries hospice approaches to pediatric care one step further by going back into the hospital and, specifically, into the neonatal unit of a children's medical center. As a general rule, such units are the epitome of advanced, high-technology, cure-oriented, "rescue mode" services. The courage to face directly the implications of dying, death, and bereavement, and the creativity to apply hospice principles in such a context speaks for itself. It applies here not only when death is anticipated, but also when death occurs suddenly, and it illustrates the value of bereavement follow-up in a setting where that might easily be neglected. Chapter 7 is powerful testimony to human sensitivity, imagination, and diligence. It clearly illuminates what can be accomplished when we take as our first priority the care and the commitment that we owe to individual children and their families. Without detracting from the sadness of death in childhood or the difficulty of this work, it is noteworthy that all of the chapters in Part II speak of the rewards, not only to children and families but also to staff, from their involvement in a hospice approach to pediatric care.

4

Home Care for Terminally Ill Children and Their Families

Belinda Barry Martin

Childrens Hospital of Los Angeles

At Childrens Hospital of Los Angeles (CHLA) it has been demonstrated that home care can be a viable alternative for every family with a dying child regardless of economic status, geographic location, type of disease, or age of child. CHLA began a home care program for children with catastrophic or life-threatening diseases in January 1980. From that time to August 1984 the program has served over 100 children and families. The ages of these children have ranged from six days to 17 years. Seventy-six percent of their diagnoses involved forms of cancer, for example, leukemia and a variety of solid tumors. However, children with noncancer diagnoses such as biliary atresia and some forms of spina bifida or multiple birth anomalies have also been served. The average length of stay in the home care program has been one month, with a range from several hours to 11 months. Of these children, 51 percent died at home, while 49 percent were returned to the hospital before death.

It is important to note that metropolitan Los Angeles is a very large geographical area, with a wide diversity of ethnic and socioeconomic groupings. In spite of such diversity, our program has been able to implement home care effectively for the terminally ill child and his or her family, and to coordinate transitions between home and hospital. In so doing, our overriding aim has been to improve quality of life for the child and for his or her family by "normalizing" daily living as much as possible in spite of the specific disease.

This chapter will describe the determination of needs and resources for a home care program of this sort, key elements in the design of such a program, its implementation and operation, and what it can mean to children, families, and staff.

Preparing for a Home Care Program

Careful preparation is essential for the introduction of services designed for a sensitive population such as families with terminally ill children (Edwardson, 1983). This should involve a determination of the numbers of such families in the local community, those who are likely to make use of the home care program, their needs, and the services they will require. Existing resources or services already operating in the community that are or might be involved in such care need to be identified. In our case, a clinical nurse specialist in the Hematology/Oncology Division of the hospital and our public health nurse conducted a pilot study in which they provided home care to 12 children and families seen over a nine-month period. Because those conducting the pilot study were themselves providing the care, they were personally aware of the time constraints and demands of this type of home care, and were able to set up realistic criteria for the establishment of such a program on a permanent basis.

Several issues were identified during the pilot study. Due to the large geographic area served by our hospital, it was more practical to use community nurses from home health agencies rather than hospital-based nurses to provide nursing care at home. This approach is one way of building upon the pioneering research of Ida Martinson and her colleagues at the University of Minnesota (Martinson, Armstrong, Geis, Anglim, Gronseth, MacInnis, Kersey, & Nesbit, 1978; see also Chapter 2 above). In a smaller metropolitan area or with other staff resources, it might be possible to operate a home care program with its own staff nurses (Lauer & Camitta, 1980). In either case, the home care nurses need to have or to develop expertise in family-centered pediatric care with specific understanding of the issues related to the care of the terminally ill child. Further, these nurses would have to be available to respond to a family's needs on a 24-hour basis seven days a week in order for that family to feel adequately supported in caring for their child at home. Our approach thus illustrates one way in which a hospital-based home care program can draw upon and help to develop resources already available in a given community.

The establishment of our program was made possible by the Medical Director of Los Angeles County Crippled Childrens Services (CCS). CCS was willing to reimburse for services provided by health personnel and for medical equipment needed at home to support the home care concept for children with cancer. The program was later expanded to include children with all types of catastrophic diseases—not just those involving hematology or oncology. At the same time, CCS expanded its geographic boundaries to include the entire state. Private insurance carriers also authorized reimbursement for home care. Horizons were broadened with each of these steps and the program expanded its involvement within the communities served by CHLA.

Designing a Home Care Program

Coordination

The fundamental element in the design and implementation of a home care program is the creation of a position designated as *home care coordinator.* At CHLA the Department of Nursing placed this position in their Office of Community Health. A pediatric nurse who was experienced in home care and had previously been involved in the implementation of a hospice home care program for patients of all ages was hired as the home care coordinator. The initial goal of the coordinator was to operationalize the program. She acted as full-time coordinator between the hospital staff, the family, and the community health team in accomplishing this goal. Together with the hematology/oncology clinical nurse specialist, the home care coordinator defined the measures necessary to establish and implement the home care program.

In order to achieve coordination of care, members of the community team must see themselves as an extension of the already-existing hospital team. The primary responsibility for care will shift between the hospital and community personnel depending on the location of the child. However, it is critical that a *continuum* of care exists so that families do not experience fragmented services or feelings of abandonment resulting from a disruptive shifting of care between home and hospital and vice versa. It is a major responsibility of the home care coordinator to facilitate this continuum through coordination of care among all the various team members.

Information

The initial contact between children, families, and the home care team is a time of great significance. In recognition of this fact, we undertook to provide community caregivers with all the information that they needed in order to care for a particular child and family. For example, names, position titles, and telephone numbers of all of the significant team members are made available in each case for resource or referral purposes. As a result, a home care nurse who identifies a financial problem can either contact the hospital social worker for discussion and resolution or, if it seems more appropriate, refer this problem to the home care team social worker where it can best be managed from within the agency. Similarly, in order to design an effective care plan the home care nurse is made aware of all past and present medical facts, as well as significant psychosocial information.

It is also necessary to identify how much the individual child and family know and understand about the child's condition. This information gives the nurse an awareness of the family's comprehension of the child's medical status in addition to that which the family may offer at the initial home visit. Thus, if a mother refers to high school plans for her 10-year-old daughter, the nurse can rest assured that the mother understands there is little chance for that future and yet allow the mother to maintain her expressions of hope. One of the main values of this fund of information is that it protects the family from having to repeat tiresome and difficult facts. Parents have repeatedly expressed their gratitude about not needing to go over such information one more time.

In preparing for our program, we designed a referral form containing the sort of information outlined above, as well as a sheet outlining a suggested format for the initial home visit (see Table 4.1). The goal of the pediatric home assessment in the initial home visit is to identify a child's normal activities in order to maintain his or her life style as much as possible. It is important for the child to be part of the family's activities and to maintain contact with friends. A careful assessment will yield an accurate concept of how the child spent his or her time prior to the illness. In consultation with the parents, this can lead to the development of a daily schedule which will parallel the previous life style as much as possible. The nurse can encourage the child to dress and be as active as his or her condition allows and even, in many cases, to plan appropriate trips outdoors, for example to a park or recreation center.

Caregivers

One of the most important roles of the home care coordinator is that of expert in community resources. Initial explorations determined that most families would require home nursing support in order to provide terminal care for their child at home. As a result of our pilot study, it was decided that the ideal choice for a professional caregiver would be a pediatric nurse who was part of an interdisciplinary hospice team. Such a

Table 4.1 Suggested Format for a Pediatric Home Visit

A. Introductions
B. Define/Specify Purpose of Visit
C. Assessment
  1. Child's Medical Condition
    a. Specific symptoms of concern
    b. Pain—type/frequency/how managed
    c. Eating/nutrition
    d. Sleeping/rest
    e. Bowel/bladder functioning
    f. Respirations
    g. Skin condition
    h. Mouth/oral care
  2. Child's Daily Activities
    a. Where does child spend most of his or her time?
    b. What does child do during the day (i.e., degree of mobility)?
    c. What does child like to do?
    d. What changes in child's activities have been observed?
    e. What is child's relationship with family members?
    f. What is child's relationship with peers? Do friends visit?
    g. Is child able to participate in school? Home teaching?
  3. Caregivers
    a. How is child's daily care managed? By whom?
    b. Are relief caregivers available?
    c. Is there support/assistance for caregivers?
  4. Family
    a. What changes have occurred in family patterns/routines due to child being cared for at home?
    b. How is life different for siblings? Working spouse?
    c. What do parents/siblings understand of child's disease, prognosis, reason for being home?
    d. How are family members managing the stress of caring for a seriously ill child at home?
    e. Do family members support/assist one another?
    f. What problems/concerns are identified by family members?
D. Plan of Care
  1. Summarize
    a. Problems/concerns identified by caregiver/family members
    b. Immediate intervention discussed
    c. Home visiting plan—when to return and why
  2. Additional Follow-Up
    a. Consultation with medical and psychosocial staff
    b. Arranging for needed medications, equipment, supplies

nurse would be skilled in the care of children, as well as being an expert in symptom control and in the hospice philosophy. Other members of the interdisciplinary hospice team would also be available: medical director, social workers, physical therapists, occupational therapists, psychologists, and trained volunteers. The home care nurse would also have full access through attendance at conferences or by telephone contact to the hospital team's consultation regarding care and support. This ideal arrangement would offer a complete and coordinated system of providing care to children and families in their homes.

In fact, however, experienced pediatric nurses and interdisciplinary hospice teams are not always available. As a result, we are often asked: What happens in smaller or remote areas where such resources are not available? Is it impossible in such circumstances to provide home care for terminally ill children or would such care inevitably be inadequate? Our reply, based on experience with many families and after providing care in a variety of communities ranging from the metropolitan area to a remote mountain town, is that it *is* possible to provide satisfactory home care anywhere by making creative use of community resources.

Each community to which we have made referrals has met the requirements of our program with some type of formal or informal hospice nursing. Often a home health agency can satisfy needs for skilled nursing services. In other circumstances volunteer nurses can be utilized or nonpracticing professionals will agree to become involved. In such cases, the home care coordinator often provides individualized in-service training and guidance related to the needs of the particular child and family. Success in such diverse situations seems to result from the fact that hospice nursing is essentially old-fashioned bedside nursing supplemented by newly developed skills, the most important of which are expertise in the management of pain and other distressing symptoms as well as the psychological support appropriate for children and families experiencing impending death. Furthermore, every family —officially or unofficially—has had a nurse who has made the commitment to be available on a 24-hour, seven-day-a-week basis. Such a commitment may appear to be overwhelming, but in reality it has not proved to be burdensome. Nurses are rarely called out at irregular hours or inconvenient times when the family has been properly educated and prepared for what is likely to happen and when support is available on a round-the-clock basis. Just knowing that a nurse can be reached if needed provides great security to families, and this availability has been recognized as the cornerstone for effective home care.

Other Participants and Needs

In addition to health care personnel, *lay volunteers* can be especially helpful in reading to or playing with siblings, in picking up medications or running other errands, and in providing transportation. However, we have not found lay volunteers to be as involved in direct care for ill children as they often are in adult hospice programs, perhaps because of the presence of parents and other family members as primary caregivers.

We do place special emphasis on the involvement of *school teachers* in many cases since being a student has usually been the child's primary role. This should be investigated by the home care coordinator, since situations will vary for different children and in different communities. If the child is well enough, he or she may attend his or her own school for all or part of the school day. Attendance at a school for the handicapped may be another option. One five-year-old child with neuroblastoma was too debilitated to walk and had never attended school. Arrangements were made for him to go to a school for the orthopedically handicapped which he attended until just days before he died. If the child is unable to go out, home teaching may also be available. Some communities have formal programs which provide teachers who make home visits. In smaller, more close-knit communities, a teacher from the regular classroom may make home visits to continue teaching the child as long as he or she is interested and can tolerate the teaching session.

In addition to the people involved in home care, there is sometimes a need for *durable equipment and supplies.* Once again, the focus must remain on quality of life. There is often a fine balance: it is best to have enough equipment to maintain optimum activity and comfort without overdoing it so that home begins to look like a hospital. In our experience, items most frequently needed are wheelchairs and hospital beds.

Obtaining reimbursement for equipment and supplies often requires some creativity. Private insurance will usually cover most items. Local children's health agencies may supply additional assistance. The American Cancer Society and similar disease-related organizations can be very generous in providing equipment for patients within their particular areas of concern. Church groups and service clubs may also be helpful in relieving families of financial burdens for items of this sort.

Implementation

Introducing the Program

A child can be identified as a candidate for the home care program in a variety of ways (see Table 4.2). At our hospital, the pediatric clinical

Table 4.2 Procedure for Implementation of Home Care

1. Identification of child for home care by: child/family; physician; clinical nurse specialist; nursing or psychosocial staff
2. Initial discussion of home care with parents by: attending physician; clinical nurse specialist; home care coordinator (HCC)
3. HCC contacts hospital staff and assesses initial home care needs
4. HCC initiates referral process
   a. Telephone referral to community home care agency or other local resources
   b. Contacts public or private reimbursement source for authorization of home care services
   c. Completes referral form signed by attending physician
5. HCC and home care nurse make joint initial home visit
6. HCC arranges team conference with hospital staff and home care nurse to discuss home care plan; documents home care plan determined during team conference; and submits for billing (conference time)
7. Home care nurse assumes primary responsibility for home care of child and family in collaboration with hospital staff. Responsibilities include
   a. 24-hour nursing coverage
      (1) Telephone availability through agency Monday-Friday
      (2) Telephone availability via beeper during evening, night, and weekend hours
      (3) Home visiting availability any time need is identified
   b. Weekly or as required home visits as indicated by child and family needs
   c. Coordination of additional home care services with community providers, e.g., equipment, transportation
   d. Provision of supplies/medications (if child has been in the hospital, an initial 10-day supply is given to family at time of discharge)
   e. Collaboration with the hospital includes
      (1) Weekly and as required telephone consultations with HCC
      (2) Referral to medical/psychosocial staff re specific concerns related to home care
      (3) Participation in additional team conferences as needed
      (4) Completion of weekly progress notes to document assessment of home care needs and implementation of service
      (5) Completion of case summary at time of child's death or readmission to hospital
8. Home care nurse follows child/family until death at home or readmission to hospital
9. Home care nurse and/or hospital personnel make a home visit at time of death
10. HCC arranges team conferences with hospital staff and home care nurse to summarize course of home care and to discuss bereavement services; documents summary of case from conference; and submits for billing
11. HCC and/or home care nurse make at least one bereavement visit approximately one week to one month following death of child
12. If child is readmitted to hospital and family decides to return to home care, implementation process is reinitiated at Step 3

specialist is most often the person to make the referral. On other occasions, referrals come from physicians, staff nurses, social workers, psychologists, other health team members, or the family itself. The child may be an inpatient at the time or receiving care as an outpatient.

Once the child is identified as a possible candidate for home care the home care coordinator is contacted. A meeting is arranged between the coordinator and the parents to explain the concepts of home care. Prior to this initial meeting, the home care coordinator becomes familiar with the projected needs of the child and family, and investigates the resources available within the community while paying attention to the financial reimbursement schedule. To date, it has never been necessary to provide care at home which has incurred an added "out of pocket" cost for a family. It is important to consider this variable when making plans for home support because increased financial commitments will all too often significantly increase the family's level of stress.

The purpose of the initial conference between the home care coordinator and the parents is to explain the option of home care versus hospitalization. Resources are identified that would be available for support if the family chooses to provide palliative care for their child at home. At this initial meeting, it is essential to stress several points to the family:

1. Home care is an alternative to hospitalization.
2. Rehospitalization is available at any time.
3. Home care does not interfere with the family's relationship with its physician or with other team members at the hospital.
4. The home care program is designed to be flexible, to adapt to, and to meet the needs of the individual child and family.

Each of these points is important to emphasize with the family. As an alternative to hospitalization, home care may not be appropriate for every family. Moreover, because home care is an addition to or extension of, rather than a replacement for the inpatient team, selecting the home care option need not significantly interrupt the family's relationships with existing caregivers and services. Often the child and family have had ongoing relationships at the hospital for months or years. A great deal of trust and security may have been built up in relationships with the hospital staff and in familiarity with its environment. It is important for the family to know that these sources of trust and security will continue to be available to them. Hospital personnel will continue contact through telephone calls, through home visits when possible, and when the child returns for clinic appointments or in the event of rehospitalization.

Flexibility regarding the frequency of the home care nurse's involvement is also an important issue to raise in the initial conference. Most of the children that we have served have had an irregular pattern of "good" and "bad" days. Families who may have expected a child to die imminently may witness improvement and stabilization. Emotional reactions can be erratic due to frequent and constant changes in the child's condition. Planning on an hour-to-hour basis is often difficult; planning days or weeks at a time is virtually impossible. Therefore, it is critical that a family know both that the support team can be flexible and will make themselves available as needs arise, and that the team is also willing to "pull back" on the good or stable days to allow the family as much normal, uninterrupted time as possible.

The home care coordinator also makes the family aware of their options within a program of home care at the introductory conference. The most significant choice is between an intermittent visiting nurse or a registry nurse who remains in the home for a selected number of hours. This choice will usually depend on the acute needs of the patient, a primary caretaker's availability and comfort in taking care of the child, and existing sources of reimbursement. A family with private insurance will usually be eligible for either nursing option, but government programs do not usually authorize ongoing nursing care.

Most families are extremely anxious at the prospect of taking their terminally ill child home for care. This anxiety can be significantly reduced through an effective conference with the home care coordinator that defines options available to each individual family according to its specific needs, resources, and situation. Careful instruction related to care of the child and time for thoughtful discussion of family fears and concerns can be critical in helping the family feel secure and comfortable with the idea of home care.

After family members have been presented with all of the options available to them, it is helpful to allow them some private time to think about and discuss alternatives among themselves. The ill child should definitely be included in this discussion in a manner appropriate for age (Jackson, 1975).

The Home Care Nurse: Options and Roles

Modes of delivering nursing support can vary greatly. One family may have a nurse available whom they will call only if they have a need. We recommend to such families that they meet their nurse at least once. Thus, if they need the nurse in a crisis they will not feel that they are calling upon a stranger. If a child is opposed to having a nurse in the home, the parents may feel adequately supported in using the nurse only as a telephone consultant. Another option is 24-hour nursing care in the home seven days a week. This is usually only implemented when a child is totally dependent and family resources are very limited in terms of caregivers in the home. Most of the children who have required this amount of nursing care have been afflicted with brain tumors in advanced stages.

The most common arrangement for nursing support is the visiting nurse. If the family agrees, the nurse will meet with them initially to discuss their needs and to set up a schedule for visits which will be most convenient for the family, usually two or three times a week. However, it is important to emphasize flexibility in such schedules. If a child is doing well and the visit seems unnecessary, the family should feel free to cancel it. If the child has a change in condition that causes concern, the family may call and arrange for an extra visit. We explain to the family that the nurse is available on a 24-hour basis. They find this tremendously reassuring. Parents have often said they were undecided about taking their child home until they were informed that someone would be available to them any time of the day or night. The importance of 24-hour availability cannot be overstated.

Parents often wonder about the qualifications of home care nurses. We respond by reaffirming our goals in caring for terminally ill children. We stress that these nurses are experts in symptom control, with special emphasis on pain management. We make clear that the purpose of home care is to maintain optimum quality of life, to normalize the individual child's life style as much as possible. Although hospice care deals specifically with terminally ill patients, the focus is not on death. Families are supported in their hope that their child will recover. However, we cannot deny that the child is seriously ill, and we recognize the importance at this time of providing caregivers who are skilled in dealing with these implications.

The family needs to understand that the home care nurse may function in a different manner than in a pediatric institution. Although the nurse may indeed do some degree of physical assessment and undertake certain procedures, he or she acts mainly as a consultant. We view the parents as their child's primary caregivers. Often, a sick child will only allow his or her mother or father to touch him. In order to respect the child's need for control and security, the nurse may guide or direct the care while the parents actually provide it. It is the parent who knows the child best and who may already be doing the best that can be done. But the presence of a skilled professional is invaluable in providing support and reassurance for the parents.

Families also need to be aware that the nurse will respect their right to privacy and control. A nurse visits a child and family by appointment only, and at the convenience of the family. The nurse respects the expertise of parents in knowing their child's needs. The nurse should never interfere with the parent/child relationship. If the child becomes comfortable with the nurse and is not threatened by direct patient care, the nurse will provide it. If the child is threatened or uncomfortable with the nurse's participation, then the nurse will work through direction of the parents. An experienced home care nurse is sensitive to the needs of parents and children, and is willing to be responsive to the best interests of those being served.

Two Key Issues

In discussions with families about taking their child home there are two issues which universally concern families most. First, they are usually fearful that their child's pain will be uncontrollable. Second, they are frightened of a sudden change in condition—usually severe respiratory distress or bleeding—which they will be unable to handle. Their profound or underlying fear is often of death itself. In an effort to reassure families, these issues are now addressed in every discharge conference.

We reaffirm continuously that the entire team will focus on the child's comfort. The child will be sent home with adequate medication to control his or her pain. If there are problems where pain is not well controlled, the home care nurse will increase the frequency of visits in order to monitor the pain and, in conjunction with the physician, will carefully adjust or increase medications until pain is once again well controlled. If necessary, as in the case of a child in distress who cannot be moved, physicians associated with the home care program or local pediatricians may visit to reassess pain management. We have found that satisfactory control of pain can usually be achieved within a 48–72 hour period. Professional confidence in this ability must be communicated to parents. It is also reassuring for parents to know that the most effective medications to control pain are now available in liquid form and can be easily adjusted for optimal relief.

The second issue, management of an unplanned emergency, usually stems from a parent's concern about how death will actually occur. As a result of experience with the deaths of children with similar diagnoses, there are some patterns that become apparent. Parents find it helpful to know that bleeding or respiratory arrest may be the cause of death, if such causes are appropriate for their specific child. It may seem unkind to deal so directly with death, but experience has shown that parents can cope more effectively with specific information rather than their fears of the unknown. Preparation before the event, when handled in a sensitive manner, can be most helpful to families in making their plans for home management.

We have also learned the value of establishing tentative plans for emergency situations or death *before the family takes their child home*. Possible situations specific to the individual child are explored and appropriate interventions are planned. The depth of this discussion can vary widely, but the value of planning ahead is undeniable. The range of these conversations has varied from families who deny or dismiss concerns and do not wish to make plans to families who plan all the way through the funeral arrangements.

It is desirable to try to assess the parents' attitude before a child's death occurs as to how much intervention, if any, they would want should their child have a respiratory or cardiac arrest. If parents are open to this type of discussion, the home care team will need to examine local options for medical intervention should it be required. Thus, if the family lives some distance from the hospital, it would be helpful if a local physician were available and familiar with the medical status of the child. Involvement of paramedics or local emergency rooms may only cause further unnecessary trauma to the child or family by providing aggressive intervention which may not be appropriate to the situation.

There are several ways to prevent unnecessary trauma. It is important to maintain ongoing discussion with parents regarding their perception of their child's medical status. Their feelings about degree of medical support desired should also be explored. If parents are in touch with their perception of their child's status, they will be better prepared to make decisions regarding medical intervention should there be a sudden, significant change in the child's condition. In addition, we encourage the family to call the home care nurse prior to local emergency personnel so that the nurse can take part in deciding what to do or in carrying out any decisions. A letter from the attending physician may also be sent home with the family containing the medical history and the names and telephone numbers of familiar health team members. The family should be instructed to present this letter to any medical person who might become involved in emergency care. The family is also advised to notify the physician or home care coordinator before the child is taken to a hospital or to any other medical facility. The proper people can then be notified and prepared for the child's arrival so the family will be spared further trauma and confusion.

Management

Bringing the Child Home

Once the family has decided to go home to care for their child it is important for the home care coordinator to plan with the hospital nursing staff to be sure all needed items are sent home with the family. These might include adequate amounts of pain medications, egg crate mattresses, or whatever other items are necessary to maintain the child's comfort. Careful instruction should also be provided to parents and staff regarding administration of pain medications. If the child is not using prescription analgesics, but pain may be anticipated, it is often helpful to give the parent a written prescription for the appropriate drug of choice. In this way, the parent can check with the physician if pain develops and have the prescription readily available for the local pharmacist if the need arises.

The next important step for the home care coordinator is selecting the community program best prepared to serve the family and making the referral. In addition to completing the referral form mentioned earlier, it is particularly useful to have direct telephone contact with the nurse who will be primarily involved. In this way the most current and accurate information can be provided which prepares the nurse thoroughly for setting up a care plan.

The next step is the initial visit to the home. An appointment is made at the convenience of the family. Whenever geographically possible, *the home care coordinator will make the initial visit jointly with the home care nurse.* The main advantage of this joint visit is to bridge the emotional gap with a familiar and credible person from the hospital who can introduce the home care nurse to the family. Parents have often expressed how difficult it is to meet a new person at this point in care, and to review and explain all that has happened since the time of diagnosis. The home care coordinator can facilitate this discussion by preparing the home care nurse with relevant information before the meeting with the family, and then by providing emotional support to the family during the visit.

During the first visit, it is essential to clarify lines of communication between the family and the health team. The family should be aware of the variety of ways to seek information or to report a change in condition. The most common pattern witnessed in this visit is that of a family who may have initially planned to call hospital personnel, but who then switch their intention within an hour's time to planning to use the home care nurse as the first contact. Ideally, the skills and sensitivity of the home care nurse will enable the family to begin to feel a sense of trust and security at the onset of home care. They realize that the nurse is by far the most accessible person to them. And they quickly begin to develop a sense of confidence in the nurse's ability to manage problems. The home care nurse's ability to help a family feel more comfortable with their seriously ill child at home is a real tribute to his or her skill and a very rewarding thing to witness.

Once the initial visit has been made, the primary management of the child's care is usually assumed by the parents with the support of the home care nurse. As can be seen from Table 4.2, the home care nurse now accepts responsibility for meeting needs identified at home.

Primary Concerns

The main concern of the home care nurse should be to help the family provide optimum quality in the child's daily life. Constant attention should be paid to the child's *physical comfort*, particularly relief from pain. The nurse should not hesitate to consult with the physician regarding pain management or other measures for comfort control. We have found that home care nurses are willing to adjust their schedules for dying children so as to be available to visit as often as necessary. In this way, the nurse can implement changes and monitor the child's condition until comfort is maintained. If a child begins narcotic analgesics while at home, the nurse should visit every day for at least three days to monitor the effect of the drug with careful assessment of toxic side effects. Simultaneously, in consultation with the physician, the nurse can titrate the drug until the optimum comfort level is maintained. This close attention to comfort measures and ready availability of the nurse gives significant support and reassurance to the family.

In addition to the physical comfort of the patient, the nurse needs to pay attention to the *psychological health* of the child. This requires a knowledge of how much the child understands about his or her disease and current condition, as this is a primary psychological concern. This understanding will vary depending on the age of the child and the wishes of the family. Our philosophy is that a child be given information about his or her diagnosis and condition as appropriate for age and developmental level. Occasionally, there are parents who do not want their child to know about his or her disease status. They may feel strongly that they do not want words like "cancer," or "tumor," or "leukemia" to be used in front of the child. Although it may be more difficult to work openly with the child and family under these circumstances, it is important to respect the parents' wishes and not betray their request to withhold information. Thus, while the nurse must always reply honestly to a child's questions, it may be necessary to limit answers according to the degree of knowledge that the parents will permit. At the same time, the nurse can work with the parents to help them see the value of a more open mode of communication (Sheer, 1977). For these reasons, it is important for the nurse to understand clearly the parents' wishes in this regard and the degree of information the child has received.

Information accompanying the referral enables the home care nurse to obtain an understanding of the child's previous *daily activities*, for example, hobbies and friends. These subjects should then be discussed with the child and the parents in order to implement measures to stimulate and interest the child. Contact with friends is very important, as is involvement with hobbies such as crafts or art work. If feasible, outings to the park or entertainment sites can become very positive experiences. Participation in school activities, whether on site or at home, is also important for normalization if physically possible. Some parents tend to be very protective and may almost isolate the child. The nurse can be helpful in reassuring them that the activities outlined above can be managed in such a way that they will actually be a positive experience, one that is beneficial both to the child and to the family.

There are other issues of care which frequently arise. One of these may be management of the child's *behavior problems.* Parents are often reluctant to use any disciplinary measures with an ill child. They may make themselves available to the child at any cost to themselves or to other family members. The nurse can consult with the parents regarding limit setting in order to further the process of normalization. Parents need to understand the meaning behind certain behaviors and to realize that it can be very frightening for a child to feel there is no control related to his or her behavior. Often a child who is acting out is asking for the security of control by his or her caretakers.

Another major issue of concern is *nutrition.* Some parents constantly encourage their sick child to eat by preparing favorite foods. They seem to imply that the child will get better if he or she will only eat correctly. Mothers whose previous major role has been to nourish their child for growth and development may become increasingly frustrated as they see these efforts become unsuccessful and insignificant. The whole issue of the child's eating patterns can create a high level of stress in the home environment. The nurse needs to help the parents understand that the body's demands for nutrients have diminished. Forcing ill children to eat usually only makes them feel worse. Instead, the nurse can offer suggestions for serving smaller portions or making food more attractive. In general, parents require assistance and reassurance in decreasing the pressure they bring to bear on their sick child and themselves around this issue.

The nurse may sometimes identify needs of the child which require the *special expertise* of another health discipline. For instance, if a child seems depressed and noncommunicative he or she may benefit from the services of an art or play therapist, a child development specialist, or a psychologist. If a relationship has already been established at the hospital, the referral should be made there. If the child is unable to come in for an appointment, a hospital staff member may make a home visit. If this is geographically impossible, a telephone conference between the hospital team specialist and the home care coordinator should occur and a referral might be made to a community specialist. Another case which requires special attention is when a child has a significant *loss of function.* In this circumstance, it may be helpful for the nurse to make arrangements with the physician for a referral to a physical or occupational therapist. The therapist can conduct an evaluation and teach patient transfer methods and activities appropriate for the situation. Interventions of this sort can significantly improve the child's quality of life.

In addition to caring for the child's needs, the nurse must also pay attention to other family members. The importance of *sibling coping* cannot be overestimated. Siblings must be given opportunities to discuss the situation in order to understand what is happening. They also need their share of parental attention during the course of the illness. Research is beginning to show that it is the siblings that suffer the most when a brother or sister is dying (Spinetta & Deasey-Spinetta, 1981). The health care team must pay attention to this in their care plan of family support. However, research has also shown that caring for the terminally ill child at home has not been detrimental to siblings (Lauer, Mulhern, Wallskog, & Camitta, 1983). In important ways, home care is helpful since the family has more time together as a unit, siblings can participate in the giving of care as appropriate, and the parents spend less time away from the home with the sick child. Parents also need guidance and support in understanding the needs of their other children, as well as realistic suggestions for giving siblings "extra attention" when parents are already physically and emotionally exhausted.

Parents' needs must also be identified and addressed. The presence of a terminally ill child puts incredible stress on any parental relationship. Preexisting problems are often exacerbated. Financial problems usually develop or increase. Working parents may feel the need to be at home with their sick child, but this may put their employment at risk. Parents often wonder if they are doing the right thing by having their child home. Many have second thoughts about discontinuing cure-oriented treatment and consider returning for experimental interventions that may have been offered as options. The nurse can serve as a sounding board in terms of listening to parents' concerns and reassuring or supporting their decisions.

At times parents' concerns are best addressed by the primary physician. The nurse has a significant responsibility in facilitating physician/parent dialogue, which often can be an invaluable means of reducing a parent's mental stress over past decisions regarding treatment and care. Also, the physician can provide the information necessary for parents to maintain an accurate assessment of the child's physical status.

The nurse must constantly assess the family's ability to cope with caring for their terminally ill child at home. If it is believed that this may be causing undue stress on them, it would be important to discuss this with the family and to consider rehospitalization, perhaps only for one or two days of respite care. This decision may also be aided by discussion with the physician.

Home/Hospital Coordination

Communication between the home care nurse and the hospital staff is extremely important. The nurse is expected to contact the primary physician after the first home visit in order to discuss the home situation and a proposed plan for care. This discussion is helpful in establishing credibility with the physician for the home care nurse and his or her assessment skills. It also opens lines of communication between the particular nurse and physician for future planning and discussion. In addition, it is essential that the home care nurse report the current status of the home situation to the home care coordinator at weekly intervals or whenever there is any significant change in condition. If other professional team members need to become involved or aware of certain conditions, it is the responsibility of the home care coordinator to direct that information to the appropriate source.

Many ill children continue to come to the hospital on a fairly routine basis during home care as long as their transport is physically manageable. Often such children will receive a course of chemotherapy or radiation for palliative purposes. Because of decreasing hemoglobin or platelet counts, they may need transfusions which are crucial to prevent bleeding episodes at home. They may also have routine clinic appointments with their physicians. During clinic visits the child and family have the opportunity to visit significant personnel such as social workers, staff nurses, psychologists, and expressive therapists or child development specialists with whom they have relationships. All of these interactions are significantly supportive to the child and family. The outcome of these clinic visits should be relayed to the home care nurse by the coordinator.

In particularly problematic or complex home situations, it has been necessary at times to schedule team conferences in which the home care team meets with the inpatient team. At these conferences, roles can be clearly delineated so the home care nurse is aware of the involvement of hospital staff. Often a child has several specialty physicians in addition to a local pediatrician and all the other members of the health team. Group discussion may be essential to clarify the overall care plan. Conferences of this sort prevent confusion or wasted efforts on the part of both the family and the home care nurse. They help identify problems, plan interventions, arrange collaboration among caregivers, and assign responsibilities or actions appropriate to each individual involved.

Conclusion of Services

Anticipating Death and Its Implications

Home care for the terminally ill child is primarily concerned with comfort care and optimal quality in each day of the child's life. *The specific goal is not for the death to actually occur at home.* This seems to cause confusion for some people due to their misunderstanding of the goal of home care. If the child is comfortable until death at home and the family is able to cope with this plan, it can be very beneficial to all. However, *rehospitalization must always be an option.* Occasionally, a child develops symptoms which are difficult for the family to manage. Such a family may feel more comfortable if their child is returned to the hospital. Often only a short stay is planned, but the child's condition may worsen and death may take place in the hospital. Some families become physically fatigued and increasingly anxious, and may need the support of the hospital environment. Children can be readmitted to the hospital and placed in a private room where they will be attended by staff who will limit care to comfort measures if this is the family's wish. The issue of death occurring at home must never be presented in a judgmental way. Team members must evaluate the individual situation on a daily basis in order to provide encouragement and support to the child and family regardless of location. If a child is readmitted to the hospital, the home care nurse is encouraged to maintain contact with the family through visits or telephone calls to the hospital.

If it has been carefully planned, the death of a child at home can be a very positive experience for a family. The home care nurse should try to anticipate the child's death and to discuss its implications with the family ahead of time in order to ascertain what their wishes may be. If they desire the death to occur at home certain arrangements should be made if the family is able to deal with them. For example, it is important to know if the family will request or consent to an autopsy. Although this seems a difficult issue to address, experience has shown that most families have already wondered about it and some may have very firm convictions related to past experiences. By at least introducing the idea to the family that has not thought about it, they will have a chance to discuss it and make a decision while they are in a stable state of mind. One might also suggest that they discuss this topic with their physician if they have questions which a doctor is best prepared to address. One reason for introducing this issue is to determine whether or not the child's body will need to be transported back to the hospital after death.

The home care nurse or social worker should also discuss the family's plans regarding funeral arrangements. Again, this is a very difficult subject. However, families who were able to make funeral arrangements prior to their child's death have repeatedly expressed their gratitude at not having to deal with those issues at a time when they felt thoroughly devastated. Those who were unable to make prearrangements have reported how difficult it was to make decisions at a time when they were so emotionally drained.

The value of a visit by the home care nurse at the time of the death of the child cannot be overstated. The nurse can confirm the family's suspicions and fears that death has actually occurred. The nurse can also provide tremendous emotional support to a family in this time of grief. The family can be encouraged to spend time with their child in whatever way they wish. They often need to know that it is not necessary to call the mortuary immediately. This can be a very significant time for a family to hold and touch their child, and to share their feelings of grief in the privacy of their own home. When the family indicates they are ready to notify the mortuary, the nurse can offer to make the necessary telephone calls for them. Often it is appropriate for the nurse to stay with the family until the mortician takes the child to the mortuary. During this time the nurse can be an important advocate for the family by answering routine questions and intervening where necessary to assure that the transport of the child is handled in a sensitive and respectful manner. For example, our experience has shown that many families do not want the memory of their child leaving with his or her face covered, and the nurse has been valuable in assuring that this does not occur.

After Death: Bereavement

It is an accepted fact that the caretakers' responsibility continues beyond the death of the child into the bereavement period. If it is possible, appropriate community and hospital staff should attend the funeral or memorial service. Families have stated how meaningful it has been to see health team members at these services. In addition, the home care nurse will also visit within one week to one month after the death. This is usually a valuable time for reflection and sharing of feelings. The nurse can answer questions parents may have at this time about their child's medical history. Families often need reassurance at this point that they provided the best care possible for their child and that nothing further could have been done to change the outcome. It is also very helpful to arrange for the family to have a meeting with the child's physician four to six weeks after the death in order to resolve questions and concerns which usually arise. One other source of help can be obtained through referrals to self-help groups, such as Compassionate Friends and Candlelighters, that may be available within the family's own local community (see Chapter 12).

Nursing Rewards and Satisfactions

Nurses who care for dying children are often asked how they can tolerate such difficult work. Numerous explanations have been offered. Some nurses have described the strength gained from the children themselves as a result of their behaviors and reactions to their illness. Others identify the personal satisfaction they feel as a result of supporting a child and family in such a way that the final days at home are full of quality time. Eugenia Waechter (1981) summarizes the feeling of reward gained from working with these children in the following way:

> Death is a part of life . . . helping children to die is as important as helping them to be born. Nurses who have really come to terms with death for themselves, and the inevitability of death really feel reward when they have accomplished helping the child to die with dignity and respect, helping parents also to see the beautiful part of dying as a part of life, helping them also to cope and to live with the death of their child. (pp. 102–103)

Conclusion

Home care should definitely be considered as an option for the dying child and family. It has been demonstrated that this type of care can be provided in any community by making use of available resources. This program must be offered to the family as an alternative method of care with 24-hour on-call nursing and rehospitalization always available. The focus is on the child's comfort and quality of life, and on support for the family. There must be ongoing collaboration between hospital and community caregivers. The emphasis is on the reestablishment of normal life style by reuniting the child and family in their own home environment. A comprehensive plan should be developed by the health team to provide the continuity of care and support necessary to enable the family to feel comfortable in being home. Families have expressed how meaningful their child's last days have been because they were at home, and how helpful it has been to allow them to feel useful. Nurses, too, have expressed their satisfaction in working with dying children and their families in the home setting. Ralph Waldo Emerson succinctly sums up these feelings: "To win the respect of intelligent people and the affection of children; to know even one life has breathed easier because you have lived. This is to have succeeded."

References

Edwardson, S. E., "The Choice Between Hospital and Home Care for Terminally Ill Children," *Nursing Research,* 1983, *32,* 29–34.

Jackson, P. L., "The Child's Developing Concept of Death: Implications for Nursing Care of the Terminally Ill Child," *Nursing Forum,* 1975, *14,* 204–215.

Lauer, M. E., & Camitta, B. M., "Home Care for Dying Children: A Nursing Model," *The Journal of Pediatrics,* 1980, *97,* 1032–1035.

Lauer, M. E., Mulhern, R. K., Wallskog, J. M., & Camitta, B. M., "A Comparison Study of Parental Adaptation Following a Child's Death at Home or in the Hospital," *Pediatrics,* 1983, *71,* 107–112.

Martinson, I. M., Armstrong, G. D., Geis, D. P., Anglim, M. A., Gronseth, E. C., MacInnis, H., Kersey, J. H., & Nesbit, M. E., "Home Care for Children Dying of Cancer," *Pediatrics,* 1978, *62,* 106–113.

Sheer, B. L., "Help for Parents in a Difficult Job: Broaching the Subject of Death," *MCN: The American Journal of Maternal Child Nursing,* 1977, *2,* 320–324.

Spinetta, J. J., & Deasey-Spinetta, P., "The Sibling of the Child with Cancer," in J. J. Spinetta & P. Deasey-Spinetta (Eds.), *Living With Childhood Cancer.* St. Louis, MO: C. V. Mosby, 1981, pp. 133–141.

Waechter, E., in "The Dying Child: Focus on the Child" (filmstrip), and accompanying handbook edited by B. Fishman, D. Miller, & R. Westphal. Irvine, CA: Concept Media, 1981, pp. 95–103.

5

Respite Care and the Dying Child

Rosalind Crenshaw Cutchins and
Barbara S. Mease

Parents will never face a more stressful event than the news that their child will die. A child's terminal illness challenges every idea, belief, emotion, and dream that a parent has. In addition, caring for a dying child is physically exhausting. If service professionals and concerned volunteers are to offer a wholistic program of services to families with terminally ill children, they must provide the necessary emotional support, as well as tangible ways to relieve parents from the continuous 24-hour care of the child.

The word *respite* means relief. This chapter will focus on ways to support parents through respite care. We will discuss the need for respite care, outline the mechanics of establishing an in-home and center-based respite program for children, and describe one program that has been successful both in providing quality services and in securing sufficient funding.

Introduction

The Family

When parents learn that their child has a terminal illness, many perplexing dilemmas automatically arise requiring difficult decisions. At the same time, the role of adult family members as parents and advocates is challenged and questioned as professionals intervene and assume some degree of control. Persons in the human service field need to be aware of the vulnerability of the family unit in this crisis period. This is a time to reinforce the parents' authority by assuring them of their rights and of their ability to make the best decisions for their family. It is a time to give the family as much control over their own lives as possible.

Perhaps one of the most critical and difficult decisions facing parents is whether and when to bring their child home from the hospital to die. At our program in Virginia—Edmarc—we have found that, for many families with terminally ill children, the time comes when the medical team and parents agree that care in the hospital is no longer necessary or advantageous. At that point, many families will consider the option of taking their child home. In order to reach the most beneficial decision for a particular child and family, the parents need to have a realistic understanding of the support services available to them.

Edmarc families have identified respite care as one of the primary measures of support for families who choose to bring their child home to die. Returning a terminally ill child to the home environment can be tremendously supportive to the family structure. It allows the parents to conduct themselves in their usual manner, it keeps the family unit located in one central place, and it permits everyone to be informed and to participate in one another's life. However, care of the dying child can become quite time-consuming. For example, we work with one family whose son's condition requires him to be tube-fed. His tube feedings must be given every four hours throughout the day and night. As a result, the mother is awakened at least twice every night to feed him. Coupled with the other care the child requires throughout the day and night, this has become an exhausting task. Fatigue is a major problem for this mother, as it is for many of the parents we serve.

Fatigue affects not only one's physical well-being, but also one's ability to cope. A routine which was once cheerfully accepted may become a never-ending grind. The misbehavior of the dying child's brother or sister may become intolerable. A difference of opinion with one's spouse may develop into a major argument. The child's illness may become overwhelming if ways are not found to relieve chronic fatigue.

The Dying Child

The foremost concern in caring for a dying child is the need to enhance the child's and the family's quality of life. Parents may need to be supported in changing the direction in the child's treatment plan from one emphasizing cure to one emphasizing pain control and alertness. This must include providing for the child's comfort through pain control medication as necessary, reinstating the child as a vital family member, and affirming the child's value and self-worth as a person.

We offer the option of home care support for families who choose to bring their dying child home because we feel that the child's needs can frequently be met more easily in the home environment. Parents are obviously the best caregivers for their own child because they know their child better than anyone else. Not only has home care proved to be better for the child, but for the family as well. One frequent fear in children is separation anxiety. Allowing the child to be with the family can allay this fear. For the family, having the child at home means, at the very least, that the parents are not being torn by two "homes" located miles apart. At least physically they are together. Very often families find that siblings are more cooperative as they participate in caring for and playing with the terminally ill child. They are able to see for themselves if the ill child is not having a good day. They begin to face the child's impending death. Anticipatory grief can be shared together. This shared experience may help the family later in resolving their grief.

If we are to encourage the family to consider the home care option, we must be prepared to offer a program which supports the parents. Parents need to go out to dinner, to go to the movies, to go to the bank, to go to the grocery store, to take a nap in the middle of the day, to do whatever they need to do, knowing that their child will receive loving, quality care. A good respite program can fulfill this responsibility. It can give the parents a chance to renew their strength and to return to a very trying situation with refreshed spirits.

A Rationale for Mainstreamed Care

At Edmarc, respite services were the first to be instituted as we developed our program. Since all of our services are solely for children, and since the parents with whom we work identified respite as their most central need, we decided that would be our first priority.

For a variety of reasons, some of them quite pragmatic, the respite program was designed to serve disabled children, including those disabled by chronic or terminal illnesses. This decision was initially dictated by our funding sources, but as a local base of funding was developed, the decision was made to continue serving a varied population for more altruistic reasons. We soon realized that parents' needs for respite were identical whether the child in question was physically disabled, mentally disabled, chronically ill, or terminally ill. It also became apparent to us that a well-run respite program could serve 50 families almost as easily as it could serve five.

It took longer to realize that a mainstreamed approach to care, serving disabled, terminally ill, and chronically ill children together with nondisabled children, would be both more efficient and theoretically sound. Educational theory indicates that mainstreaming disabled and nondisabled children in a structured setting has the potential to create a more demanding and stimulating environment for the disabled or terminally ill child (Guralnick, 1979). Parents and teachers are likely to become more realistic in their expectations of the "special" child. Likewise, peers are likely to encourage behavior which will be most beneficial to the disabled child. Additionally, we have found mainstreaming a way to help fund a respite program; an issue we shall explore in greater detail later.

In-Home Respite

The Families

Throughout this chapter, a broad definition of developmental disability will be used which includes both the dying child and the chronically ill child. One benefit in serving a variety of children with respite services is that it allows the inclusion of terminally ill children whose life expectancy is unknown or who may live several years with a chronic or degenerative condition. Thus a family may be supported throughout their time of need, not just during a final crisis period. At Edmarc this more extended period has allowed us to develop a relationship with the family. This relationship has, in turn, enabled us to be more effective supporters and counselors during the child's final illness.

It is important to develop an admission policy so that the population to be served may be defined. However, an admission policy will not replace the need for individual assessments. At Edmarc, the staff has some flexibility in deciding which children to admit to the respite program, with the primary criterion being the family's need for respite care.

Referrals to a respite program may be received from many sources. Program staff must decide which referral sources are acceptable and appropriate. At Edmarc referrals from all sources are accepted for an initial evaluation. Some referrals are clearly inappropriate and the family is not contacted. Some families are contacted but not admitted for services. We feel that the screening time that may be lost on an inappropriate family is more than compensated when a previously unknown family is identified. Appropriate referrals will most frequently be received from physicians, health departments, social service agencies, school systems, and community mental health and mental retardation boards. Sending notices to these professionals and service organizations should be one of the first steps taken in publicizing a respite program.

Once the eligibility requirements have been established, the screening process can begin. As mentioned earlier, programs that accept referrals from any source may occasionally receive inappropriate referrals. On one occasion Edmarc received a referral of a 70-year-old man with prostate cancer. Since our program serves only children, we were unable to accept the referral. On the other end of the spectrum, we received a referral through a public speaking engagement stated in these terms: "I know of a pitiful little boy who barely has a leg to stand on." With some reluctance, we located the family and screened the child, a severely disabled, dying child who had never received services from any service organization. We have become a vital part of this family's life.

Accepting referrals from the general public may present problems. Many organizations justifiably refuse such referrals. Any investigation of nebulous referrals must proceed cautiously. Staff members must be extremely tactful and have an inherent respect for the family's right to privacy. With all of the preceeding limitations, we have nevertheless found that pursuing such referrals has brought us into contact with families who need and welcome our care.

We use a variety of techniques for screening, depending upon the referral source and the child's history. A home visit by a staff member gives good insight into the family's situation. For some children, medical records are obtained before finalizing the registration. A third method is a telephone call to the family in which enough information is shared to determine if the child is eligible and if the family is interested. Depending again upon the source of the referral and the diagnosis, the screening process may be deleted and the child automatically registered.

The registration process will necessarily vary from program to program. Our registration has changed over the years as we have refined and adapted it to meet our needs. We expect it will continue to change. Most respite programs, including our own, are willing to share registration forms with other programs.

Our registration form includes family information, such as the name of the child, parents, siblings, or others living in the home, their ages, the address, home and business phone numbers, and two emergency contacts. Also included is the name and phone number of each doctor and hospital with whom the child is involved. It is particularly important when working with dying children that a parent can be reached at all times. This is reassuring to the parent and to those caring for the child. All concerned need to know that the parents could be reached immediately to come home should their child need them or be at the point of death.

The nature of the child's disability is listed along with a brief description in lay terms. There is also a brief description of any serious medical problems of close relatives.

A section is included on the child's general health history including immunizations, any seizure activity, and routine medications. Registration forms are revised semiannually. They do not replace the more detailed instruction given by the parent to the care provider at the time the child is being given care.

The section on activities of daily living includes such items as equipment used, motor abilities, visual ability, hearing ability, and eating habits. Additional information is obtained regarding the child's favorite foods, dislikes, and allergies. A typical menu and times for each meal and snack during the day is available for reference. Should there be an emergency in which a care provider is called on short notice, this extensive information allows the care provider to adapt to the child's routine easily.

Sleeping habits, bedtime and morning routines, toilet habits, and hygiene are included. A brief description of the child's speech is also noted. Favorite activities, toys, and television programs are recorded.

Information on any behavior problem or emotional problem the child may have and how to handle such problems is also available. Parents are encouraged to describe disciplinary measures which work best for them. We are very firm, however, in refusing to use any type of corporal punishment. We do encourage parents to continue to require the ill child to conform to expected behavior patterns, as this is both reassuring to the child and to the entire family.

Liability is an issue which no program can afford to ignore. The mere fact that a beneficial service is being provided does not negate legal liability. Nor will consent forms relieve the care provider and the program staff of the responsibility to act prudently and responsibly. Liability insurance is discussed later in the chapter.

Despite their lack of legal significance, we do require the following forms for parent signature: waiver of liability, waiver of transportation liability, permission for emergency medical attention, publicity/picture release, and a financial agreement form. Parents are not required to sign the publicity/picture release forms, but are merely asked to indicate whether or not they wish to participate in publicity events.

One valid concern about the registration process is the length of time required to complete it. Generally, registrations can be completed in one hour during a home visit. One factor which influences this is the type of forms used. Ours have been adapted to a check list whenever possible. In addition, a certain amount of the information can be ascertained before the visit, thereby speeding up the process. Once the procedure is completed, the registration form is taken back to the office. There it is typed and copied. A file is kept on each child including all of the registration information. A copy of the registration form and a medical authorization form are then sent to the parents. They are advised to make these available to care providers. Also included in the child's file at the office are pertinent medical records. These are obtained by sending a request for information to the physician or hospital with a release of confidential information form signed by the parent. All of the registration materials are treated as confidential information and are divulged to others only if a signed release accompanies the request.

One major decision for a respite program is whether or not to care for siblings when providing respite. Our philosophy is based on the fact that parents need some time alone, including time away from their other children. We would only refuse to provide care for siblings if that would mean jeopardizing the care of the disabled child. Frequently, too, parents choose to use respite periods in order to spend special time with their nondisabled children. Therefore, at Edmarc siblings are often included in respite care. Parents have reported this to be very supportive. We anticipated many problems, but few have developed.

Care Providers

At Edmarc, the persons we send into the home to care for the child are called care providers. Recruitment of these individuals has been through classified advertisement, contacts during community speaking engagements, personal contacts, and family contacts. All of our care providers are required to take a formal 20-hour training session sponsored by Edmarc. The training session gives us the opportunity to become acquainted with the care provider, assess the skills and knowledge base of the person, and match up their specific interests and personalities with registered families. One of the important, yet intangible, qualities we seek in a care provider is the desire to work with disabled children. Another is the ability to be an empathetic listener. A third quality is the capability to work independently while functioning as a team member. It is important, especially when working with dying children and their families, for care providers to maintain open communication lines and to seek support for themselves as well as for the families they are serving.

One major issue to be decided in designing a respite program will be whether to use paid or volunteer care providers. Many programs have had success with each method. Edmarc uses both paid and volunteer care providers in the respite program. However, we do require that all care providers—paid or volunteer—complete the training course and adhere to all policies and procedures. It has worked most successfully in our program to use volunteer care providers for routine respite care—those respite visits which take place at the same time each week. For example, one family has routine respite each Wednesday from 1:00 to 3:00 P.M. The mother uses this time to grocery shop and run errands. A volunteer care provider goes into the home each week and provides care for the disabled child. Sporadic respite, one-time respite visits, have been staffed by paid providers. Usually, there is shorter notice for such respite and the duration of the visit is often longer. For example, a family will call on Wednesday to arrange for a care provider on Saturday from 6:00 P.M. to 12:00 midnight. The parents would like to go out to dinner and to a movie. This type of respite request has generally been easier for us to fill with a paid provider.

All care providers have annual evaluations. The evaluation forms are the same ones used for full-time staff employees. Evaluation information is routinely sought from the families that care providers serve, as well as from their supervisor. At Edmarc, evaluations are used to compliment the provider on any outstanding characteristics and to explore those areas which may improve quality of service. The care providers also evaluate themselves, and their comments are documented as a part of the evaluation. In addition, annual evaluations have provided an ideal time to work out any recurring difficulties together.

Mechanics

The coordination of respite care may best be described through the family illustration which follows. John is a 14-year-old boy with severe brain damage. At birth his parents were told he would not live to be four years old. Throughout his life, he has had many physical problems which have required hospitalization over 50 times. Presently his prognosis is guarded. His parents understand that he could die at any time. He frequently has pneumonia. His feeding problems have necessitated the insertion of a gastrointestinal tube. Therefore, he receives all nutrition and medication through the gastrointestinal tube. Although John does not require constant supervision, he does need to have someone nearby at all times. John has an older brother, who is married and has one child. The father is John's primary provider and the mother works in the home.

This family requested one full day of respite care each week. A care provider was contacted who agreed to work with John each Monday for eight hours. She is responsible for his entire care. She bathes him, feeds him, plays with him, does his range of motion exercises, gives his medication, and provides any other care he needs. Once this routine respite was established, the care provider was expected to care for John each week unless other instructions were received from her supervisor. This family also expects her each week unless otherwise contacted. The parents may use this time in whatever way they choose. One advantage in this particular situation is that the care provider also provides companionship to the mother, who is virtually confined to the home.

When John is hospitalized, the care provider continues to provide respite in the hospital. John's mother usually stays with him when he is hospitalized. Relieving her to go home for eight hours is respite in its truest form!

On one occasion, John's mother had to be hospitalized on short notice. At this time John's family made use of emergency respite. This dimension of the respite program is available to all of the families we serve on a 24-hour, seven-day-a-week basis. John's father wanted to be with his wife, and we were called to provide respite. We were able to send in a care provider who took care of John until other arrangements could be made. Families who have children with special needs such as John's frequently do not have the luxury of calling on neighbors to care for their child. Fortunately, the combination of training, experience, and registration information allows our care providers to take over on short notice.

At the birth of their grandchild, John's parents wished to travel to their older son's home and spend some time with his family. However, they did not feel that John could tolerate the trip. We provided them with extended respite. A care provider was assigned to provide care from Friday afternoon through Sunday afternoon. The care provider was familiar with John and his care. Throughout the weekend, phone numbers were available for her to reach John's parents, a relative who lived nearby, John's physician, and an agency staff member. John's parents checked in by telephone each day, as did a staff member, to assure that everything was running smoothly. As a result, the weekend was a success. John's parents returned refreshed and satisfied that he had been given quality care.

This is a family with a high potential for "burnout." John's care is overwhelming at times and must result in a high degree of chronic fatigue. We have been able to allow this family to experience regular times for renewal, as well as the chance to meet family emergencies and to participate in a family celebration.

Employee Issues

Despite the waiver of liability form that parents sign when being registered into the program, the agency must consider its legal responsibilities in the event of a lawsuit. Care providers need to be aware of the ramifications of their actions while in the home. Liability insurance is a necessity both to protect care providers and to protect the agency. Our policy covers both paid employees and volunteers.

Strict documentation is required of volunteers and care providers. On each occasion service is rendered, a written report must be submitted to a supervisor. This serves as a vehicle for billing as well as for the care provider's accountability. In the event that an accident occurs, the care provider is instructed to contact the supervisor immediately. The care provider and agency also have the responsibility of serving as advocate for the overall well-being of the child. This includes the referral needs, physical or emotional, of the child, as well as the legal responsibility to report suspected child neglect or abuse. These are legal and moral responsibilities for any agency offering service to children.

Center-Based Respite Care

The Children

Another option in providing respite care is the development of a center-based program. Such programs are well recognized in geriatric circles and have recently been described as a valuable component of adult hospice services (Wilkes, Crowther, & Greaves, 1983; Cockburn & Twine, 1982). For our purposes, center-based respite care may be used as an alternative to home care or in addition to an in-home program. The selection of appropriate families is somewhat more difficult in a center-based program. We have successfully combined terminally ill, disabled, and nondisabled children in a somewhat innovative program of both drop-in and scheduled respite care. We have certainly experienced many benefits by mainstreaming all of these children and have been able to offer a more extensive, cost-effective respite program to families. Children must be registered with our respite program to be eligible for our center-based program. The nondisabled children are a combination of staff members' children and board members' children. These nondisabled children are charged the full cost of day care services. This enables us to have full-time, drop-in respite available while covering the costs of a full-time child care worker without compromising sliding fee scales for the disabled children. Because siblings are allowed to use the service, the disabled and nondisabled children are naturally integrated. Mainstreaming allows the nondisabled children involved to become aware of children with different needs, to become friends with these children, and thus to become their advocates.

The disabled children's need to be with nondisabled children can be met through a center-based respite program. The developmentally disabled child needs role models as well as the opportunity to interact in those areas in which he or she is not delayed. The terminally ill child also needs to be with peers to interact socially and educationally.

A consideration in planning such a program is the medical needs of the children. It may be necessary to have a nurse available to consult or provide medical assistance. It is also necessary to have pertinent information on the children which identifies any special needs, medication, equipment, and so on, that they may require. Again it is important to have medical releases, waivers of liability, and emergency contacts signed and available to the staff.

One drawback to center-based respite care for certain children will be their exposure to disease. Even with monitoring to prevent ill children from attending the center, there will necessarily be a certain degree of exposure to whatever the prevalent virus happens to be. Parents will need to take this into consideration as they weigh the merits of center-based versus in-home respite.

Staff Requirements

Staff members who work in a center-based program primarily need to enjoy working with children, have a thorough understanding of their developmental needs, and be effective in planning and implementing daily activities. Supervisors need a background in early childhood education to enable them to plan appropriate activities and to understand the behavior of the children being served.

Adequate staff coverage can be a major scheduling problem. One guideline to use is the state's day care licensure requirements. It may also be that a program needs more coverage during certain times of the day, such as at lunch time. Adequate coverage helps reduce staff burnout and allows for a more interesting and varied program that includes special activities and field trips.

At Edmarc, paid staff are scheduled to meet our own determination of "minimum" coverage in a ratio of one staff member to five nondisabled children over the age of two, one staff member to two disabled children over the age of two, or one-to-one depending on the level of disability. Generally, these are higher staff-child ratios than those demanded by licensure requirements. Staff members are also supplemented by a stable group of volunteers who are assigned, usually on a one-on-one basis, to the same children as much as possible.

Mechanics

Because our program has staff coverage at all times, we are able to offer drop-in respite. Registered parents may phone in the morning if they want to bring their child by for a couple of hours that day. Drop-in day care is particularly popular with parents as it allows them some freedom and spontaneity. Another advantage, from the staff's point of view, is that the children in day care are varied; frequently they include children who would not otherwise attend. This is also a fairly simple program to operate once it has been established. The disadvantages of drop-in respite are that it becomes difficult to plan specific activities and it sometimes means bringing in additional staff on very short notice.

The daily schedule for the children is generally the same each day. Specific activities are determined according to the group for which we are planning. There is time in the schedule to work individually with children. For instance, a child with cystic fibrosis may need percussive therapy during the day. Another child may need to be catheterized or tube-fed. Scheduling must be flexible enough to meet these needs. Staffing patterns must also be flexible enough to meet the children's individual needs, as some children require individual attention. Volunteers can be used at busy times to work with children individually or to work with a group of children while a staff member attends to a child. At Edmarc, program staff with other duties may be called upon for specific children for brief periods of time. For instance, a registered nurse from our home health agency may be asked to administer a child's medications or take care of a tube feeding.

One hazard in providing drop-in respite to such a varied group of children is the tendency to become complacent in scheduling activities. Field trips may seem insurmountable obstacles. It takes a lot of planning and energy to sponsor a successful field trip, especially when dealing with children requiring special equipment. However, the benefits received by the children make the work involved worthwhile. Dying children, chronically ill children, and disabled children need to be exposed to new experiences, to enjoy what nondisabled children enjoy. Volunteers may once again be extremely helpful in providing a high ratio of staff to children for one-time events.

Precise documentation is essential for center-based respite. At Edmarc we require recording of eating habits, toilet habits, sleeping habits, and any special events during the day. This enables the parents to continue to be informed of their child's schedule and to feel more a part of the daily routine.

Facility equipment requirements will be determined by the type of program offered. If the program is licensed by a governmental agency, certain pieces of equipment will be mandatory. There may also be the need of medical equipment, depending on the children's disabilities. Of course, the developmental age of the children served will determine which equipment will be needed, as will the nature of the children's illnesses and disabilities. Beds, cribs, cots, high chairs, mats, therapeutic equipment, and play equipment will all be necessary for most programs.

Outdoor play equipment may need to be modified to serve disabled children; however, by doing so, a more normalized life style is provided. Every effort should be made to include all children in outdoor activities. Offering sufficient time for play gives children opportunities to express themselves and to deal with their feelings. This is particularly appropriate for the dying child.

Another program option for center-based respite is an extended care program. This type of facility can offer overnight respite for several nights. One agency in our state offers only extended care. Registered families have access to the program for three nights every two months. The families bring the children in and leave them for three consecutive nights. The agency transports them to any day program or schools they attend. This gives the parents a periodic break from their responsibilities. We do not have this program at Edmarc, but recognize that it is beneficial, particularly if offered in conjunction with the program described above.

Parent Involvement

At Edmarc, parents are recognized as vital elements in planning and implementing all of our programs. Parents are involved in our home health agency and our infant intervention program, as well as our respite program. Our philosophy is based on the premise that parents are the best and most knowledgeable caregivers for their own children and that children will respond best to care that is provided in the home.

Of course we recognize that parents do not usually have the expert knowledge needed to manage specific issues relating to their child's physical illness or disability and that certain types of care can only be provided in a hospital or other institution. However, we are committed to supporting the parents' role as parents. We encourage parents to continue to make parenting decisions even when the child's medical condition may be managed by professionals.

Parent Support Groups

Our agency offers parent groups as a part of the respite program. The purpose of a parent group is to provide education and emotional support. We have a morning parent group and an evening group. The morning group consists mainly of mothers with young children. The evening group is attended by both mothers and fathers. Each meeting has a planned program with scheduled free time for socializing. Educational programs have included such topics as physical therapy techniques, occupational therapy techniques, speech and language development, behavior management, depression, communication, and children's understanding of death. We have also had such social events as cookouts, pot-luck dinners, and Christmas parties, for the entire family. Social events have been perhaps the most therapeutic times for some of the families we serve. Parents of dying children need the companionship of other parents with similar experiences. They need to know that the multitude of feelings they experience have been felt and survived by others. Other parents' experiences can be most helpful and comforting. Parent groups also help staff members become aware of and be more sensitive to the needs of parents.

One staff member in our agency is responsible for parent groups. With the help of a parent advisory board, topics are selected for meetings. The staff member is then responsible for finding a speaker, arranging the meeting place, and notifying parents. Before each meeting, a notice is sent to the family as a reminder. It has been our experience that families under stress need reminders each month. They also need encouragement to make the effort to attend. Frequently, one family will provide transportation for another, thereby offering incentive to an overburdened parent.

Parent Advisory Board

Parent advisory boards are made up of parents in the program. They meet to give feedback to staff on the various aspects of the program. They have helped decide what information is needed on the registration forms, what topics should be covered in care provider training, and what programs would be most appropriate for parent group meetings. They also serve as evaluators for the program, advising staff members on all aspects of the program. Perhaps the greatest error an agency can make is to develop a program without first asking parents what they need. A parent advisory board, properly used, can help prevent such an error.

Bereaved Parents

Edmarc also sponsors a Bereaved Parents Group for parents who have experienced the death of a child. This parent group has become a vital part of our bereavement follow-up service, an essential part of any program serving seriously ill and dying children. This group includes parents in our program with children who have died, as well as families in the community whose children have died of accidental or other causes. A monthly meeting is held to provide a time for sharing and an occasion for mutual- and self-help. Parents continually tell us of the benefit of having a time to be with other parents who share their experience. Each month a brief program is planned which focuses on an aspect of bereavement. However, most of the meeting time is used to give parents guided "talking time."

Because our program serves a large rural area, many parents must travel an inconvenient distance to attend meetings. When bereavement groups offered by other agencies are more conveniently located, we make referrals to those other groups. But we always offer to attend the first meeting of the other group with the parent. We feel that a bereaved parents group is so beneficial that extra efforts need to be made to give parents the least stressful opportunity to attend.

Funding Sources

Funding for a respite program will depend on the type of program being developed, the client population to be served, support staff and programs already in existence, and the local resources available in each community. This section will discuss funding sources Edmarc has used as a means to prompt ideas which may be applicable in other communities.

Federal and State Sources

In the United States, federal and state funding sources should not be overlooked. Our respite program was developed with a grant from our state Department of Mental Health and Mental Retardation, Developmental Disabilities Unit. We were able to acquire the grant funds because we were willing to serve disabled children. Under the federal government's definition of developmental disabilities, terminally ill children are developmentally disabled.

Focusing on disabled children, including dying children, has also given us access to state funds. In Virginia, respite services are "core" services which local community services boards are required to provide. At this time we are a contract agency for our local services board, providing respite care which they help to fund.

Many programs will also have access to Title XX money for day care respite services. Title XX funds will depend upon the individual state and community plan for use of such funds.

Community Support

Community support is a nebulous and shifting means of supporting any program. At Edmarc, we have relied upon it heavily, despite the disadvantages inherent in such dependency. To be effective, community support must be linked to community education and public relations. If the community does not know what is being done, does not understand why it is being done, or disapproves of the methods used, it cannot be expected to lend financial support.

At Edmarc, community education has relied heavily on two distinct avenues: newspaper coverage and speaking engagements with clubs and churches. We have also received exemplary support from local television and radio stations. Frequent positive newspaper articles have had the effect of making the community at large recognize Edmarc as an established and helpful agency. Likewise, speaking engagements provide a captive, receptive audience, and many groups are seeking ideas for service projects.

The local United Way fund drive should also not be overlooked in determining means of community support. Most United Way programs are searching for organizations that can spark the community into higher levels of giving. Even if the initial grant is small, United Way funding can provide a comparatively stable item in an agency's revenue budget.

Local foundations will vary from community to community both in number and in resources available. While most foundations will not support general operating funds, they will frequently make an annual gift, particularly if requests are written for specific items or specific events.

At Edmarc, private, unsolicited contributions and memorial donations have formed the backbone of our revenue budget. Repeated contributions can be encouraged by prompt, accurate acknowledgements, including acknowledgements to the bereaved family in the case of memorials. Positive media coverage is very often the reason we receive initial donations.

One method we use to encourage repeated donations is the development of a membership organization. Members may be frankly but tactfully "reminded" when they have not made a donation during the previous year. The formation of a membership group may also provide the foundation for an annual dinner and meeting, and the number of people participating is useful information to provide to potential funding sources as validation of the agency's general support.

No discussion of community support would be complete without mention of the use of volunteers. Some respite programs have been successful using only volunteers, including a volunteer coordinator and volunteer care providers. Some programs use only paid staff. There are certainly advantages and disadvantages in the use of volunteers. The most critical disadvantage is that volunteers do what they want to do when they want to do it. This does not mean that volunteers are unreliable; we have found the opposite to be true. It may, however, be difficult to find a volunteer willing to work on Friday or Saturday nights, a time many parents would appreciate a few hours of respite.

The benefits of using volunteers are numerous. In addition to the special feeling they bring to their work, volunteers help to encourage a broadening base of community support. At Edmarc, it is often volunteers who encourage their clubs to invite a speaker or make a donation, and it is volunteers who involve a whole church in "adopting" a family for Christmas or Lent.

At Edmarc, we use a combination of paid staff and volunteers. Volunteers are used to coordinate other volunteers, to provide refreshments at parent group meetings, to transport children to the respite center, to supplement child care staff at the center, and to provide some of the scheduled in-home respites.

The use of professional volunteers should not be overlooked both for the skills they possess and as a means of offsetting program expenses. We use professional volunteers primarily for our training programs. We have found many talented local physicians, nurses, psychologists, and educators more than willing to participate in training sessions for care providers. This group can be a rich resource for initial training and subsequent in-service education.

Parent Fees

Edmarc uses a sliding fee scale based upon family income. We do not require proof of income and the scale may be adjusted due to unusual expenses. Many programs take a stricter approach to setting fees. Our own approach is to view the payment of fees as an opportunity for the family to feel they are purchasing a service and thus have the right to make certain demands. We also view the determination of fee assessment to be an interpersonal process with the staff member and parent together determining an appropriate fee.

Fees are a minor source of support for our respite program. We believe that parents who qualify for respite should not have to pay more than other parents in the area pay for babysitting. But since care providers are paid at least minimum wage, fees—even from middle income families—do not meet the direct cost of the care providers.

At Edmarc, parents are billed monthly for the services they have received during the preceeding month. Care providers are paid, along with other program staff, on a biweekly schedule. The two events are not related. That is, care providers are paid whether or not parents pay for the service.

Some respite programs use an alternative means of paying care providers by supplementing the amount paid by the family. That is, the family pays the care provider, as they would a babysitter, and the remainder is paid by the program according to a predetermined schedule. The care providers are considered employees of the family, whereas the program subsidizes the family's payments. This is evidently a viable alternative because many programs use it. We prefer to separate the two for several reasons. The main benefit of direct payment is that we prefer to have everyone involved recognize that the care providers are employees of and responsible to Edmarc. This allows us to make certain demands upon care providers for in-service education, written reports, confidentiality, and quality of care. It also clarifies such issues as staff evaluation and staff medical records. Another benefit of this approach is that of confidentiality. How much a parent pays and whether a parent is up-to-date on payments is not information available to care providers.

Many programs have had success with realizing a substantial portion of program costs through direct fee payments. At Edmarc, we have not. This may be in part due to the general low income of the area we serve or to factors in our own program. We have, however, not found funding a respite program to be difficult.

Conclusion

At Edmarc special services are offered for special children. Some of the children we serve are dying, others are chronically or terminally ill. Our services include respite, early intervention, home health, and rehabilitative therapy. Because we serve such a broad range of children, we are able to offer each family a specially tailored program to meet their needs.

Programs that specialize in other areas, such as hospice services for a broad age range, may find it more costly or difficult to develop the type of respite services described in this chapter. However, respite care is a critical area in serving the needs of families with a terminally ill or chronically ill member, and it is especially important in cases involving children.

Programs may need to broaden their sights in seeking funding opportunities. Respite is not primarily a medical/nursing issue. Agencies with a concern for the disabled may be more appropriate resources for help in planning and funding a respite program.

Finally, programs seeking to provide pediatric care must be willing to share experiences and resources. At Edmarc, we have found other agencies and individuals more than willing to share knowledge, forms, problems, and successes. Parents with dying children deserve to have professionals working together to support them in every possible way.

References

Cockburn, M., & Twine, J., "A Different Kind of Day Unit," *Nursing Times*, 1982, *78*, 1410–1411.

Guralnick, M. G., *Early Intervention and the Integration of Handicapped and Nonhandicapped Children*. Baltimore: University Park Press, 1979.

Wilkes, E., Crowther, A. G. O., & Greaves, C. W. K. H., "A Different Kind of Day Hospital—For Patients with Preterminal Cancer and Chronic Disease," in C. A. Corr & D. M. Corr (eds.), *Hospice Care: Principles and Practice*. New York: Springer; London: Faber and Faber, 1983, pp. 308–316.

6

Helen House: A Hospice for Children

Mother Frances Dominica

Introduction

Terminal Illness, Chronic Illness, and Respite Care

Helen House, a hospice for children, opened in November, 1982, in Oxford, England, offering *respite care and terminal care* on a home-away-from-home basis to children with life-threatening disease. It is thought to be the first home of its kind in the world.

Starting from the belief that home is almost always the best possible place for a child who cannot benefit further from attempts at curative therapy, Helen House aims to ease the strain for those families who care for their child at home by offering respite care at intervals. Also, Helen House helps make it possible for other families to have their child at home, who, without the offer of respite care might find it necessary to leave the child in full-time residential care. The Helen House team offers support and friendship to children—as well as to their families—who have life-threatening or profoundly handicapping disease. We try to be sensitive in responding to individual needs, thereby enabling both child and family to achieve the optimum quality of life. We want to help the child to die with dignity if and when the time comes, and then to help the family live on after the death of their child.

Helen House was not a carefully formulated hospice programme planned, as it were, in the abstract. Rather, it is the actualization of an idea which grew out of the tragic illness of one small child. For this reason, it seems important to describe Helen's history at some length because each detail has bearing on the vision and ideals out of which Helen House has grown and now functions.

Helen

In August, 1978, a small child was admitted to an acute-care hospital in Oxford with a three-week history and signs of raised intracranial pressure. Helen was then 2½ years old and had previously been a bright, happy child. Investigations showed evidence of a massive cerebral tumour which was surgically removed the day following admission. Postoperatively Helen haemorrhaged and began convulsing.

A chance encounter a few days after Helen's initial surgery led to my growing friendship with her family. As a trained nurse, it was a new experience for me to be deeply involved with a child during hospitalization, not this time in a professional capacity, but simply as a friend of the family. This afforded an opportunity of seeing things through their eyes, sharing their anxieties and their hopes, feeling both the gratitude and the frustration of being heavily dependent on professionals within the hospital for the well-being of Helen and for such information as they might choose to impart or withhold concerning her condition and prognosis. One saw a gradual change between an all-out attempt to promote recovery, whether it be total or partial, to the reluctant acceptance that Helen's condition was not responding and would not respond to treatment. It was hard for everyone concerned, professionals as well as parents, to adjust from an attitude of hope for cure to one of knowing that she would never get well. There is always a danger of saying in a situation like this, whether with words or manner, "There is nothing more we can do."

A brain scan six months after surgery showed sufficiently conclusive results to convince Helen's parents that nothing useful could be achieved by prolonging her stay in hospital; it had become an inappropriate environment for her. With her neurosurgeon's full agreement, she was taken home where she has been cared for by her parents ever since. She was then just three years old and her sister had been born one month before Helen left the hospital.

However competent and intelligent parents are, it can be a frightening and isolating experience to leave an acute-care hospital with the round-the-clock skill and support it offers and to find oneself alone at home with a gravely ill child. Even frequent home visits of doctors, nurses, and other members of the health team leave the parents on their own with the child for the major part of the 24 hours of every day and particularly through the long, lonely hours of the night. Helen suffered frequent convulsions and often seemed distressed, but she had no means of communicating the cause of her distress. She frequently had very disturbed nights. The physical strain of caring for her day and night, as well as that of caring for a newborn child, began to tell on her parents, but this was nothing in comparison with the exhaustion from the prolonged grief they were suffering.

Very tentatively, I asked if they would trust me enough to "lend" me Helen sometimes. Over the next three years, she came to our convent in Oxford on a number of occasions. We would put up her cot or a small bed in my room and I would look after her for a few days about six times a year. Because I knew the nursery rhymes she had loved before she was ill and which her parents continued to sing to her, because I knew that she had hated baked beans before she was ill and that they still taste of baked beans even if they are put through a liquidiser, and because they believed that I loved her as a person with a spirit and with feelings as well as a body, Helen's parents were content to entrust their daughter to me. This enabled them to have the luxury of a few unbroken nights' sleep, the chance to concentrate on the other children (three and five years younger than Helen), or to take an occasional holiday. There was also the relief of knowing that if Helen's mother was herself unwell, there was somewhere that Helen was known and could be cared for.

On one of Helen's early visits the idea occurred of extending what had by then become a very special friendship with Helen and her parents to other gravely ill children and their families. We would not be offering a long-term facility but rather supporting families who wanted to care for their sick child at home. With encouragement and advice from many people concerned with the well-being of such children and their families, plans for Helen House were drawn up and a leaflet giving information and asking for financial help was printed in 1980. Within a year the general public had given the necessary £500,000 to build, furnish, and equip the hospice and construction began, the site being in the grounds of our convent in Oxford. Building took one year to complete and during this year a further £500,000 towards an endowment fund for future running costs was given through voluntary sources. Helen House received its first young visitors in November, 1982, just three years since the original concept of the idea; Helen, herself, was then almost seven years old.

Facilities and Program

The Building

Helen House is set on three acres of well-established and beautiful gardens. It is a minute's walk from shops and a bus route to the city centre which is 1½ miles away. The house has accommodation for eight children at any one time and provision is made for parents and siblings to be resident too if they so wish. Of the eight individually designed and furnished children's bedrooms, two pairs of two have intercommunicating double doors, making it possible to have two double rooms in place of four single rooms. Advantage is taken of this when two children of the same family visit or if children make friends with each other and choose to share. It is interesting to note that most children consider their bedroom as their territory and seem to enjoy the security and the privacy it can provide. Six of the bedrooms have a window seat which converts to a comfortable divan where a parent may choose to sleep, but most parents prefer the apartment designed for their use upstairs, with its two double bedrooms, sitting room, kitchen, and bathroom.

The main playroom has glass doors opening out into the garden. A small hobbies room has easy-clean surfaces for messy activities, and another playroom is used for reading and listening to tapes or as a day room for a child confined to bed. The jacuzzi, a gift from the Royal Air Force, is not only a pleasure to children who are mobile and alert, despite their disease, but is also of tremendous benefit to those suffering varying degrees of paralysis, immobility, or emaciation. It often evokes delighted response from children rarely known to respond to any kind of stimulus. The kitchen with dining area is designed in farmhouse style and is a natural focal point of the house—children, parents, and staff eat together and often share in the preparation of meals and the washing of dishes! A room resembling an ordinary bedroom, but with a cooling system, is available for use when a child dies in Helen House, and parents and relatives are able to spend time there with their child.

The staff of Helen House are all nonresident. This is a deliberate policy, as it is felt to be important that they live away from what is inevitably emotionally taxing and often draining work.

Every possible emphasis has been laid on making the house resemble home rather than hospital or institution, both in architectural design and in the choice of fabrics and furniture. The house is carpeted, each room has different curtain fabric, and much of the furniture, including the beds and cots, was designed and made in ash by a local craftsman. Machine-washable continental quilts with attractive covers are used for all children. Light, colour, and space were of prime importance in the minds of the design team.

The Team

The team caring for the families in Helen House consists of 20 people with widely varying experience and qualifications. They work together as a team with a Head Nurse and her Deputy and a Medical Director, but with minimal emphasis on hierarchy. These people together with other registered nurses with specialist paediatric training, nursery nurses, teachers, a social worker, and a part-time physiotherapist with several others comprise the team. No one is employed specifically as a cook or cleaner; each person shares in these activities. Those without specific qualifications are mostly mothers with experience of their own children or, in one case, a girl waiting to go to university whose brother was killed in a road accident and who is a greatly loved "big sister" to some of our children.

Our Medical Director is in General Practice, based in the immediate vicinity. He visits the house regularly once a week, with frequent shorter visits during the week and otherwise by request. With only a small number of our children suffering from malignant disease and requiring pain relief and symptom control, part-time medical input is sufficient.

Members of the staff do not wear uniforms and are known by their first names. In selecting the team, it was recognised that it was essential to have people with the right qualifications and experience, but the greatest emphasis was on their personal qualities and on whether they "spoke the same language." The final selection relied heavily on the intuition of the selectors.

Liaison with Other Agencies and with Families

One member of the staff, a trained social worker, is employed to work half-time in the house on the ordinary duty rota and half-time in the community, visiting children and their families at home or in hospital, and liaising with other agencies involved in caring for the families. Where, for example, a family doctor, home tutor, or physiotherapist who cares for a child when at home is willing to continue to be involved on a practical level during the child's visits to Helen House, they are encouraged to do so; continuity is seen as vitally important for both child and family. However, distance and other practical difficulties often make this impossible.

Specialists in many fields of medicine offer their services free of charge on a consultancy basis and although Helen House is a freestanding facility, we work closely with National Health Service facilities where this is appropriate.

Home Care

A home care service has not yet been developed on a formal basis and at present we work in liaison with the existing domiciliary paediatric nurses employed by the National Health Service.

Where distance permits, members of our team do give help and support in the child's own home when the need arises, but this is on an informal basis.

Staff Support

A consultant child psychiatrist acts as enabler at a weekly staff support group, offering an opportunity for open discussion among members of the team about matters of mutual concern with the chance to share some of the joys and sorrows, perplexities and misunderstandings which inevitably occur. Everyone recognises that despite the genuinely happy and informal atmosphere which prevails in the house, it is inevitably linked with grief in its many forms and considerable emotional demands are made on the staff day by day. An essential attribute for members of the team is a sense of humour! It is vital to care for the carers.

Administration and Finance

An administrator and a secretary handle the administration of Helen House. The annual running costs amount to £125,000, government sources supplying one-sixteenth of this. The remainder comes from the endowment fund and from voluntary gifts. We do not employ anyone as fund raiser, but nationwide support and interest continues to grow throughout the United Kingdom. No charge is made to families using Helen House, either for the children or their relatives, as it is felt that many of them have already suffered very considerable financial strain through the sickness of their child.

"Hospice" and "Terminal Illness"

It seems important to define the word "hospice" at this point. The *Oxford English Dictionary* definition is: "A house of rest and entertainment for pilgrims, travellers or strangers—for the destitute or sick." A petition to Henry VIII in 1538 reads: "For the ayde and comforte of the poor sykke, blynde, aged and impotent personnes . . . whereyn they may be lodged, cherysshed and refreshed" (Clay, 1966, p. 236). Hospices have been in existence in one form or another since about A.D. 475 and were particularly in evidence in the Middle Ages, during which time they were places where pilgrims and travellers could receive refuge and sustenance. The religious orders who were responsible for the hospices started caring for the sick and dying, and gradually the term "hospice" came to be associated more with this aspect of the work. In England in the nineteenth century the charitable hospitals were refusing to take in incurables and workhouse infirmaries catered solely for the destitute, so hospices came to provide an alternative to either of these.

Latterly, hospices have been associated mainly with the care of the terminally ill. One of the forerunners in the specialist care of the dying was St. Joseph's Hospice in East London, and it was here in the 1950s that Dame Cicely Saunders began to develop her methods of pain control in the terminally ill and chronic sick and to pioneer the modern hospice movement. In 1967, under her leadership, St. Christopher's Hospice was opened. Here, as in some other hospice units, it is deliberate policy to care not only for those in the last weeks or months of life, but also to offer respite (or in some cases long-term) care to those with chronic illness.

Despite the efforts of many working within the hospice movement, the popular idea amongst the vast majority of the general public is that all hospices cater exclusively for the dying. If the term were not so cumbersome, "continuing care units" might perhaps be the more appropriate designation for such programs.

Six months before Helen House opened, a father asked if we could help care for his three-year-old son who was "terminally ill." Explaining that Helen House was not yet open and that very regretfully, therefore, we could not help, the father replied that this was all right; he was in any case thinking in terms of the time when the hospice would be open. "My son has been terminally ill for two years," he said. At the age of one, the little boy had been diagnosed as having a life-threatening condition with a prognosis of not more than five years. From that time on, his parents understandably described him as terminally ill.

The Children

Those To Be Served

Priority is given to children in the final stage of illness. Statistics show that, in the West, a high percentage of children who die do so in the hospital. In cases of acute infection or accident this is clearly the right place, with all the facilities for saving life where this is possible and appropriate. But in other situations it is very often the wish of the family to have their child at home to die and, given the right kind of support, this is both possible and desirable. However, it is important that we do not generalise when assessing the best course of action for any individual family; each one has different reactions and different needs. No family should be coerced into having their child at home to die against their wishes or made to feel that they are "bad" parents if they decide not to. Sometimes parents feel they could not bear to continue to live in the house where their child has died and would have to move out of the house if the child died at home. Others may have seen other people's children with the same disease as their child dying by haemorrhage or in convulsion or with pain, and may prefer to be in an environment where they feel totally supported and surrounded by people who will know how to meet all eventualities. Sometimes children themselves will feel more secure in a place where they know there are doctors and nurses. We have known each of these situations to exist, even where home care support has been available, and the feelings of each child and family must be respected.

When a child who is in the final stages of illness comes to Helen House, we welcome and encourage any members of the immediate family to stay with us too, and to be with their child and care for him or her as much as they feel willing and able.

Babies in the first weeks of life are sometimes referred to us from special care baby units of hospitals. If it is recognised that a baby has a condition which is not compatible with life and curative therapy is either not attempted or is abandoned at an early stage, it is conceivable that an intensive care unit ceased to be the appropriate environment for the infant and parents. However, the parents may not feel sufficiently confident to take their baby home, and the solution can sometimes be a halfway house such as we are able to provide.

Children in the final stages of illness, however, form a minority of those who come to Helen House. The majority are those in varying stages of chronic, life-threatening disease, for example, cystic fibrosis, muscular dystrophy, biliary atresia, pulmonary atresia, Batten's disease, Trisomy 18, and the mucopolysaccharide diseases—Sanfillipo's disease, Hurler's disease, Hunter's disease, and so on. Children who come suffering with malignant disease most often come towards the end of their life and therefore come into the category mentioned above, but a common exception to this is children with cerebral tumours where curative therapy has been abandoned but where the disease then spans a considerable length of time.

A third category consists of children with a profound handicap whose condition appears to change little, if at all, but who need total care. These children frequently live on with an uneventful history and then die suddenly of respiratory infection, kidney failure, or major convulsion, sometimes with the onset of puberty. One of our biggest problems is selection of the children in this third category; we try to take into account not only the severity of the child's condition but also the needs of the family as a whole.

Many of the children who come to Helen House have diseases which cause brain damage and mental retardation along with other effects. Others, however, are mentally alert and active, though restricted in their physical activity. In planning the children's visits we try to arrange for mentally alert children to have the companionship of others equally alert so that they can provide stimulation for each other. Loneliness, boredom, and frustration, through an inability to join in with the activities of their siblings and peers, are often among these children's greatest problems and they look to us when they visit for stimulation, entertainment, and company. "I am bored at home and I've fallen out with my parents. Would you book me into the Snoopy room for next week, please?"

Parents and siblings of all children are welcome to stay for part or all of their child's visits. We particularly encourage this on the initial visit, so that the family can teach us how best to care for their child, especially if the child is unable to communicate himself, for without doubt they are the people who know their child best and we have much to learn from them. It also gives us the opportunity of getting to know them and gives them the opportunity of getting to know us, in the hope of establishing a relationship of friendship and trust.

Irrespective of race or belief, children who can benefit from our type of hospice care are welcomed, in an age range from birth to 18 years. Our catchment area covers the United Kingdom.

Pattern of Visits

Children coming for respite care either come at regular intervals (for example, two weeks in every two months, one week in every six weeks, alternate weekends) or by arrangement with the family. Some ask only for occasional help in order to cover a holiday or a period of crisis at home. A child would not normally come for more than a month on any one visit unless in exceptional circumstances, and we do not provide long-term institutional care. It is important for the child to believe that he or she belongs at home with his or her own family and just comes to visit us from time to time, as one might visit friends.

Referrals

Initial enquiries come from many sources including the family, doctors, nurses, social workers, and others in the health team—and sometimes from teachers. All we require when we have decided that this is a family to whom we can offer help is that the parents wish to accept our offer and that the doctor responsible for the child's care is in agreement.

Case Histories

The spirit of Helen House and its objectives are best illustrated by the case histories of several of its young visitors.

Susanna

Susanna's parents are first cousins. They produced an apparently healthy daughter who progressed normally for the first six years of her life. At the age of six she had her first grand mal convulsion followed by frequent petit mal attacks. Her parents were reassured that she would probably "grow out of it," but during the next year her schoolteacher complained that she was not making progress and the child herself complained that she could not see very well. Over the next three years her sight deteriorated, as did her mental age. At the age of nine Susanna was diagnosed as having juvenile Batten's disease.

Susanna attended a school for the blind as a weekly boarder, but when she was twelve the staff no longer felt able to handle the problems she presented. By now she was severely mentally and physically handicapped and totally blind, able to do very little for herself and with limited comprehension. She was still continent but could walk only a few steps with help and was virtually wheelchair-bound. Susanna went through a very distressing stage with bouts of dementia and frequent hallucinating. She had periods of hyperactivity followed by uncontrollable sobbing, and to some extent this pattern continues some months later.

Susanna's father is an Air Force pilot, necessitating frequent absences from home, so the burden of caring for Susanna, their only child, fell largely on her mother and this placed an immense strain on her. She is of slight stature and her daughter is considerably heavier than she is herself. At the time that Helen House opened, four months after the school ceased to be able to help with Susanna, the only alternative respite care offered was a bed in a psychogeriatric unit, so her parents chose to drive the difficult six-hour journey to bring her to Helen House for two weeks in every two months. Usually they stay with us themselves for several nights of the visit. They quickly built up an exceptionally trusting and loving relationship with members of the Helen House team. During her more lucid times, Susanna also enjoys many friendships, especially with male members of the team and with the Helen House puppy! She loves babies and delights in holding one, stroking and cuddling him. She almost always responds to her parents' voices. Thus, if they are not actually present, we often play her tapes of them talking to her and reading her stories.

In the last few months, Susanna has become doubly incontinent and unable to walk even with help. On several occasions she has been in status epilepticus and we have thought that she could not survive more than hours, or at most a few days, but each time her condition has improved. This proves a devastating experience for her parents each time it happens. They prepare themselves emotionally for what looks like the inevitable outcome, and then have to adjust to a further prolongation of their daughter's tragic illness. Susanna's condition has deteriorated considerably over the nine months we have known her and her visits to us have become longer and more frequent, her parents spending more time here with her.

Mark

Mark is eight years old. At fourteen months he was found to have congenital pulmonary atresia and at the age of six he had surgery. However, this was not successful and Mark remains with severe central cyanosis and is very limited in his exercise tolerance. He frequently exceeds his limitations and as a result loses consciousness. He often complains of his "puff pain" which is thought to be anginal and which causes him great anxiety and fear. He often talks about his own death in connection with this pain and has a marked reluctance to fall asleep, sometimes having quite disturbed nights.

Mark is an intelligent child, quick-witted and lively in temperament but constantly frustrated by his physical limitations. His parents find it difficult to agree about his management and upbringing, his father accusing his mother of overprotecting him and his mother accusing her husband of being insensitive and brutal. The marriage suffers seriously as a result. Mark attends an ordinary school part-time, but this is a further cause of anxiety to his mother; the child does not enjoy school or enter fully into relationships with his peers and the mother feels he is not achieving his full potential academically. Mark comes to Helen House for about one week in every six, and one day a week between visits for teaching purposes. When he stays here, his mother and seven-year-old sister remain throughout the visit, the latter going to her school during the day in term time. His father accompanied them on the first visit and occasionally comes for a few hours during subsequent visits, but seeing

Mark among other seriously ill children depresses him and makes him realize the gravity of their own situation which he is reluctant to think about or discuss.

Mark and his sister enjoy each other's company, despite frequent arguments and fights, but they do not play easily with other children. Mark enjoys the stimulation and entertainment provided in Helen House, as much as anything else, though it is difficult to hold his concentration for any length of time. His mother looks forward eagerly to each visit, with the opportunity of talking to people, mostly about her anxieties and the difficulties the family faces, but also just enjoying the company of others as a relief from the loneliness and isolation she feels at home.

Sammy

Sammy was diagnosed at the age of four as having a Stage IV non-Hodgkin's lymphoma involving the ileum with secondary deposits in the bone marrow. At the time of diagnosis he had a six-week history of intermittent abdominal pain with severe occurrences ten to twenty times a day, associated with vomiting one to five times a day. He underwent a course of chemotherapy, but in view of the high likelihood of disease relapse on standard chemotherapy, it was felt that the only possibility of long-term survival would be with bone marrow transplantation following total body irradiation. However, it proved impossible to find a perfect match and he therefore underwent an autologous bone marrow graft. Initially he did well, apart from two brief episodes of right facial palsy, but one month later he complained of headache, vomiting, and lethargy, and lumbar puncture revealed numerous blasts. It was concluded that there had been a focal deposit of lymphomatous cells which resisted radiation treatment and rapidly recurred.

Sammy's young parents were fully involved in discussion about his prognosis and future management. His central nervous system relapse during the period of marrow regeneration was only partially controlled with intrathecal chemotherapy and a course of palliative cranial irradiation. Acute care hospital ceased to be the appropriate environment and it was suggested that the family might like to visit Helen House to see if it was a place they would choose to come to if the situation became unmanageable at home. Sammy, his parents, and three-year-old sister spent a day with us. Sammy often asked if they could have a holiday, but his parents had never been able to afford this. When he saw Helen House for the first time, he exclaimed: "It's a real holiday camp! Can we stay here?" He cried miserably when his parents told him that they could not stay here this time. His condition deteriorated rapidly over the next few days and the whole family returned to us for the last five days of his life.

Pain control was one of the most urgent problems and this was achieved fairly satisfactorily after a day or two. Sammy improved a little and was able to enjoy playing and being taken out in a push-chair. There were many moments of real pleasure interspersed with the times when he clearly felt very ill indeed. His parents took turns being with him day and night. He developed minor nose bleeds and haematuria, and was given platelets to prevent fatal haemorrhage—the form of death witnessed by his parents in another child and which they dreaded more than anything. Sammy died suddenly and peacefully the following morning, having been fully conscious to the end.

Sammy's grandparents came the next day to see him for the last time, to be with his grief-stricken parents and little sister, and to see the room and "holiday camp" that they knew Sammy had loved. At the end of the day, they took the little girl home with them and Sammy's parents asked if they could stay with us during the last three days until the funeral. Sometimes alone together and sometimes with us, talking of Sammy before he was ill, of his illness, of the future without him, crying with us, sharing meals with us, and sitting up with us late into the night, they now talk of those days as a time when the healing began. Two of us went with them to their home town on the South Coast for Sammy's funeral. We knew that returning home was hard for them. We keep in touch with fairly frequent telephone calls, and they, like all our other bereaved families, accepted our invitation to visit us and plan to spend part of their summer holiday in Helen House.

Joanne

Joanne is eleven years old. She was born following an uncomplicated pregnancy, but at birth the umbilical cord was said to be around the baby's neck and she did not establish spontaneous breathing for some minutes. In her first weeks of life Joanne was difficult to feed, and at two months old she was admitted to hospital because she was suffering from episodes of generalized convulsions with cyanosis. Over the next few years she had frequent periods of hospitalisation. A diagnosis of cerebral palsy with epilepsy was made and it became obvious that she was grossly mentally retarded. Joanne did not respond to any known anticonvulsant therapy and she continued to suffer numerous grand mal convulsions. At the age of six her anticonvulsants were stopped by her parents without any obvious change in the frequency or severity of her fits.

Joanne moves her head from side to side, but has no spontaneous movement in her limbs. She occasionally seems to respond to her mother's voice, but to little else. Over recent years she has developed a marked kyphoscoliosis and flexion deformities of the limbs. She has repeated chest infections, sometimes severe, which, at the request of her mother, have been actively treated with antibiotics and physiotherapy. In addition, over recent months, she has developed very noisy respirations with episodes of apparent intermittent partial airway obstruction.

Joanne had been nursed at home continuously, apart from the periods of hospitalisation in her early years, until Helen House opened. Her mother felt she had to be 100 percent responsible for the care of her daughter and would not countenance separation from her, often it seems to the detriment of her own health and of the well-being of the rest of the family—Joanne's father, brother (three years older), and sister (two years older). Her mother feels guilty about the other two children who, she says, "have missed out on a lot."

On Joanne's first visit, her mother stayed throughout. Initially, she did everything for her daughter and we were able to learn a lot from the mother, but after a few days she began to go out shopping or walking, leaving Joanne in our care. On Joanne's second visit, her father had persuaded his wife to leave her with us and she agreed, somewhat reluctantly. Afterwards, she told us that she had found it almost impossible to relax and kept catching herself going to Joanne's bedroom to get her up in the morning or starting to prepare the next meal for her. With each visit, Joanne's mother has become more relaxed and happy about entrusting her daughter into our care. Now, Joanne comes for a visit varying in length from about five days to two weeks every two months or so. This summer the whole family are taking a holiday abroad—the first proper family holiday since Joanne was born—while Joanne stays with us.

Principles Underlying Care

Children and Their Families

The physical care of a child who has a life-threatening disease is only a small part of the care he or she needs (Mother Frances Dominica, 1984). The child's emotional and spiritual needs and those of the family are of equal importance. Caring for such a child is about caring for the whole child and family, helping them to achieve the optimum quality of life throughout, even though the life span may be short, enabling the child to meet diminishment of health or death with dignity, and helping the family to live on. We must be sensitive to the very different needs of each person and be ready to respond in the way which is most appropriate to each individual.

Although families in previous generations faced the same kind of tragedy much more often, the existence of the close-knit extended family and the greater involvement of the local community provided a kind of support which is lacking today. Today's nuclear family, not infrequently a single-parent family, can suffer terrible feelings of loneliness and isolation. One of our tasks in a children's hospice is to try to supply some of the missing elements by offering active friendship on a regular and reliable basis, often extending over many years.

Our children are a part of the family to which they belong and they cannot be seen other than in that context. Some of our families face immense practical problems, but these are seldom the worst of the difficulties. However imaginative and understanding we may be, we can only begin to be aware of the strain and anguish which the family experiences physically and emotionally. With an acute illness or accident followed by death, the grieving process and mourning have the potential of being resolved over a period of time. Objectively, at least, others accept this process. With chronic sickness the grief is terribly prolonged and may often begin from the moment of diagnosis where it is recognised that there is no known cure and there is not the same possibility of resolving or completing the mourning. Every stage of diminished ability or independence, every loss of function, and each new sign of deterioration is a further cause of mourning to the family and needs the acknowledgement of those around, not least those professionally concerned.

We need to recognize that father and mother may react in very different ways to their distress. Their relationship may become strained because of the difficulty of one partner in understanding how or why the other is behaving in a certain way. Sheer physical exhaustion may affect communication, so that things go from bad to worse. One or both partners may feel ashamed or guilty about their child's disorder and their own inadequacy in coping with it. It is generally easier and more acceptable for a woman to show her emotions than it is for a man and it is particularly difficult for him in the social or work context. It is also traditional for her to perform the nurturing, caring role which reinforces the bond between mother and child, sometimes to the apparent exclusion of the father. Either parent may have periods of time when they distance themselves from the child as a form of self-protection. Arguments occur about the treatment and management of the child. It is not for us to take sides, but rather to be sensitive to the difficulties which each faces and to make positive suggestions about activities they and their child may be able to enjoy together.

There is a temptation for relatives to overindulge a child by showering him or her with material gifts or allowing antisocial behaviour. We have to try to help them see that this often adds to the child's feeling of bewilderment. Children need a recognised structure for their own security in a world where many things have deviated from the norm. The principal need is for physical and emotional love and strength, rather than material possessions. The disruption of family life inevitably affects other children in the family who may feel neglected in favour of the sick child, and in some cases this can lead to strong resentment, resulting in disturbed behaviour. Their sorrow may manifest itself in many ways and may not always be recognised. Siblings may have fears that they themselves may suffer the same illness or even die. Nevertheless, they may well feel that they must protect their already overburdened parents from this and from other anxieties or strong emotions. Siblings who do in fact suffer from the same condition, for example, inherited progressive disorders, as some of our children do, have their own very special needs. We try to be here as friend and confidante to the siblings. Explanation and involvement appropriate to the age and temperament of each child may help to overcome some of the difficulties.

Grandparents and other relatives, as well as friends and neighbours, are affected by the child's suffering and we have to be aware that as well as being a potential source of help they can be potential casualties in the unfolding of a particular tragedy. Brothers and sisters need to be encouraged to enjoy their own friendships and not to feel guilty about this.

As we come to know members of a family well, it is sometimes possible for us to help them encourage their sick child to enjoy such independence as is possible, even though it may be minimal, rather than cling to what is so often the instinctive approach—to protect at all costs. Gradually, we try to build up a relationship of mutual trust and acceptance with the child by behaving consistently and responding honestly at all times. Sometimes a child trusts us enough to be able to relax and share some of his or her worst anxieties. "Mum and Dad think I don't know, but I have got cystic fibrosis, and when you've got that, you don't live long. I'll probably be dead in a year or two. What do you think it is like when you are dead?" "I am frightened, 'cos if I die my Mummy can't come with me." "What will my parents do when I die? I musn't die."

It is vital to listen carefully to what the child is actually saying or asking. Adults easily fall into the trap of assuming that children are asking a more complex question than they really are. Our cardinal rule is never to lie to a child. This does not mean to say that he or she must be given the whole stark truth in one blow. One is often able to give truthful reassurance and allay the child's fears about the actual process of dying and death itself—always, of course, using terms which the child understands and being careful not to contradict beliefs held by his or her family.

We find that the small child has a natural capacity for being able to live for the present moment; recognition of this can be used to advantage by those giving care. If children are free of pain and discomfort and are surrounded by people they love and trust, they are less likely to be fearful for the future. The older child will have taken on more of the fears and complexities of an adult in facing dying and death. It must be categorically stated that there are no hard and fast ways of answering questions or set methods of helping a child come to terms with the truth. So much depends on our own ability to absorb the impact of the emotional and spiritual implications and cope with them ourselves. Platitudes and pat answers are less than helpful. At times when there seems to be nothing to say, it is better not to use empty words but rather try to communicate reassurance through physical presence—just being there alongside through it all. We often remark how protective sick children feel towards their parents and to what great lengths they will go to spare them further pain, whereas someone they trust who is less closely related, but has some authority, may be taken into the child's confidence.

The family may well feel inadequate in caring for the child as his or her condition deteriorates. They need constant reassurance and encouragement to be involved on every level as far as they are able. Too often, they have fears and fantasies as to the mode of dying which are unrelated to reality. If these can be expelled, a little of the anguish may be removed. Through all the strain of caring for a chronically sick child, there will almost inevitably have been moments when parents have wished it would all end. When the end of the child's life is actually in sight, this may result in great feelings of guilt. With the actual death of the child, the family needs to be helped through the appalling confusion of a mixture of relief and grief.

If the relationship has been one of trust and friendship, it will follow that it does not end with the death of the child. Bereavement, particularly when it centres around a child, is often a very lonely time. Friends and even relatives may find it an impossibly difficult task to be faced with the family's grief in all its varying forms of expression. They may be afraid of their own emotional reactions and the instinctive response is to stay away, hoping that the family will find support from others. Behaviour and remarks indicating that it is time the family "got back to normal" can be devastatingly hurtful. We must remember that a family never gets over the death of their child, even though in time they may adjust. Their greatest need is to have a friend or friends who are prepared to stay alongside, not only through the tears, but through the anger and accusations, the guilt and denial, and all the bleak, inexpressible grief.

It is sometimes hard for us to understand why anger can be directed against those who have genuinely tried to offer help and friendship. We realise as time goes on that in situations where we do not honestly feel the anger or accusations are justified, we may have a role to play as scapegoat.

Practical Care of the Child

Caring for children with life-threatening disease needs a great degree of flexibility and creative use of imagination. Children may well contribute some of the best ideas themselves, and it is important to consider these, even though commands and instructions may be issued in a demanding and cheeky manner. Necessary changes in treatment sometimes bring parents face to face with the harsh fact of further deterioration in their child's illness and we have to be sensitive and understanding in meeting their response and gaining their cooperation.

Meticulous attention must be given to the basic physical needs of the sick child, avoiding or relieving discomfort or distress wherever possible: attention to skin, hair, mouth, diet, and bowel function, as well as the more specific pain relief and symptom control. Our children sometimes enjoy cooking or helping to choose and prepare a meal. Shopping expeditions in the neighbourhood help to make it feel more like home. Attractive clothes that are easy to wear will boost the child's morale as well as that of those around.

Conclusion

It is an immeasurable privilege and a humbling experience to be allowed to share in the care of a very sick child. We are alongside members of a family at a time when they are at their most vulnerable. We are there not just as professional caregivers, but as fellow human beings who must be able to be trusted implicitly and with whom there need be no pretence. There are often times when we have nothing wise to say and when all we can do is stand by, not trying to set ourselves up as having the answers. Simply by sharing in the pain we may help to dissipate it a little.

Helen House is an attempt to offer an ordinary kind of friendship to people facing an extraordinary kind of grief. It is the friendship with one little girl and her family extended to other gravely ill children and their families.

References

Clay, R. M., cited in *The Mediaeval Hospitals of England*. New York: Barnes & Noble, 1966.

Frances Dominica, Mother, "Nursing Care of the Chronically Sick or Handicapped Child," in G. T. McCarthy (ed.), *The Physically Handicapped Child: An Interdisciplinary Approach to Management*. London: Faber and Faber, 1984.

Bibliography

Bluebond-Langner, M., *The Private Worlds of Dying Children*. Princeton, NJ: Princeton University Press, 1978.

Stinson, R., & Stinson, P., *The Long Dying of Baby Andrew* Boston: Little, Brown, 1983.

Zorza, V., & Zorza, R., *A Way to Die*. London: Andre Deutsch; New York: Knopf, 1980.

7

A Hospice Approach to Neonatal Care

Roberta Siegel, Susan H. Rudd, Cindy Cleveland, Linda K. Powers, and Robert J. Harmon

Introduction

This chapter outlines an intervention program for families whose infants die in a neonatal intensive care unit. Included are descriptions of the neonatal intensive care unit (NICU), the hospice principles upon which this program is based, and, more specifically, the program as it has been implemented at The Children's Hospital in Denver, Colorado. The chapter also discusses our clinical and research experience with family grieving processes, as well as the influence of our program on staff effectiveness.

The hospice program described in this chapter was developed in the Department of Perinatology at The Children's Hospital, Denver, Colorado. This program is supported in part by grants from the Department of Perinatology, the McArthur Family Foundation, the Little John Fund, the Anderson Foundation, the Rocky Flats Employee Donate-Once Club, the Williams Family Foundation, and private and memorial donations. The authors wish to acknowledge the staff of the Newborn Center at The Children's Hospital, including Dr. Jacinto Hernandez, and Drs. L. Joseph Butterfield and Jonathan M. Whitfield for their help in establishing the Neonatal Hospice Program. We also wish to acknowledge R. Comfort, D. Freeland, E. Goldson, A. Glicken, L. Huntington, and M. McCord for their assistance in various aspects of the program.

Neonatal Intensive Care Units

Over the past 20 years, advances in medical knowledge and technology have dramatically improved the outcome and survival of infants born either prematurely or with birth defects (Hernandez et al., 1981; Koops & Harmon, 1980; Jonsen & Garland, 1976; Fitzhardinge et al., 1976). Despite progress in the care of these infants in neonatal intensive care units, there are a significant number of infants whose deaths are inevitable because of either their terminal condition or poor prognosis. These deaths can occur early during the initial phase of treatment or as late as many weeks or months after a prolonged course in the NICU. Because of the intensity of activity and the complexity of care provided in the NICU, families of these infants experience extreme stress resulting both from their own situations and from the unusual environment of the NICU. Such families require a significant degree of attention from staff members "who must provide not only complex treatment but also adequate medical explanations and emotional support" (Whitfield et al., 1982, p. 421). The emotional effect of neonatal loss on families, as well as their particular experiences in the neonatal nursery, both have a significant impact on family functioning and maternal grieving (Harmon, Glicken, & Siegel, 1984; Klaus & Kennell, 1982; Borg & Lasker, 1981; Cullberg, 1972). Facilitation of parental grieving is strongly influenced by the NICU environment and the attitudes and actions of staff (Benfield, Leibs, & Vollman, 1978; Rowe et al., 1978).

In addition to the grief experienced by families who have suffered a neonatal death, the health care professionals who work in a NICU also experience their own grief reactions. The caregivers in this setting are primarily concerned with neonatal survival and are oriented to a "rescue-mode" approach to therapy (Solnit & Green, 1959). When death does occur, they often suffer from a great sense of helplessness and failure (Luxton, 1979). Members of the staff frequently experience difficulty in accepting this situation and may not be able to assist families who are struggling with the same feelings of loss and helplessness (Benfield, Leibs, & Vollman, 1978; Easson, 1968). Even though tertiary care neonatal units are becoming increasingly attuned to the dying child and the importance of family support, the rescue-mode orientation of the staff and the crisis nature of the environment have made it difficult to provide optimal care for dying infants and their families.

Hospice Principles

In order to help both families and staff deal with the complex issues related to the care of the dying infant, a comprehensive program, The Neonatal Hospice Program, was developed in 1979 at the NICU of The

Children's Hospital in Denver. The basic aim of this program is to provide a private, comfortable, and supportive environment for families and their dying infant, thereby creating an atmosphere in which parents have the opportunity to deal with their infant's death in a personally meaningful way. The program is based in part on a modification of the principles of the adult hospice movement (Saunders, 1978; Krant, 1978). The authors feel that many of the concepts from the hospice movement can be readily adapted to specific needs of the NICU.

Our clinical work with families led us to make the following observations about families who had experienced a neonatal death in our NICU: (1) the chaotic nursery environment offered little privacy and comfort; (2) the staff was often insensitive to the individual needs and wishes of families at the time of their baby's death, that is, wishes to hold their infant, requests for visits by relatives or friends at the time of the infant's death, and the unfamiliarity by staff of options related to autopsy and funeral arrangements; (3) some families reported significant family disruption including marital difficulties, separation, or difficulty dealing with their other children; (4) families experienced feelings of isolation and a lack of understanding on the part of their relatives and friends; (5) many families had significant financial difficulties related to their infant's hospitalization; and (6) families frequently did not receive adequate autopsy and/or psychosocial follow-up.

As a result of these observations, it seemed appropriate to apply to our NICU the following basic hospice premise: the setting where most people with a fatal illness die may be insensitive to the physical, psychological, social, and spiritual needs of the patient and family (Krant, 1978). The hospice philosophy promotes an approach that is responsive to these needs and there is a recognition that at times the patient may no longer benefit from a "rescue mode" of treatment. This approach at times involves a revision of medical care to include less aggressive forms of treatment and to provide a more comfortable physical environment; there is also an emphasis upon seeing the patient within the context of the whole family system (Whitfield et al., 1982). This approach to "palliative care" embodied by these hospice principles has become the basis for the Neonatal Hospice Program. A guiding premise of the program has been to recognize the importance of a more sensitive individualized approach for each dying infant and his or her family, whether the child's death is anticipated or the infant has died suddenly.

On the basis of the hospice principles discussed above, the following adaptations were made to the NICU: (1) recognition of the need for a specially-trained staff educated both to be more knowledgeable in the issues of death, dying, and bereavement, and to accept death as a tragic but nevertheless positive outcome for some infants and their families; (2) provision of a more formalized system for mutual support among staff members through regularly scheduled meetings; (3) acknowledgement that at times a rescue mode of treatment has its limitations and that palliative care often resulting in death may be a positive option in some situations; (4) creation of a more homelike environment (the Family Room) which allows for privacy and comfort in contrast to the busy NICU environment; (5) opportunity for meaningful involvement of family members with their infant at the time of or immediately following the death; and (6) recognition of a need for an organized and systematic follow-up protocol for all families suffering a neonatal loss. In our view, the conjunction of these six points constitutes a comprehensive hospice approach to neonatal care.

The Children's Hospital, Denver

The Newborn Intensive Care Unit at The Children's Hospital is a regional referral center for infants transported from a nine-state area. The nursery contains 33 intensive care beds which are primarily situated in one large room. During 1983, of the 671 admissions, 32 percent of the infants weighed less than 1500 grams, 25 percent had severe congenital malformations, and 12 percent died. This last figure (12 percent) has remained fairly constant since 1978.

The NICU has a busy transport service bringing infants in from both large cities and small rural communities throughout the Rocky Mountain area. These infants are brought in by ground ambulance, helicopter, or fixed wing aircraft. In addition to the actual separation and family disruption that occurs after an infant is transported to the hospital, parents must make cultural and financial adaptations in traveling to visit their infant in a large, possibly unfamiliar, city at a sophisticated medical center. If parents are not able to visit the hospital (because of family responsibilities, financial constraints, or mother's physical condition), further emotional turmoil must be dealt with.

Since 1976 a program of family-centered care has been offered to all of the families served by our NICU (Siegel, 1982). In addition, since 1980 all of the families whose infants have died in the NICU have had available to them the hospice approach to neonatal care described in this chapter. In cases where families live far away from Denver and are not able to be with their child at the time of death, the staff maintains close telephone communication with them. The family, although not present, is still offered emotional support and follow-up services.

Elements of the Neonatal Hospice Program

Staff Training and Support

The education and training of the neonatal staff has become the cornerstone of the Neonatal Hospice Program. In order to equip the staff with the skills and understanding necessary to deal with the personal, emotional, ethical, and moral issues that arise from caring for critically ill and dying newborns and their families, a training program was implemented. The goals of this program were to foster an interdisciplinary approach, increase knowledge and self-awareness in the areas of grief and loss, enhance communication among the professional team, and sensitize staff members to their unique role with dying patients and families. To enlist the support of the staff, they were surveyed as to their educational and emotional needs in working with dying infants and their families. A course curriculum was formulated and is offered periodically to the neonatal staff (physicians, nurses, social workers, chaplains, and hospital volunteers). The course content includes an overview of hospice concepts, the effects of a sick or dying infant on family functioning, normal and pathological grieving processes, psychosocial support and counseling techniques, medical and legal aspects of death and dying, ethical issues involved in the decision-making process of terminating cure-oriented care, and information on autopsy and funeral arrangements. The course provides didactic information with an emphasis on group discussion in an attempt to facilitate communication skills. The course helped the staff more clearly define their role with families by increasing their knowledge and acceptance of death. Staff members who attend the course are designated as the Hospice Team or are identified as a Hospice-trained staff member. These individuals are available to provide direct care to the dying infant and family, to serve as a resource person to other staff members in these situations, and/or to coordinate discussions (both formal and informal) regarding management of the dying infant as well as reactions and feelings of the staff.

In order to provide support to staff, interdisciplinary team meetings are held twice a month. Each infant's death which occurred during the previous month is reviewed from medical, nursing, and psychosocial perspectives. This case review serves several purposes. It offers the staff an opportunity to discuss individual concerns and feelings about these deaths and how each patient was managed. It provides an opportunity for the perinatal social worker, the family care coordinator (a neonatal nurse who works directly with families and staff), or the chaplain to share information about the family that they have from their follow-up contacts. This feedback is very helpful to staff members (often nurses) whose involvement was extensive before the death, yet minimal afterward. An additional purpose of the meeting is to discuss the overall functioning of the Neonatal Hospice Program so that necessary adaptations and modifications can be implemented. The meeting also serves as a forum for continuing staff education in the areas of grief and loss, through periodic in-service programs.

Although the discussion in these regular hospice team meetings is facilitated by a social worker, the cases are presented by any staff member who was involved with the infant (neonatologist, nurse, perinatal social worker, family care coordinator, or chaplain). Minutes from the meetings are distributed along with the names of the cases to be discussed at the next meeting. The minutes help notify staff members, who can then attend meetings that are relevant to their needs. Meetings are open to all staff members. This helps reduce the risk of hospice team members being viewed as having "special group" or "elitist" status.

The Decision-Making Process

The advances that have occurred in technology in NICUs have created many moral and ethical dilemmas regarding the initiation, continuation, and termination of certain forms of treatment for critically ill newborns. While the prognosis for many infants has been greatly improved by progress in the field of neonatology, there is a group of unfortunate infants whose conditions are either incompatible with life or whose eventual outcome and prognosis for quality of life is extremely guarded. The health care providers who work in NICUs must be able to apply the available technology to their patients, but must also appreciate its limitations, understand the ethical implications, and maintain a concern for the psychosocial needs of the patient and his or her family.

Decisions about care are extremely sensitive and complex, and require a great deal of thoughtful consideration by the perinatal health care team. In recent years, the literature concerning these issues has greatly expanded. It is our recommendation that within the context of the current medical-legal climate, each perinatal health care team develop its own philosophy regarding medical intervention and establish guidelines for approaching these situations when they arise.

Our NICU uses a team approach to decision-making with an emphasis on family participation and involvement—a family-oriented, decision-making ethic (Duff, 1979). This involvement of families is encouraged not only in discussions about medical intervention, but also in all aspects of care regarding their infant, as will be described in the next section. It is our particular philosophy that when the prognosis is clearly very poor, noninitiation or discontinuation of certain forms of treatment may be appropriate options for some infants and some families. Palliative care, often resulting in death, can be regarded as a tragic but positive option in some situations (Whitfield et al., 1982). We believe that with a thoughtful clinical assessment of the patient and the family situation, the neonatologist, with consultation from the health care team, can give the family advice and recommendations regarding treatment options. The family then is encouraged to share their thoughts, values, and feelings about the recommendations. The primary responsibility for decision-making rests with the neonatologist, although all members of the team are involved. The health care team in our NICU consists of a bedside nurse, a nurse manager, perinatal social worker, family care coordinator, resident in pediatrics, training fellow in neonatology, attending neonatologist, and respiratory therapist. We feel that most parents—with the advice, recommendations, and support of this team—are capable of discussing and arriving at an optimal decision about the care of their infant.

Involvement of Family Members

In order to help facilitate a successful resolution of the grieving process, we make every effort in our role as caregivers to provide an opportunity for families to have personally meaningful involvement and contact with their dying infant. Our goal is to help parents deal with the reality of the loss, insure that grieving begins, and be sensitive to the individual needs of the family (Klaus & Kennell, 1982). The grieving process involves reviewing the attachment with the infant and the memories of events associated with the infant's life. This helps prepare for and come to terms with the impact of the child's death. To facilitate this process, frequent family conferences are held during the hospitalization in which parents are encouraged to discuss their infant's birth, their own feelings about the current situation, and how they wish to participate at the time of their infant's death. These discussions usually develop over a period of time and occur both formally and informally with staff members. This approach often helps families master their situations, provides them with emotional support, and is specifically tailored to their individual needs, personality, and availability (Siegel et al., 1983).

A number of options for involvement are offered to families with an emphasis always on individual differences and preferences. These are available to families both when a death is anticipated or when a death occurs suddenly (e.g., in surgery or during a resuscitation). Either before, during, or after the death of their infant, parents are given the opportunity to see, touch, hold, and talk to their infant alone or with the support of family, friends, clergy, or staff members. They may wish to bathe and dress the infant. Some parents want a lock of hair, a foot print, or a picture of the infant. They may also desire a religious adviser to be present for a blessing, a baptism, prayers, and/or support. Parents are given the infant's personal belongings (i.e., clothes, stuffed animals, and hospital tags) when desired.

Involvement of significant people is encouraged if the parents feel this would be helpful. They may wish that a sibling see the infant in order to help him or her better understand the reality of the loss. This should only be done with careful evaluation and preparation of the sibling. The presence of family members such as grandparents, aunts and uncles, friends, or religious advisers may be helpful to the parents not only to provide emotional support at the time of death, but later as the parents proceed through the grief process when the hospital staff is not as available. If parents initially choose not to see their infant or are not able to be present at the time of death, they may see and hold the infant at a later time (as long as several days later). These arrangements are usually made by the parents through the social worker or the family care coordinator. It is our policy to take pictures of each infant at the time of death, and offer them to parents. If parents initially prefer not to take the pictures, they are filed and kept available in case the parents change their minds—as is often the case. The pictures are not kept as part of the infant's medical record, but are attached to the Infant Death Data Sheet (see Appendix 7–1) and kept in a "Hospice Notebook."

Funeral arrangements, autopsies, and organ donations are all areas in which parents can participate in decision making regarding their infant. Funeral and memorial services or other burial alternatives are beneficial for families because they serve to finalize the loss and to acknowledge the importance of the child. The process of making the necessary decisions and arrangements can help parents begin to appreciate the reality of the death and aid them in mastering their situation. Various options including hospital burial, private burial, cremation, and memorial services are discussed with families. If they need assistance in making these arrangements, the social worker or family care coordinator is available.

Autopsy requests are made in situations where it would be beneficial to understand the reasons for the infant's death and possibly in planning for future pregnancies. Requesting an autopsy is a sensitive area, but with openness it can be approached honestly. Before parents agree to an autopsy, the procedure should be adequately explained to both of them. Parents are then given an opportunity to ask questions and are provided time to discuss and consider their options. Because some parents feel reluctant to put their child through further procedures, they can specify that limitations be made on the extent of the autopsy.

Organ donations or the donation of the body constitute another way some parents wish to bring meaning to their infant's life and death. These options are mentioned to families if appropriate.

The Family Room

Because the NICU is busy and noisy with an abundance of high technology equipment and limited space, it does not lend itself to an event as sensitive as the death of an infant. As a result, the Family Room was created—a quiet room furnished with comfortable chairs, tables, carpeting, drapes, pictures, a telephone, and a "call" button. The room offers a more home-like atmosphere that permits privacy and comfort for families to be with their terminally sick or dead infant. The room is adjacent to the intensive care area of the nursery and is equipped to allow for continued life support of a critically ill newborn (see Figure 7.1). In addition, the

Figure 7.1 NICU Floor Plan

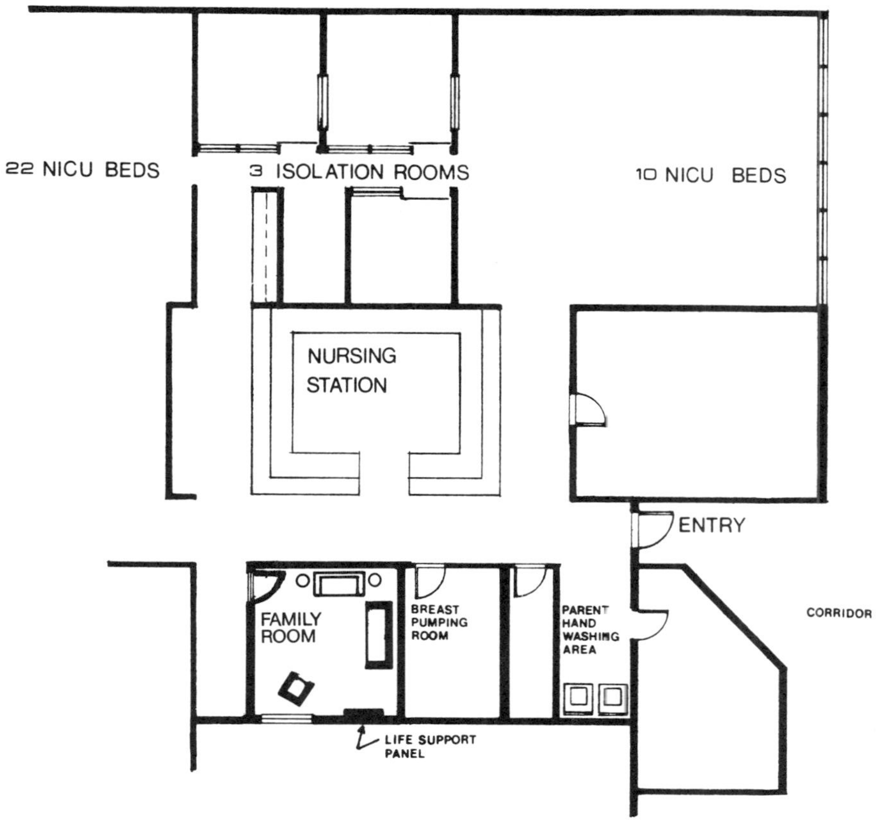

room is used for family conferences, staff discussions, parent-infant privacy, and breast feeding. Priority for use of the room is always given to the family of a dying infant (see Table 7.1). Guidelines have been formulated for the use of this room with an emphasis on flexibility to meet the individual needs of families. The average length of stay of a family with their infant in the Family Room is two to three hours although it has been used for as much as 12 hours at a time. The charges to the family are the same as for a regular NICU bed.

The Family Room is used for infants who are in the process of dying, as well as for babies who have already died. When infants die unexpectedly in the NICU or in surgery, their families may use the room afterwards to see or hold their infant. This can also be arranged when parents are not able to be present at the time of death. In addition, the room can be utilized by staff members to hold a dying baby when the family is not present. This has been helpful to give the infant's death a sense of peace and dignity, as well as to offer the staff an opportunity to express their own personal feelings related to the death of an infant to whom they have become attached. In some situations, when the family and/or staff may choose not to use the room, the infant dies in the NICU. In these cases, the staff can use screens around the infant's bedside to allow for privacy. The potential of assuming that the Family Room is the optimal setting for all families in all situations has serious implications. As is often true with any new intervention program, generalizations about the Family Room's exclusive usefulness have been observed in our staff. Some members of the staff have expressed the feeling that the Family Room is the most comfortable setting for parents with a dying or dead infant. This has resulted in some families not being offered the option of remaining in the NICU with their infant. Some families may feel overwhelmed or isolated in a private room.

Table 7.1. Priorities for Use of the Family Room

1. Used primarily for the family of the dying infant.
2. May be used for a family whose infant has already died and wishes to be with their dead infant (e.g., infant died during surgery or prior to parents' arrival at the NICU).
3. May be used for the dying infant and staff when family is not present.
4. When not being used for 1, 2, or 3, the room can be used for breast feeding, as a predischarge room for the family taking home an infant that requires special care, or as a conference room for staff and family members. A family with a dying infant always has priority to use the room.

Every time an infant dies, a formal record is completed by the nurse involved (see Appendix 7–1). This record includes important medical data such as mode of death and medications given, as well as important psychosocial information such as who spoke with the family about the death, questions asked by the family, their responses to the infant's death, records of photographs taken and received, discussions about autopsy and funeral arrangements, who was present at the time of death, any problems encountered by the family or staff, and the location of the infant at the time of death (i.e., Family Room, NICU, surgery). These data have proven useful in furnishing a comprehensive picture of the events surrounding an infant's death, as well as the family's and the staff's involvement in this process. This record of events has resulted in a sensitive and thorough approach to our follow-up contact with the family. The Infant Death Data Sheet is also used as the basis of discussion about each case in the hospice team meetings. These Death Data Sheets (along with any pictures or name tags) are kept in a Hospice Notebook.

Follow-Up Services for Families

It is well recognized that follow-up services are essential to a family's understanding of their infant's death, as well as helpful in facilitating their grieving process (Klaus & Kennell, 1982; Schreiner, Gresham, & Green, 1979; Rowe et al., 1978). As a result, we attempt to provide all families with the opportunity for follow-up discussions with our staff (physicians, nurses, social worker). The purpose of these conferences is to discuss the infant's medical course, review autopsy findings when appropriate, provide genetic counseling if indicated, offer emotional support, and assess the family's responses to the death and their need for further counseling. These discussions usually include an explanation of the grief process, questions about future pregnancies, and recommendations about the needs of other children in the family. Since our Newborn Center serves a large geographic area, the referring physician collaborates with our staff in providing the follow-up whenever possible. The perinatal social worker and family care coordinator have assumed responsibility for coordinating these services (see Appendix 7–2). In addition, they routinely have telephone contact with families (or in-person contact, if desired) at three and nine months following the infant's death. In reviewing and evaluating the family's functioning, it may be determined that additional emotional support could be beneficial. Referrals are made either to our own psychosocial support team or to resources in the family's community (i.e., loss support groups or bereavement organizations and self-help groups such as Compassionate Friends). Our involvement with these families at the time of death frequently establishes valuable relationships such that families have found it easier to request additional counseling if they have subsequent difficulties.

Effects of the Program: Families

Effects of the Neonatal Hospice Program for families can be illustrated in two case studies, and are also evident in the results of our follow-up study which interviewed mothers after the death of their child.

Case 1: When Death Occurs Suddenly

Molly Jones was admitted to the NICU at two days of age with an admitting diagnosis of a cardiac defect—Coarctation of the Aorta. Mrs. Jones was 21 years old; this was her first pregnancy with no complications although a Caesarean section was necessary due to a long labor. Mr. and Mrs. Jones lived out of state and were planning on visiting the NICU as soon as Mrs. Jones was released from the hospital.

Molly's condition deteriorated on the second day of admission and immediate surgery was recommended. Her parents were notified by phone and consented to the surgery. Mrs. Jones' private physician said she could be released the next day and Molly's parents made plans to travel to our unit.

Unfortunately, Molly died in surgery. Her parents were called by the cardiac surgeon and were told the devastating news. They also talked with the nurse who had been taking care of Molly. The nurse offered the parents the option of coming to our NICU to see their daughter. Mr. and Mrs. Jones said they could be there in 2½ hours. While the parents were traveling to the hospital, the nurse went to surgery and brought Molly's body back to the NICU. She took the body into the Family Room and bathed, dressed, and wrapped it in a blanket. Another nurse helped her take pictures of Molly and collected her few belongings—name bracelet and bed tag.

The nurse sat in the Family Room and began filling out information on the Death Data Sheet. She knew this would be extremely important to the social worker who would be making follow-up calls with the family, but who was not available that evening to meet the family when they came to the hospital.

When Mr. and Mrs. Jones arrived at the unit, they were met by the nurse who had cared for Molly. She explained to them how Molly looked at this time and offered them the use of the Family Room to see and hold their daughter. The mother clearly wanted to see her daughter, but the father was very undecided. The nurse supported each of their feelings; she offered to take Mrs. Jones into the Family Room while Mr. Jones waited in the parent lounge.

When Mrs. Jones entered the Family Room, she immediately picked up her daughter's body, rocked her, and cried. The nurse sat with her, only talking with Mrs. Jones when she asked questions. After being with Mrs. Jones for 15 minutes, the nurse said she would like to talk with Mr. Jones to see how he was doing. Mrs. Jones said she wanted to stay with her daughter and would appreciate the nurse checking on her husband.

The nurse found Mr. Jones very anxious and afraid. He was concerned about the way his daughter's body would look and was afraid of being with a dead baby. The nurse answered his questions openly and honestly, explaining exactly how his daughter would appear. Mr. Jones finally decided that he wanted to see his daughter, but asked the nurse to stay in the room with him. Mr. Jones sat with his wife and touched his daughter, but did not want to hold her. He stayed for ten minutes and then left the room. Mrs. Jones was concerned that her husband did not hold their baby and had only stayed with her a short time. By contrast, Mr. Jones was concerned that his wife was spending too much time with their baby and that the stress might be too much for her to handle. The nurse approached this by helping the parents understand that each person grieves in his or her own individual way, and that one way is not better than the other. This seemed to relieve the concerns of each parent. Mrs. Jones stayed in the Family Room with her daughter for more than an hour. She was able to say goodbye to Molly and to give her body back to the nurse.

The parents then met with the neonatologist and the nurse. A request for an autopsy was discussed and the parents readily agreed because they wanted to know if there were other problems with Molly.

The nurse offered Mr. and Mrs. Jones the pictures she had taken of their daughter. Mr. Jones refused them and Mrs. Jones was unsure. The nurse said the pictures would be kept on file in case they changed their minds. The nurse also stated that the NICU social worker would call them in the morning to discuss options for funeral arrangements.

When the parents left, the nurse finished filling out the Infant Death Data Sheet, including questions and concerns the parents had and how each had responded. This information was left in the unit in the Hospice Notebook which contains Infant Death Data Sheets.

The social worker called the parents the next day with options for funeral arrangements. The parents had several questions regarding cremation and finally decided on that option. The social worker reiterated that the pictures of their daughter would be kept on file in case they decided they wanted them. She told the parents she would be calling back in three months with a follow-up interview.

Mrs. Jones called the social worker one week later to request the pictures of Molly. At the three month follow-up call, the social worker again talked with Mrs. Jones. The mother discussed how important the time was that she spent in the Family Room with her daughter. Both parents were glad they had the pictures of Molly. Mr. Jones especially felt the pictures were valuable because he had spent such a short time with his daughter. In the end, Mrs. Jones felt she and her husband were more open in discussing their feelings and she felt closer to her husband.

Case 2: When Death Is Anticipated

Timothy Brown was born at 26 weeks gestation and weighed 630 grams (1½ pounds). He was admitted to the Newborn Center at two hours of age with the diagnosis of severe Hyaline Membrane Lung Disease and a serious prognosis. Timothy's mother was 32 years old, had three other living children, and had had two previous miscarriages. The other children were: Mandy, 10, Sara, 9, and Lindsay, 4. Timothy's siblings had been very involved with the pregnancy and with Timothy's birth. There was no extended family locally, but some close friends of the family were supportive and visited Timothy occasionally. The family visited the NICU often.

Timothy continued to gain weight and his respiratory status improved until two days prior to his death when he was diagnosed with severe gastrointestinal disease (Necrotizing Enterocolitis). Timothy was rushed to surgery twice in order to remove the diseased bowel. During these times, the surgeon, attending neonatologist, bedside nurse, chaplain, and family care coordinator held several conferences with the family to discuss Timothy's condition, to explore his prognosis, and to offer emotional support. When it was found that Timothy did not have enough of his gastrointestinal tract to survive, and that he would die despite any medical or surgical efforts, it became apparent that a shift to palliative care for him was appropriate. Various options about his continued care were discussed with the family.

The family requested privacy with Timothy so they could hold him and take pictures. Since Timothy was in an isolation room because of an infection, the Family Room could not be offered to his parents. However, the hospice concepts were applied for the family in the isolation room. It was important to this family that the siblings be involved at the time of death, although the parents needed and requested guidance on how to proceed with the siblings. Friends and family all held Timothy. With the assistance of the family care coordinator, his two older sisters went to the hospital gift shop to buy him something to wear. Lindsay became restless, so the staff suggested she play in the Creative Play Center which is a child care facility within the hospital. Timothy was baptized by the chaplain upon the parents' request. Timothy's sisters had many questions so they were given a coloring book, *The Frog Family's Baby Dies* (Oehler, 1978), with the parents' permission. This coloring book explains death in children's terms. After Timothy's death, Mrs. Brown bathed Timothy, and Mandy and Sarah helped their mother dress him in his "special outfit." The family stayed with Timothy for more than two hours after his death to hold him and say their goodbyes.

The parents had many questions about funeral arrangements, so the attending neonatologist and family care coordinator reviewed the funeral alternatives and discussed the option of having an autopsy performed. The family care coordinator called the Browns the following day to inquire about their decisions regarding funeral arrangements and an autopsy. Finances were a concern, so the family care coordinator helped them make funeral arrangements at a minimal cost. The family was informed about what they may experience emotionally during the next few months. They requested and were given the booklet, *When Hello Means Goodbye* (Schwiebert & Kirk, 1981), which is a guide for parents whose infant has died. Some members of the staff attended Timothy's funeral, which the family found supportive. They considered some of the staff Timothy's "family" since the extended family did not have the chance to meet him. They proudly showed the pictures of Timothy at the funeral which was their attempt to enhance their family and friends' appreciation of Timothy's life and death.

This case was discussed one week later at the hospice team meeting. The siblings were discussed because there were some concerns about their involvement at the time of death. In addition, some staff had difficulty accepting the family's need to be present for several hours after Timothy's death. As a result of this discussion, staff realized the importance of individualizing our interventions to meet the family's needs.

The family care coordinator and neonatologist met with the family three months after Timothy's death to: (1) discuss the autopsy results; (2) evaluate the family's functioning; and (3) provide emotional support and counseling. It was found that Mr. Brown was functioning well, while Mrs. Brown seemed to be having some difficulty performing her daily tasks at home. Sarah was having behavior problems at school. The family care coordinator and neonatologist explored counseling options for Mrs. Brown and Sarah, and a referral was made to the school psychologist for Sarah. Mrs. Brown did not wish to pursue counseling at this time. Mr. Brown was supportive of both decisions. During this meeting, the parents also expressed their desire to have a memorial plaque for Timothy placed in the NICU, which we later arranged to have done.

At the follow-up appointment at nine months, the family was coping well. They were more accepting of Timothy's death and functioning well in their everyday tasks. Sarah was doing better in school and Mrs. Brown had started back to work. Both parents stated their relationship was closer since Timothy's death and they expressed a greater appreciation of their other children. The parents were discussing future pregnancies and they spoke fondly about their memories of Timothy.

Follow-Up Study Results

A research study was done to investigate maternal grieving and to examine the effects of the Neonatal Hospice Program on this process (Harmon, Glicken, & Siegel, 1984). A total of 38 married women were interviewed (by telephone) at three and nine months following their infants' deaths. The interviews were conducted by health care professionals who were unaware of the circumstances surrounding the infants' deaths and who had no previous contact with the mothers. The mothers were similar in social class, level of education, causes of their infants' deaths, and length of hospitalization for the infants. An interview format was developed consisting of questions designed to elicit information about: (1) the effects of the loss on the mother; (2) her relationship with her husband and family; and (3) how she experienced the neonatal staff's interventions both during and following her infant's hospitalization and death.

The findings supported the observations of other researchers who describe a heightened potential for long-term ill effects on families suffering a neonatal loss (Borg & Lasker, 1981; Speck & Kennell, 1980; Cullberg, 1972). Most mothers did feel that the death of their infant had a major impact on their functioning (Harmon, Glicken, & Siegel, 1984). At three months 80 percent and at nine months 74 percent reported that their lives had changed as a result of the loss. At three months following the loss, only 23 percent described life as "OK" or going reasonably well for them, whereas at nine months 68 percent felt this was the case. The general trend seemed to be that the impact of the loss was greatest at three months and began to decrease at nine months. A majority of mothers felt that the period between two and four months was the most stressful because there was an expectation on the part of relatives and friends to "get back to normal" and these support people were less emotionally available during this time.

In terms of grieving, at nine months 74 percent of the mothers were still having feelings of depression, 42 percent reported episodes of crying, and 53 percent still described themselves as irritable. Sixty-eight percent of the mothers at three months reported feeling angry (specifically at health care professionals) about their infant's death, while only 37 percent felt this way at nine months.

Both at three and nine months, approximately 50 percent of the mothers described their relationship with their husbands as closer as a result of the loss. At nine months, only 10 percent reported marital difficulties. In addition, 65 percent of the mothers reported at nine months that they appreciated and loved their other children more as a direct result of the loss. Relationships with extended family were reported as closer by 45 percent of respondents at three months, and by 29 percent at nine months. Mothers also reported significant financial difficulties (at three months, 53 percent, and at nine months, 52 percent) directly related to the infant's hospitalization.

With regard to an evaluation of the effects of the Neonatal Hospice Program, of the 38 maternal interviews obtained, 19 were conducted after the program was in effect. We were interested in comparing staff involvement and effectiveness between the mothers in the two samples. We also looked at specific interventions parents found useful. In general, the Hospice Program mothers seemed to be more positive about their experiences in the NICU than were the mothers who had not had the benefit of the Hospice Program. In addition, the follow-up contact and the subsequent grieving process was also more favorable on comparison (Siegel et al., 1983). For example, 92 percent of the Hospice intervention mothers were contacted about autopsy results, as compared to only 60 percent of the mothers interviewed prior to initiation of the program. This contact was more likely to have come from a staff member in the hospice group (75 percent), while only 33 percent of the prehospice mothers were contacted by a hospital staff member. The mothers who were contacted expressed an appreciation that someone from the hospital cared enough about them to speak with them about their loss. This is especially important in view of the fact that friends and relatives became less emotionally available to them after the death. The Hospice Program mothers (92 percent) reported that this contact and the explanation of autopsy results had helped them in their understanding of the reasons for their infant's death, as compared with 33 percent of the prehospice mothers. The Hospice mothers also described less irritability and fewer sleep difficulties, which could be related to a better understanding of why their infants had died. It might also explain why a significantly higher number of mothers in the Hospice group who were not pregnant at nine months wanted to get pregnant again.

The interviews also demonstrated that the hospital staff members were more likely to speak to families about funeral and memorial services after the Hospice Program was implemented, and that these services were more likely to have religious or personal significance. We believe this has occurred because staff members are more familiar with the various options available. It is also reflective of our belief that some type of service is beneficial to families to help them finalize the loss. The data also underscored the importance of taking pictures of the infant at transport, during hospitalization, or shortly after death. A majority (86 percent) of mothers either received pictures or would have liked them. Our recommendation is to take a picture of every baby near the time of death because parents who initially did not desire pictures often change their minds months later.

An analysis of the data seems to indicate that by making some significant programmatic changes in our approach to neonatal death, namely the Neonatal Hospice Program: (1) maternal grieving has been facilitated; (2) staff awareness and knowledge of the complex issues regarding the care of the dying infant have increased; and (3) staff follow-up and psychosocial support have improved (Harmon, Glicken, & Siegel, 1984).

Effects of the Program: Staff

The Hospice Program has had a significant positive impact on our neonatal staff—physicians, nurses, social worker, and family care coordinator—in the areas of increased knowledge concerning death and grieving, positive attitudinal changes, and reinforcement of the interdisciplinary team approach.

The staff have grown in their *knowledge* of both the decision-making and grieving processes. They are now more familiar with the psychodynamics of normal and abnormal grieving responses, and are better able to assess both their own reactions and the reactions of a family. An increased capacity to appreciate the wide range of grief reactions in families has enabled the staff to deal with and tolerate their own feelings of frustration, helplessness, sadness, and anger when faced with a dying infant. On the whole, the staff has a greater understanding of how to intervene in these situations, coupled with an appreciation of the differences and preferences of individuals. Not only has their repertoire of supportive techniques expanded, but their information about resources for families has grown. For instance, staff members are now more likely to "listen" to a family as they talk about the impending death of their infant, to include significant others, to offer pictures, and to be more familiar with the options regarding autopsy and funeral arrangements.

Attitudinal changes in the nursery have included an improved acceptance of death and a feeling that it can be a positive growth experience for both staff and families involved. This has enabled the staff to be more supportive of each other and more sensitive to their particular roles as they interact with each other and with families. Through the hospice training course and ongoing case conferences, the staff has been given the opportunity to examine their own ethical, moral, and personal views regarding death. This increased self-awareness has encouraged openness in expressing one's own feelings of grief, given permission to share these feelings with others, and fostered a willingness to give and accept support.

The program has reinforced our *interdisciplinary team approach* especially by opening up new channels of communication among the professional team. Improved communication and a more effective team approach have involved staff more in the decision-making process. This has been facilitated through the systematic use of conferences with staff and/or families (around the time of the infant's death). These staff and family conferences deal with issues related to the treatment and care of the infant and family, together with the effects these decisions have on the staff. Many staff members have expressed a new sense of involvement and relief at the opportunity to discuss both personal and professional feelings surrounding the care of these infants.

The increase in the use of the team approach has led to a decrease in interdisciplinary tension and conflicts. These conflicts usually have arisen when individual team member roles and responsibilities have not been clearly defined (Marshall & Kasman, 1980). The opportunity to work together closely on difficult situations seems to have renewed each staff member's respect and appreciation for the expertise of other professionals and individuals. For example, physicians seem to have a greater acceptance of the assessment skills of the social worker and family care coordinator as the physician struggles with ways to approach a particular family. Likewise, the physicians are more likely not only to solicit a nurse's clinical assessment of a patient, but also to give her or him a greater role in treatment decisions. Volunteers are more often used to hold a dying infant (if the parents cannot be present) or to babysit siblings of the dying infant. The team has also had closer involvement with local referring physicians as they collaborate on providing appropriate follow-up for families.

Staff conferences and meetings have reinforced the team approach by providing an ongoing support system and an opportunity to share problems and solutions. Although not formally evaluated, it is our impression that this process has had a beneficial effect on staff morale and a decrease in the well-known phenomenon of burnout in NICUs (Marshall & Kasman, 1980).

Conclusion

Death is a significant event. Its impact can be substantial, both in anticipation during the dying process and in retrospect during bereavement. In our experience, one context in which this impact is felt most keenly is when death involves newborn infants and when it occurs in the neonatal intensive care unit. In such situations, death sharply reminds family members and caregivers alike of their finitude and vulnerability. But even though death may not be avoided, there are ways to render its impact less harmful and to find in its presence opportunities for constructive growth. This chapter has described one such way through an application of hospice principles to the high-technology, rescue-mode environment of the NICU. This approach identifies the needs of infants, families, and staff members who are faced with death in the NICU and responds to these needs in a way that is legitimate, healthy, and humane. Our experience has demonstrated that this type of individualized and family-centered program of palliative care which specifically addresses issues related to death can be meaningful for all concerned. We encourage others to consider applications of the principles underlying this approach to their own local situations and needs.

References

Benfield, D. G., Leibs, S. A., & Vollman, J. H., "Grief Response of Parents to Neonatal Death and Parent Participation in Deciding Care," *Pediatrics,* 1978, *62,* 171–177.

Borg, S., & Lasker, J., *When Pregnancy Fails.* Boston: Beacon Press, 1981.

Cullberg, J., "Psychosomatic Medicine in Obstetrics and Gynecology," in *Proceedings of the Third International Congress, London, 1971.* New York: S. Karger AG, 1972, pp. 326–329.

Duff, R. S., "Guidelines for Deciding Care of Critically Ill or Dying Patients," *Pediatrics,* 1979, *64,* 17–23.

Easson, W. M., "Care of the Young Patient Who is Dying," *Journal of the American Medical Association,* 1968, *205,* 203–207.

Fitzhardinge, P. M., Pape, K., Aristikaitis, M., Boyle, M., Ashby, S., Rowley, A., Netley, C., & Swyer, P. R., "Mechanical Ventilation of Infants of Less Than 1,501 Grams Birth Weight: Health, Growth, and Neurologic Sequelae," *Journal of Pediatrics,* 1976, *88,* 531–541.

Harmon, R. J., Glicken, A. D., & Siegel, R. E., "Neonatal Loss in the Intensive Care Nursery," *Journal of the American Academy of Child Psychiatry,* 1984, *23,* 68–71.

Hernandez, J. A., Lazarte, R. A., Goldson, E. J., Honeyfield, P. R., & Butterfield, L. J., "Mortality and Early Morbidity in Infants Less Than 1,000 Grams Birth Weight" (abstracted), *Clinical Research,* 1981, *29,* 118A.

Jonsen, A. R., & Garland, M. J. (Eds.), *Ethics of Newborn Intensive Care*. Berkeley, CA: University of California Health Policy Program and Institute of Governmental Studies, 1976.

Klaus, M. H., & Kennell, J. H., *Parent-Infant Bonding* (2nd ed.). St. Louis: C. V. Mosby, 1982.

Koops, R., & Harmon, R. J., "Studies on Long Term Outcome in Newborns with Birth Weights Under 1,500 Grams," in B. Camp (Ed.), *Advances in Behavioral Pediatrics*. Greenwich, CT: JAI Press, 1980, Vol. I, pp. 1–28.

Krant, M. J., "Sounding Board: The Hospice Movement," *New England Journal of Medicine*, 1978, *299*, 546–549.

Luxton, R. W., "The Modern Hospice and Its Challenge to Medicine," *British Medical Journal*, 1979, *2*, 106–112.

Marshall, R. E., & Kasman, C., "Burnout in the Neonatal Intensive Care Unit," *Pediatrics*, 1980, *6*, 1161–1165.

Oehler, J., *The Frog Family's Baby Dies*. Illustrated by K. Shelburne. Raleigh, NC: Duke University Medical Center, 1978.

Rowe, J., Clyman, R., Green, C., Mikkelsen, C., Haight, J., & Atiade, L., "Follow Up of Families Who Experience a Perinatal Death," *Pediatrics*, 1978, *62*, 166–170.

Saunders, C., "Hospice Care," *American Journal of Medicine*, 1978, *65*, 726–728.

Schreiner, R. L., Gresham, E. L., & Green, M., "Physician's Responsibility to Parents After Death of an Infant," *American Journal of Diseases of Children*, 1979, *133*, 723–726.

Schwiebert, P., & Kirk, P., *When Hello Means Goodbye*. Portland, OR: University of Oregon Health Sciences Center, 1981.

Siegel, R., "A Family-Centered Program of Neonatal Intensive Care," *Health and Social Work*, 1982, *7*, 50–58.

Siegel, R., Henneberry, S., Harmon, R. J., Cleveland, C., & Glicken, A., *Handbook on Neonatal Hospice*. Denver, CO: The Children's Hospital, 1983.

Solnit, A. J., & Green, M., "Psychologic Considerations in Management of Deaths on Pediatric Hospital Services," *Pediatrics*, 1959, *24*, 106–112.

Speck, W. T., & Kennell, J. H., "Management of Perinatal Death," *Pediatrics in Review*, 1980, *2*, 59–62.

Whitfield, J. M., Siegel, R. E., Glicken, A. D., Harmon, R. J., Powers, L. K. & Goldson, E. J., "The Application of Hospice Concepts to Neonatal Care," *American Journal of Diseases of Children*, 1982, *136*, 421–424.

Bibliography

Duff, R. S., & Campbell, A. G. M., "Moral and Ethical Dilemmas in the Special Care Nursery," *New England Journal of Medicine*, 1973, *289*, 890–894.

Duff, R. S., & Campbell, A. G. M., "On Deciding the Care of Severely Handicapped or Dying Persons: With Particular Reference to Infants," *Pediatrics*, 1976, *57*, 487–493.

Fletcher, J., "Humanness," in *Humanhood: Essays in Biomedical Ethics*. Buffalo, NY: Prometheus Books, 1979, pp. 7–19.

Fletcher, J., "Pediatric Euthanasia: The Ethics of Selective Treatment for Spina Bifida," in C. A. Swinyard (Ed.), *Decision Making and the Defective Newborn.* Springfield, IL: Charles C. Thomas, 1978, pp. 477–488.

Fost, N., "Counseling Families Who Have a Child With a Severe Congenital Anomaly," *Pediatrics,* 1981, *67,* 321–324.

Fost, N., "How Decisions are Made: A Physician's View," in C. A. Swinyard (Ed.), *Decision Making and the Defective Newborn.* Springfield, IL: Charles C. Thomas, 1978, pp. 220–230.

Fost, N., "Ethical Problems in Pediatrics," *Current Problems in Pediatrics,* 1976, *6,* 2–31.

Appendix 7–1
Infant Death Data Sheet

Date________________

1. INFANT DATA:

NAME:____________________________ SEX:______________

DATE & TIME OF ADMISSION______________________________

AGE ON ARRIVAL AT NBC:______________________________

DATE OF BIRTH:______________________________

DATE & TIME OF DEATH:______________________________

HOSPITAL OF BIRTH:______________________________

HOSPITAL NUMBER:________________ TYPE OF DELIVERY:__________

PROBLEMS WITH PREGNANCY:______________________________

____

WEIGHT:__________ APGAR:______________ G.A.:____________

MAJOR DIAGNOSIS ON ADMISSION:______________________________

PROGNOSIS ON ADMISSION:______________________________

COMPLICATIONS LEADING TO CURRENT TERMINAL STATE:______________

____

ATTENDING NEONATOLOGIST:______________________________

2. FAMILY DATA:

FATHER'S NAME:______________________________

MOTHER'S NAME:______________________________

ADDRESS:______________________________

PHONE: (Home)________________ (Work)________________

FATHER'S OCCUPATION______________ MOTHER'S OCCUPATION__________

ADDRESS/PHONE OF NEAREST RELATIVE________________________

____

MARITAL STATUS______________________________

RELIGION______________________________

INSURANCE______________________________

(continued)

INFANT DEATH DATA SHEET
PAGE 2

3. FAMILY HISTORY:

MOTHER'S AGE:________GRAVIDA:__________TAB:_________SAB:____________

STILLBIRTHS:_________L.C.:__________

FATHER'S AGE:__________

PLANNED PREGNANCY (IF KNOWN): YES__________ NO__________

OTHER CHILDREN AND AGES: (Including previous to this relationship)

____

PREVIOUS FAMILY EXPERIENCE WITH DEATH:____________________________

4. DEATH OF THE INFANT:

HOW WAS INFORMATION ABOUT THE IMPENDING DEATH COMMUNICATED TO FAMILY? (i.e. in person conference, telephone call)__________________________

WHO PROVIDED THIS INFORMATION?____________________________________

HOW DID INFANT DIE?: (i.e., while still on support, in surgery, during a resuscitation, support discontinued)______________________________

WHO WAS PRESENT?: (i.e., physician, nurse, social worker, chaplain)

____

TIME OF DEATH:____

IF SUPPORT WAS DISCONTINUED, HOW?:__________________________________

WHO DISCONTINUED?:____

MODE OF DEATH (i.e., agonal breathing, seizures, calmly)______________

LENGTH OF TIME FOR INFANT TO DIE:__________________________________

DRUGS USED:____

5. FAMILY INVOLVEMENT:

WHERE DID THE INFANT DIE: (i.e., NICU, Family Room, Isolation Room, surgery) ____

FAMILY:	PRESENT:	HELD BABY:
BEFORE	________	__________
DURING	________	__________
AFTER	________	__________

INFANT DEATH DATA SHEET
PAGE 3

WAS THE FAMILY ROOM USED? YES__________ NO__________

IF YES, LENGTH OF TIME:______________________________

IF NO, WHY?______________________________

WHO SPOKE TO FAMILY ABOUT USE OF THE FAMILY ROOM AND WHAT WAS THEIR REACTION?______________________________

ANY OTHERS PRESENT AT TIME OF DEATH? (i.e., extended family, siblings, friends, clergy)______________________________

WAS BABY BAPTIZED?________________

BLESSED? ________________

PHOTOGRAPHS TAKEN? YES__________ NO__________

GIVEN TO PARENTS? YES__________ NO__________

WHO SPOKE WITH FAMILY ABOUT FUNERAL ARRANGEMENTS?____________________

WHAT WERE THE ARRANGEMENTS?______________________________

WHO SPOKE WITH FAMILY ABOUT AUTOPSY?______________________________

WHAT WAS THE DECISION?______________________________

PARENTS' QUESTIONS: (i.e., is my baby suffering; have other parents held their baby; how will brother or sister react; what caused my baby's problem, etc.)______________________________

____

ANSWERS GIVEN:______________________________

____

PROBLEMS ENCOUNTERED BY FAMILY (i.e., parents had great difficulty being in room, but wanted to, parents could not contact significant other persons, i.e., minister, grandparents; disagreements by family about autopsy/funeral arrangements; marital discord etc.)____________

____

PROBLEMS ENCOUNTERED BY STAFF (i.e., could not reach family; difficulties with transfer; use of room):______________________________

____

____

Appendix 7–2

Neonatal Death Follow-up

BABY'S NAME:____________________SEX____BIRTHDATE:________________

PARENT'S NAME:________________________GESTATIONAL AGE:__________

_______________________________________BIRTHWEIGHT:_____________

DIAGNOSIS:____________________________HOSPITAL #:______________

_______________________________________ADMITTED:________________

EXPIRED:________________

SUPPORT DISCONTINUED: Y__N_

	AT TIME OF DEATH	CURRENT
ADDRESS		
HOME TELEPHONE #		
WORK TELEPHONE #		
NEAREST RELATIVE TELEPHONE #		

RELIGION: ________________________________

INSURANCE: ________________________________

PHYSICIANS:

OBSTETRICIAN ________________________________

PEDIATRICIAN ________________________________

NEONATOLOGIST ________________________________

SOCIAL WORKER/FCC ________________________________

MOTHER'S AGE _____ GRAVIDA _____ PARA ____ SAB ____ TAB ____ LC___

FATHER'S AGE _____ SIBLING'S AGES________________________________

	DATE REPORT RECEIVED	DATE REPORTED TO FAMILY	REPORTED BY WHOM	REPORTED TO REF. PHYSC.
AUTOPSY REPORT:				
PROVISIONAL	________	________	________	________
FINAL	________	________	________	________
NO AUTOPSY	________	________	________	________

COMMENTS:

	DONE (Specify in person/phone)	DATE
3 MONTH SOCIAL WORKER/FCC FOLLOW-UP	____	____
9 MONTH SOCIAL WORKER/FCC FOLLOW-UP (OPTIONAL)	____	____

COMMENTS:

III

Symbolic Interactions with Dying and Bereaved Children

In recent years heightened prominence has been given to the significance of noncognitive modes of communication and to the therapeutic value of symbolic interactions. Caregivers have long recognized the importance of what has lately been called "body language"—expressions of attitude and affect through posture, gestures, clothing, and the like. By extension, the potential of art, music, crafts, poetry, play, and other modalities has increasingly been appreciated as vehicles for communication and for constructive intervention. Similarly, the role of animals or pets has been seen as quite special in providing comfort and support, especially in long-term situations. Based on these realizations, therapists have learned to apply media and related resources to patients of all sorts with good results. Undoubtedly, such resources are of unique consequence for those who do not possess well-developed cognitive and/or interactive skills, such as young children, the retarded, and some among the elderly.

In Part III, we address symbolic interactions especially as they apply to chronically ill, dying, and bereaved children. Dying, death, and bereavement touch human beings to the core, whether they are the protagonists or are coping in some other way. These events resonate with the fundamental heartstrings of our own mortality and bring forth unexpected feelings. Often what emerges exceeds our cognitive grasp and is difficult to articulate. For these reasons, symbolic interactions are an essential consideration in chronic and terminal illness and in bereavement.

Both Barbara Schmitt and Molly Guzzino, on the one hand, and JoAnn Zimmerman, on the other, give witness in their work and writings to these lessons. Schmitt and Guzzino are professionally trained in this area, while Zimmerman is self-taught. Yet, their chapters speak in unison on all of the key points. Both proclaim that children feel deeply the events and the emotional climates within and around them; that, even so, they may not always know or be able to say what they feel; that, in particular, children may sense anxiety or pain in concerned adults and family members, and may act to control or suppress overt communications so as to "protect" these others from added burdens; that symbolic interactions may open new windows for identifying and ameliorating such underlying or hidden feelings; that there are a variety of modalities which might be selected for such interactions and a multiplicity of levels at which they function; and that therapeutic intervention as simple as a bear hug or as easy as a drawing can do much to restore or increase quality of life in vulnerable individuals. It should be noticed that while our focus in Part III is on symbolic interactions with children, we do not thereby neglect or dismiss their import for and use with parents or other adults.

One final note: these two chapters have been marked off here from those in Parts I and II—on caring for ill children prior to death—and from those in Part IV—on support for survivors. Quite clearly they belong together, but it is equally evident from the chapters themselves that symbolic interactions and expressive therapy have applications throughout the living-dying-grieving spectrum. In our judgment, these two chapters are particularly appropriate as a bridge between the first two and last sections of this book. More importantly, their presence here is a kind of testimony to the fundamental continuity of hospice principles both for pre- and post-death care and for children and adults. In each case, services are offered to the living and the goal is to heighten quality of life as much as possible in the present moment.

8

Expressive Therapy with Children in Crisis: A New Avenue of Communication

Barbara Bouton Schmitt and Molly Hardy Guzzino

Children confronting death, whether it is their own or that of a family member, are children in crisis. They have many questions, thoughts, and feelings which, when adequately addressed, enable them to cope better with death. Though caregivers may effectively address these needs in a variety of ways, the use of expressive therapy has been found to be of particular value in such crisis situations. Expressive therapy serves as a vehicle through which these children can communicate their needs, pose their questions, and express their thoughts and feelings.

It is the purpose of this chapter to introduce expressive therapy and, in particular, art therapy,[1] to the reader, explaining its premises and general application. Art therapy will then be discussed in terms of its application to terminally ill and grieving children.[2] Case examples are included.

[1]The authors recognize the contributions of all forms of expressive therapy. This discussion, however, will focus on the therapeutic use of art, as that is the primary expressive modality utilized in their work. In some contexts, expressive therapists are known as child life or child development specialists.

[2]For the purposes of this chapter, the grieving child is identified as one who is anticipating loss as well as one who has experienced loss.

Introduction to Expressive Therapy

Expressive therapy incorporates nonverbal (creative art) and verbal (psychotherapy) communication. Its use provides outlets to the panorama of thoughts and emotions experienced—for the purposes of this chapter—in a crisis situation. Expressive therapy exists in various forms: art, music, dance/movement, poetry, prose, puppetry, and play. Each of these modes of self-expression offers a new means of communicating thoughts and feelings.

A basic premise of all expressive therapy is that the created product mirrors inner feelings. The creation is an extension of oneself and serves as a concrete representation of one's inner world. Expressive therapy, then, allows the communication in alternate form of that which may be difficult or impossible to put into words.

An externalization of strong emotions frequently occurs as one creates a painting, a melody, or a dance. When these expressions are combined with more traditional modes of verbal therapy, personal attitudes, ideas, and feelings about oneself and one's environment may be explored.

The Therapeutic Art Process

Media

Art therapy involves the use of a wide variety of media, each of which lends itself to a different type of creation. An expression of the emotional state "depression" in clay, for example, would be rendered in an entirely different manner than if paint were utilized and would likely produce different responses by its creator. The art therapist considers such media properties and variables, and encourages use of those that will best facilitate a particular child's expression (Kagin & Lusebring, 1978). A child confined to a hospital room can experience a sense of freedom and independence if provided paint and large sheets of paper. An angry child can experience a great sense of release and revenge if given clay to prod, pound, or throw. Children with poor self-concepts can feel better about themselves if provided a medium over which they have control and can master, resulting in products that are pleasing to them. Conversely, introducing a medium that is difficult to control to children who already feel things are "out of control" will only further frustrate and agitate them.

Levels of Expression

A child may use a particular medium in any number of ways. There are various levels on which media may be explored and experienced, each of which serves a different purpose for the child (Kagin & Lusebring, 1978).

On one level, for example, a lump of clay might be thrown or beaten. The child's action upon the medium occurs through his or her movement which provides a release of energy. Such release can be especially therapeutic for the angry child, as the clay serves as the vehicle through which angry feelings may be expressed.

On another level, the child may use the clay to create a form. The child's action upon the clay becomes more controlled. As form is given to the clay, it is given also to the child's inner feelings.

On still another level, the child may name the clay form. The child has now given cognitive meaning to the image which may be further understood as a story is created about it.

These levels are important in developing a therapeutic design. The art therapist may provide media and activity that facilitate expression on a particular level to best meet a child's needs. This structuring of the therapeutic art process enables children to express their inner worlds, release their feelings, and derive meaning and growth from them.

Art Therapy with Children

Children are "natural" artists and can express themselves with few inhibitions. A child's art is an extension of his or her world. The images produced may reflect the child, his or her perceptions of position within the environment, and areas of question, concern, conflict, or need (Lowenfeld & Brittain, 1975).

The child may be unable to talk about these feelings as he or she may lack the conceptual development or verbal skills necessary to do so. A child's unwillingness to talk about such feelings may be the result of fears or having learned that such expression is unacceptable.

The child's art communicates what words cannot. The art therapist is provided with a concrete picture of the child's inner state. Then, by talking with the child about the art work, the therapist assists in bringing greater understanding and integration to the experience.

Understanding the Created Expression

Understanding the images produced by children is of crucial importance in determining areas of normalcy, need, and appropriate therapeutic intervention. The therapist must first be familiar with developmental levels of artistic expression.

As children mature in cognitive development, they develop patterns of artistic expression (Lowenfeld & Brittain, 1975). Toddlers express themselves in increasingly complex scribbles which become more refined as manual dexterity and fine motor control are developed. Children of three-and-a-half to four years of age begin to create form, producing drawings of greater complexity. As children mature, their art work becomes more realistic, logical, and sophisticated. An awareness of a child's graphic development helps the therapist to recognize regressive tendencies (which are common in the art work of children in crisis) and prevents the therapist from misinterpreting developmentally-related data.

Further, each object and form should be identified by the child. Persons represented should be named and their relationship to the child explained. Obvious omissions are significant. Has the terminally ill boy excluded himself from his "family portrait"? In a terminally ill girl's drawing of herself, are body parts missing or represented in an unusual manner? Does a grieving boy represent himself in a "groundless" environment?

Children's feelings are often released as they talk about their creations. The request to "tell a story about your drawing" allows a child to project himself or herself into the art work (Oaklander, 1978). A child may be able to "become" one of the forms in the expression and speak for that form, as did Gina, a 13-year-old bereaved child whose two-year-old sister had recently died. Gina drew a large, dark blue and purple pond bordered by a lone tree in the distance on a hill. When requested by the therapist to "become" the pond and speak for it, Gina replied, "I am a blob." She continued, "I am happy when people, fish, and birds swim in me. . . . I am angry when people throw garbage into me." A child can also express inner feelings by describing how a picture and its story relate to a present situation. Children's emotional responses to their creations and their decisions about what to do with their art work provide additional information for the therapist.

There is, at present, research that attempts to provide a psychological "picture" of children based on their drawings or paintings (Burns & Kaufman, 1972; Koppitz, 1968). The presence of "heavy clouds" in a drawing, for example, is believed to indicate environmental stress or pressure. Such research can be most valuable to the art therapist when placed within the context of the child's experience and his or her perceptions of that experience. However, interpretation of the child's work must come primarily from the child. The therapist must avoid personal projections which may lead to inaccurate conclusions. Stereotypical interpretations are not employed by the serious art therapist whose desire is to enter into the world of the individual child. Collection of a series of the child's art products, which are executed with a variety of media, is helpful to both therapist and child. The therapist is thus provided with a rich sample to aid in understanding the child, and the child is able to further develop his or her own creativity.

Environment

In work with terminally ill and grieving children, art therapy sessions usually occur within the home or hospital. Each environment presents the therapist with unique and often challenging factors that are inherent to a particular location.

Home

Though the child at home, whether terminally ill or grieved, is in a familiar and secure environment, the home is generally not conducive to free expression. Activities and behaviors which are acceptable during art therapy sessions may not be permissible in the home. Space sometimes presents a problem, as few homes have areas that allow dribbled paint or clay throwing. Disruptions are common and may lead the child to focus attention on other activities. When in the home, we have found it helpful to request a quiet space in which to work with the child where disruptions are unlikely. Sessions outdoors, which provide freedom of space, often facilitate greater participation on the part of the child.

In spite of these and other obstacles, productive art therapy sessions are possible in the home environment. Of particular value to the art therapist working with the child at home is the opportunity to observe family interactions and to learn about the child's environment.

Hospital

Most hospitalized children welcome the opportunity to express themselves through art. Art therapy sessions provide a period of "normalcy" for the terminally ill child who faces frequent examinations, tests, and treatments. Sessions may occur in children's rooms, at their bedsides, or in the hospital's playroom. Disruptions are much more frequent in the hospital than in the home environment. Space and opportunities for free expression may be limited.

Group art therapy, by providing an opportunity for terminally ill children to communicate and socialize, may decrease symptoms of withdrawal and feelings of isolation. Additionally, such groups help children to learn about and understand their disease, as well as to express their feelings about it (Bluebond-Langner, 1978). Further, communication and understanding are enhanced when family members participate with the child in art therapy sessions.

Children receive recognition and reinforcement when their creations are displayed in their rooms and throughout the hospital. Their self-esteem and self-worth are enhanced when their achievements are noticed.

Art expressions of particular significance to the child's care should be recorded and related to the medical staff. Such information is valuable to staff who are concerned with the wholistic care of the terminally ill child (Furth, 1981).

The Terminally Ill Child

Terminally ill children can exhibit a multitude of psychological responses to illness which require attention. Such responses, which are varied and may fluctuate widely, include acting out, depression, guilt, fear, and withdrawal (Blom, 1958). These responses are, to a great degree, the result of the children's grief over their losses of well-being, mobility, control, physical integrity, independence, and, inevitably, loss of life. Art therapy or other forms of expressive therapy are an effective means of therapeutic intervention for the terminally ill child who is experiencing these thoughts and feelings. Their use promotes a greater sense of self-control, independence, and self-esteem for children whose illness and hospitalization result in their dependence upon others.

A terminally ill child often expends emotional energy in a dysfunctional or unproductive manner during illness. Such energy, when appropriately channeled through art and other forms of expressive therapy, can positively affect the child's ability to cope with illness.

Acting out, a common response of seriously ill children, may be exhibited in disruptive, impulsive, or demanding behaviors. Frustrations caused by illness and repeated hospitalizations may be translated into anger and rebellion (Plank, 1962). Children may not be afforded means of discharging energy and emotion through movement and activity, particularly if they are restricted to bed. Such restriction may heighten feelings of helplessness and lead to increased hostility, struggle, and overactivity (Blumberg, 1978).

The art therapist can channel acting-out behaviors into more appropriate behaviors by providing a means of discharging energy through movement. "Scribble chases" on mural paper or manipulation of clay by slapping, throwing, or pounding are excellent means of channeling such behaviors and they provide release of tension and energy. Dramatic play with puppets, and drawn or sculpted figures, allows a child to express feelings of helplessness and rebellion.

Children need to express their conflicts and concerns, perhaps repeatedly in physical and verbal ways—though such behaviors often concern caregivers, they generally represent a healthy response to illness (McCollum, 1981). If these children are permitted and encouraged to confront the powerful feelings that accompany their illness, they can experience, practice, and acquire alternative coping behaviors.

Fears are another common response of terminally ill children, the greatest of which are those of pain, abandonment, isolation, and the unknown. These fears must be acknowledged, accepted, and respected by the therapist. Children may be encouraged to portray particular likes and dislikes of their present environment. Depicting a fear-producing object or procedure helps the child to feel in control of his or her fears and thus to become better able to cope with the illness. The therapist and child can work on alternative coping skills and realistic expectations. Misconceptions may also be identified and corrected.

Feelings of depression in terminally ill children may result from the physical pain of illness and treatment procedures, as well as from the many losses that are caused by the illness. Such reactions are also likely to occur in children who believe that illness is a punishment for their misbehavior (McCollum, 1981). Depression is exhibited in the child's flattened affect, activity, perception, and cognition. The expressions of depressed children often center on negative images and experiences (Blumberg, 1978). The art therapist emphasizes with such a child significant areas of the child's life that promote a positive self-image. Caregivers may participate in art therapy sessions with their children. This often promotes greater understanding, communication, and closeness, and it may combat symptoms of depression.

Group sessions are especially valuable for depressed children, as they may reduce feelings of isolation. When children participate in a group painting of the hospital or of a special place where they can live, they begin to share themselves with others.

Terminally ill children may withdraw by internalizing their feelings, increasing their isolation, and decreasing communication. Lack of spontaneity, apathy, and despair may result as a child confronts his or her helplessness to change the situation. The terminally ill child who responds in this way desperately needs the support, care, and comfort of caregivers. Unfortunately, such behavior often discourages caregivers, who may decrease or limit their contact with the child (Blumberg, 1978).

Low self-esteem and poor body image are common feelings of withdrawn children. These may be addressed by suggesting body tracings, self-portraits, or drawings of "how others see me." A child's self-esteem and sense of control will increase if the child is allowed to decorate his or her room.

Critically ill children benefit from art therapy even though they are unable to participate actively themselves. The therapist can create an environment of peace and comfort by drawing beaches, mountains, sunsets, home, or other images that are meaningful to the child.

The art work of terminally ill children has been found to share common features and to follow particular trends. In her work with the terminally ill, Susan Bach (1966) found that patients' art work changed as their illnesses progressed. Bach's empirical research showed that objects and forms tend to move toward the upper left quadrant of a page as a patient's death approached.

An awareness of disease progression, sometimes before its discovery by the medical staff, has been exhibited in the figure drawings of the seriously ill. An unusual treatment of a particular body area, or a significant omission, has corresponded to new areas of disease (Bach, 1966).

Additionally, pictures that depict extreme weather conditions have been noted frequently in the art work of terminally ill children. Clouds, heavy rain, or snow indicate feelings of anxiety, uncontrollable conditions, or feelings of being overwhelmed (Bach, 1966). These extreme weather conditions are often portrayed with a brightly shining sun nearby.

Color choices may also change during the course of an illness. The decreased use of bright colors (which are often associated with energy) may reflect the child's decreased physical stamina and emotional energy as his or her disease progresses (Bach, 1966). Grove (1978) exemplifies this in her short account of a terminally ill child's depictions of a ship—which became smaller and darker as his illness progressed.

The following case examples illustrate the value of art therapy for the terminally ill child.

Ann

Five-year-old Ann, diagnosed with neuroblastoma, Stage IV, drew a figure she labelled "The Devil" (see Figure 8.1) during an art therapy session. In describing the devil, Ann stated that he was bad and that he lived under the ground, that his pets were snakes, and that he came to get bad children. She also believed that "he steals people's souls," though she admitted that she did not understand what that meant. She was, however, afraid of him. To enable Ann to gain some control over this fearful image (which may have served as a personification of death), she was asked what she would like to say to him. In a whispered voice, she immediately replied, "You'd better leave me alone." The child was asked to repeat her message several times in an increasingly loud voice to enable the devil to hear her. Such repetition enabled Ann in the end to relay her message with great conviction and control. When she felt that the devil had received her message, Ann began a drawing with a much different theme. Ann left the session with an appearance of confidence and control.

John

John, a five-year-old child, was introduced to the art therapist eight months after his diagnosis of Wilms's Tumor, Stage IV. During their first session, John seemed shy and refused to draw. When he returned the following week, John presented the therapist with five drawings. One of

Figure 8.1 Ann's Drawing of the Devil

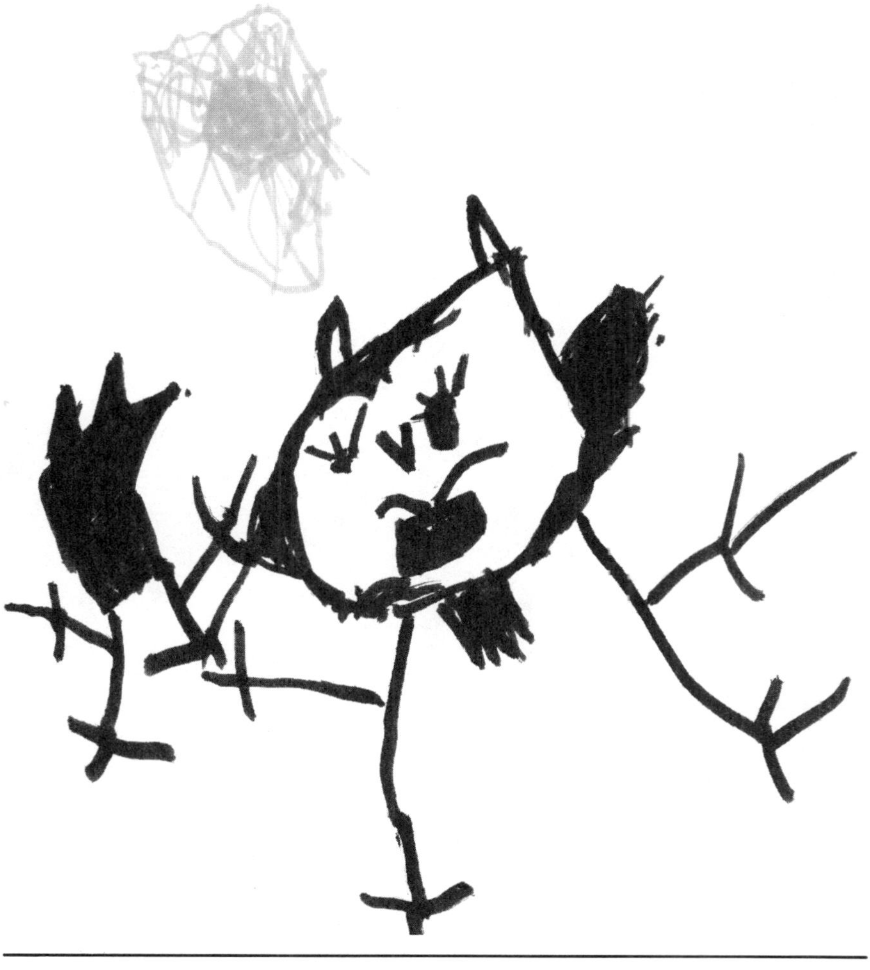

these is reproduced in Figure 8.2. He briefly explained that his drawing was of monsters who had baby monsters with tumors inside of them. Of the monsters, he said only that they were "sad," "bad," and "mean."

The monsters' tumors which John drew corresponded to his own disease process and suggested his identification with the disease and

Figure 8.2 John's Drawing of Monsters and their Tumors

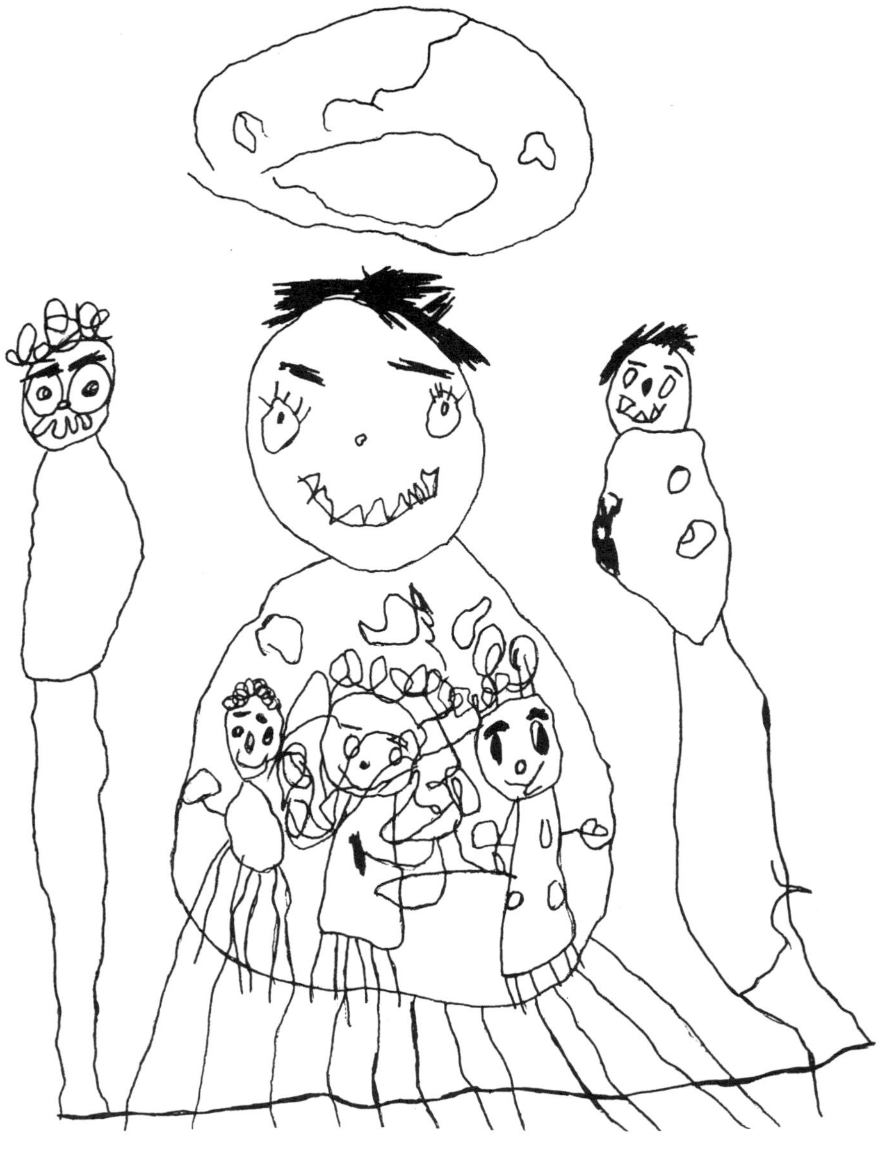

with a monster self-image. This drawing, and similar ones of this series, allowed John to relate his understanding that "bad" things were happening inside his body. Through these drawings, John was able to draw his feelings about his illness and to indicate the disease's progression inside his body. Such expression would have been most doubtful on a verbal level alone. John continued to participate in art therapy until his death five months later.

Jane

Jane, a ten-year-old child with multiple cardiac abnormalities, produced Figure 8.3 the day prior to her heart surgery. The emphasis on weather conditions (sun and rain) tends to indicate feelings of anxiety. Jane was physically unable to participate in active play and so spent much of her time alone. The roof-like shape of her house suggests an emphasis on fantasy in her life and may have been a compensation for her aloneness. The orientation of most elements of the drawing toward the left indicates downhill trends and exiting from life. Jane's upcoming surgery was apparently cause for much anxiety and feelings of being overwhelmed by forces outside her control. Jane's ability to draw these feelings provided an emotional release for her. She was assured of support and comfort from the therapist and her caregivers.

Billy and Carrie

Billy, age five, with a diagnosis of Wilms's Tumor, Stage IV, and Carrie, age five, with a diagnosis of cystic fibrosis, created the following story in response to Billy's drawing of "The Doctor and Skinny Boy."

> Skinny Boy is five years old and he has to have heart surgery and he keeps throwing up. He can't get up and he has to get a shot. He has to get it in his behind. Skinny Boy says, "Don't give me that shot. If you do, I'm going to punch you straight out of the hospital onto the street and let the car drive over you and let God take you."
>
> Then the doctor died. And Skinny Boy said, "Good grief!" Then Skinny could go home. Then he gave the doctor a shot and the doctor said, "Weeee—did that hurt!" Then the doctor left and he broke his collar bone. Then he had to go in the hospital and he had to have surgery and get a shot. The doctor said, "Give it to me, give it to me, but don't do it hard." He blinked his eyes and said, "Ouch."

In this example, the use of art and creative storytelling provided an outlet for these children's fears, frustrations, anger, and desire for re-

Figure 8.3. Jane's Drawing prior to Heart Surgery

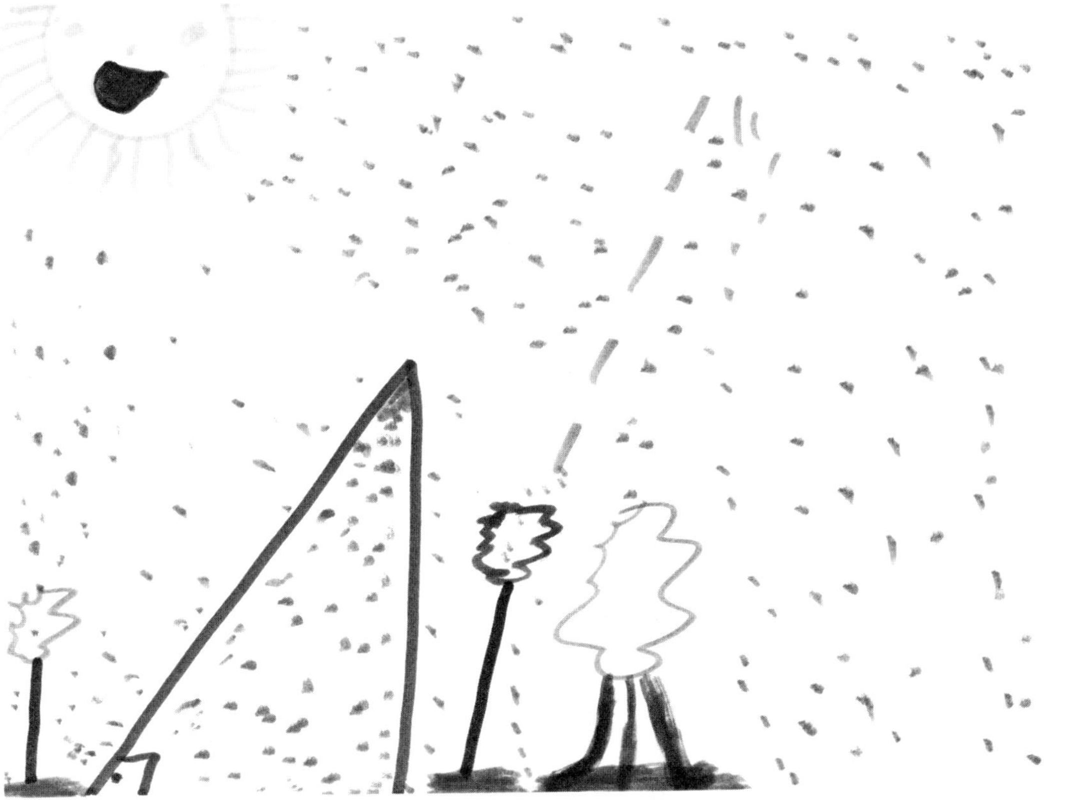

venge. Their powerful feelings were expressed in a safe and appropriate manner. They gained control and mastery through their identification with the hero created in Skinny Boy. Their references to death suggest an awareness, perhaps on an inner level, of the gravity of their illnesses.

The Grieving Child

The reactions of a child to the death of a significant person are determined, in part, by the child's developmental level, previous losses, the importance of his or her relationship to the deceased, and by observations made of others' responses to loss. Children's questions about death and its meaning or about their own roles in a changing situation are frequent. Fear of one's own death or that of another is a common theme of grieving children. Feelings of intense sadness, anger, and guilt, as well as damaging fantasies and misconceptions about death, are common. As with terminally ill children, grieving children may respond to loss by acting out, by becoming depressed, or by withdrawing (Jewett, 1982; Grollman, 1967).

For children anticipating the death of a family member, art therapy or other forms of expressive therapy help to prepare them for the loss. By providing experiences that encourage children to express questions and concerns, the therapist can assist them in their understanding. Fears and emotions can be addressed prior to the death, thereby assisting the child in a healthy resolution of his or her grief. This support enables children to gain control in a situation that may be perceived as uncontrollable.

Following a death, expressive therapy supports children through the grieving process. The therapeutic experiences help the child to place memories of the deceased into a realistic perspective.

As the child learns about a family member's terminal illness, a multitude of questions may arise. These questions may be expressed verbally or nonverbally either to the therapist or to family members. Parents are encouraged to be open and honest in their feelings and in their answers to children's questions (Grollman, 1976). It is particularly important that questions regarding God and religion be addressed by parents within the context of their own religious beliefs.

An eight-year-old child, who was being seen in art therapy prior to the death of one of her parents, wrote out a number of questions she wished to have her mother and father address. The questions sought to confirm her parents' love for her, which she doubted since much of their attention had been inevitably withdrawn from her. By writing the questions down and providing space for her parents to respond in writing, the child was able to gain emotional distance from the questions.

Other questions may be more concrete and directly related to the situation. Often these occur as the child is involved in the art process. A young child stated during one session, "My dad is on medicine all the time now, but it is making him sicker. He should stop taking it." It was necessary for the therapist to help the child understand that: (1) the disease, not the medicine, was making his father "sicker"; (2) the medicine took away some of his father's pain; and (3) if his father stopped taking the medicine, he would not get better. A related issue for this child was his belief that the doctors who had prescribed the medicine were responsible for his father's illness. The therapist, in this and similar situations, is able to alleviate the child's misconceptions and promote better understanding.

Another child was able to communicate a special need through a painting of her mother's hospital room. Though only the child, mother, and grandmother were depicted in the painting, she talked about the many people who were in the room when she visited. She was then able to relate her wish—and need—to visit alone with her parents. The child's father was alerted and the three were able to spend important time together prior to the mother's death.

The involvement of the art therapist seems to be particularly important to the terminally ill parent. The parent is assured that the child will be helped to cope with and resolve the loss in a healthy way. It seems that the parent is able to begin the process of "letting go," once assured that the child will be supported after his or her death.

Art therapy provided to the child anticipating loss also helps the child in "letting go." Art experiences that allow a review of the relationship with the dying family member and that encourage the child to imagine the dying family member and himself or herself in the future help the child to understand and integrate the experience. A child's drawing of past vacations with a dying parent, a painting of games previously played with a dying sibling, and drawings of a child's ideas about what occurs after death all facilitate the grieving process.

Art therapy also strengthens the grieving child. The therapist is perceived as one who is there for the child—one who may be more attentive than other family members are able to be. This affirms the child as a significant person and communicates that his or her questions and feelings are important. The child is assured of an objective, open, and caring person who will provide support through the death and afterward. This relationship is stable and consistent at a time when family relationships may not be. When death occurs, the therapist again may be able to respond to the child's needs when other family members, themselves grief stricken, cannot.

Fears of the grieving child are also apparent through the child's art work. Four- and five-year-old siblings of an older brother who had died drew and expressed fears that their brother was watching them and that he might choose to take them away. Dreams related to their fears were also depicted, which alerted the therapist and the parents to their needs for reassurance.

Anger toward the deceased or surviving family members is quite common (Jewett, 1982). People, animals, or other symbols and the child's action upon them, as well as what is said about them, provide a vent for otherwise unacceptable feelings. Such expression also provides an opportunity for the therapist to assure the child of the normalcy of such feelings. Five-year-old Laura was overtly angry following her father's death. She symbolically communicated her feelings by throwing stones at her house and by speaking of her intense anger through a stuffed lion.

Grieving children may misconstrue reality as they try to understand death. Children may experience feelings of guilt if they believe they are responsible for a death. "Magical" thinking is often apparent during art therapy sessions. One young child remembered that her deceased mother had become angry when she left marks on the wall with her hands. The child then began to press her hands all along the wall in a symbolic effort to bring her mother back to her, as well as to seek revenge on her "deserting" mother. The child and therapist discussed how good it might feel right then to hear her mother yell at her, yet how impossible that was. The finality of death was reiterated and the child was perhaps better able to understand that, regardless of her wishes, thoughts, and behaviors, her mother could not return.

Experiences that permit symbolic expression are generally less threatening to grieving children than experiences that confront the death. One child who was unable to talk about her mother's death was easily able to express her longing through her drawing of a "Mama" tree. She was further able to release her feelings in a nonthreatening way as she acted out a story about the drawing. Her tree, which "lived" in a park, was dug up, brought to her home, and planted in her back yard. It was "the best tree in the world," and she wanted no one else to have it.

The following case examples serve to illustrate the value of art therapy for the grieving child.

Kellie

Nine-year-old Kellie was referred to the art therapist two-and-a-half weeks prior to her mother's death in the hospital. At the time of the therapist's first visit, Kellie had not been told of the impending death. One of her drawings of that session, however, clearly indicates an awareness of the events occurring around her. Upon being invited to draw or paint, Kellie drew a large "cloud" (see Figure 8.4). As a story was imagined about the cloud, Kellie drew a person, rain, and provided

Figure 8.4. Kellie's Drawing of a Child Under a Cloud

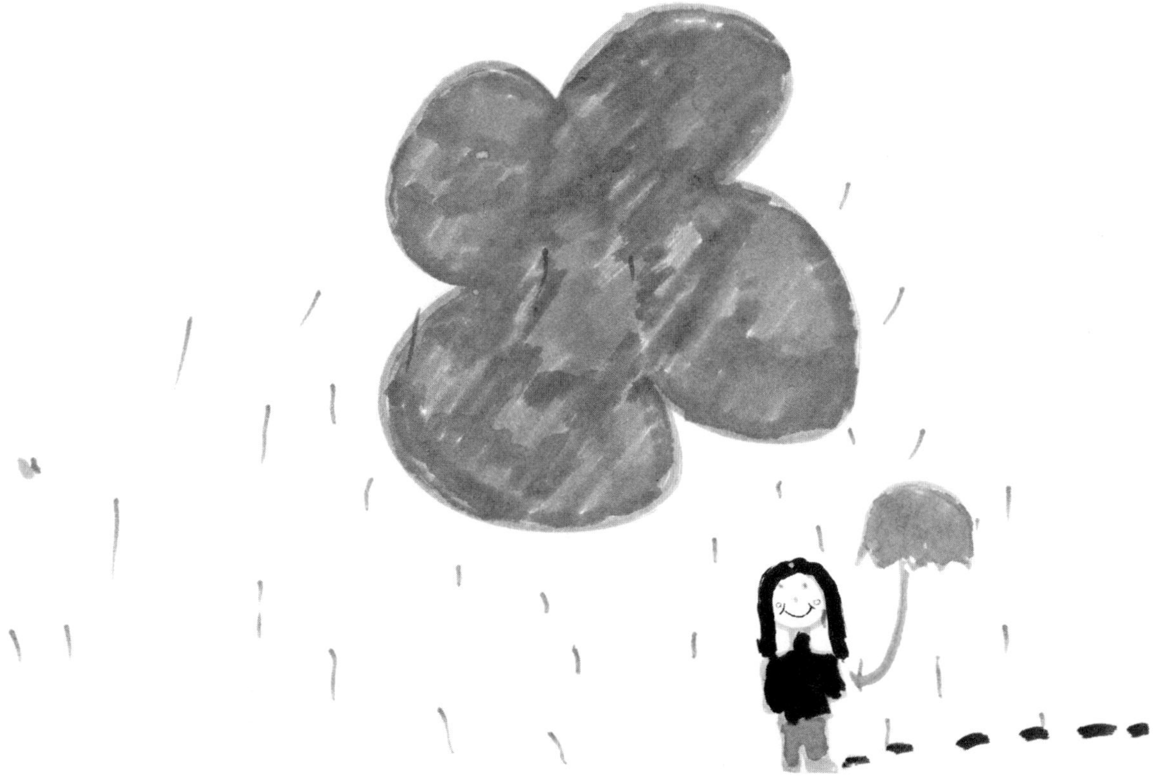

an umbrella for the figure. The clouds and rain suggest that Kellie was aware of the stress within her environment and that she was experiencing it. Though her figure is not protected from the rain by the umbrella, Kellie said that there was a "world" underneath the figure and that, being caught in the rain, "she would go home." Kellie's story suggests that, though there was great stress in her life, she felt supported by a world and could find relief at home. A painting "about being sad" (see Figure 8.5), produced in a subsequent session, provided an opportunity for Kellie to express and release her strong feelings. She first painted "a dead plant" which became erased by the lines and forms which covered it. "Snow" was included, which was sad because "it keeps Mom from coming home" (Kellie had still not been informed of her mother's approaching death). "Dead grass" was painted and words communicating her fear and dislike of "going to the dentist" and "surprise parties" (she recalled one where her mother had cried) were written. The resulting painting is a confusing jumble of lines and words that symbolically represent Kellie's inner confusion and the feelings she was experiencing.

After her mother's death, Kellie frequently chose to express herself in words. When asked to depict the feelings she experienced when talking about her mother, Kellie wrote, "sad and sometimes mad." In an effort to promote a better understanding and release of these feelings, the therapist asked Kellie to "show me how the mad and sad feels inside your body." Kellie immediately tensed her body, gritted her teeth, grimaced, and clenched her fists. Further exploration enabled Kellie to imagine telling her mother, "I am mad because you left me." During this period Kellie also frequently drew geometric forms—particularly squares—which served as indications of her desire to control and "hold in" her feelings. Figure 8.6 shows this most clearly. Kellie referred to her mother as "her," perhaps in an effort to protect herself. The box around her words also may have served a similar safeguarding purpose. Kellie was unable to say much about this drawing, though she did relate that she did not know what the question marks were about. The therapist assured Kellie that even though her mother had died, Kellie's love for her remained. Perhaps her questions involved her anger: How could I be so angry with someone I love so much? Or perhaps she wondered: How could my mother have left me when I loved her so? In any event, Kellie was able to express herself through a very powerful drawing.

Jessica

Jessica, a child of eight, utilized the therapeutic art process in a very different manner. A child who was desperately trying to understand the events leading to and following her mother's death, Jessica produced

Figure 8.5. Kellie's Painting "About Being Sad"

Figure 8.6. Kellie's Geometric Expression of her Feelings of Grief

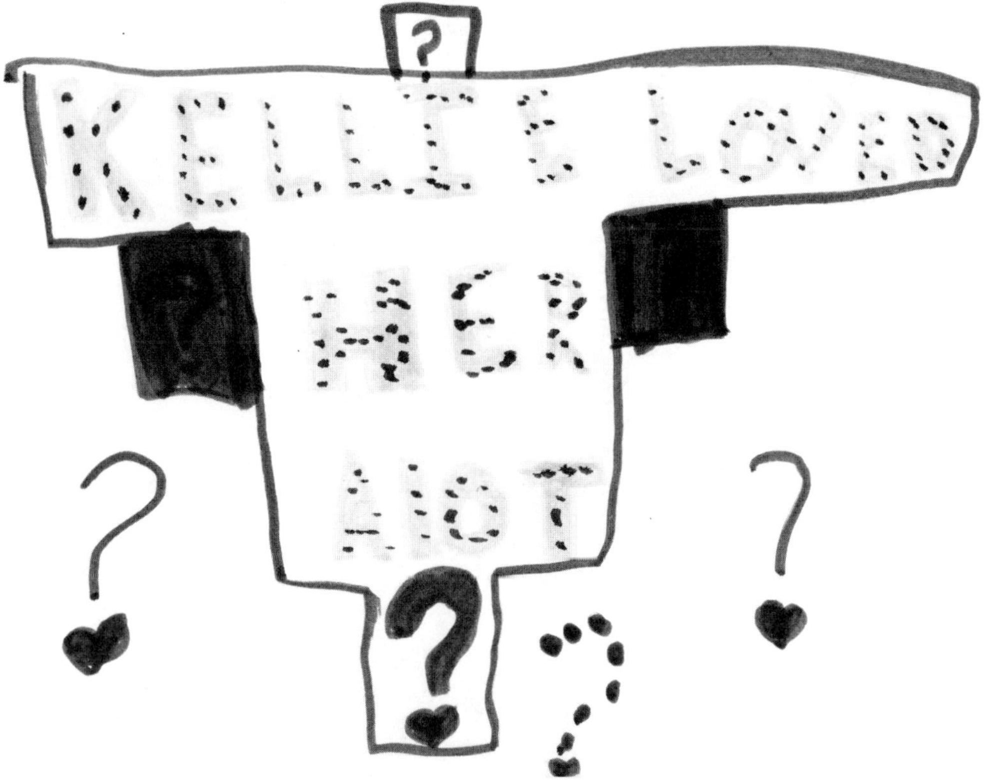

many drawings in an attempt to integrate her experience. Jessica is a very religious child, and many of her drawings were produced in an effort to concretize, and thus make understandable, the abstractions of her religious teaching. Approximately one week prior to her mother's death, Jessica produced a series of drawings about God, heaven, and the soul. These works, along with her descriptions and a drama she enacted, helped her prepare for the death. "This is what happens when you die," she told the therapist, as she lay down on the floor. "Then your soul leaves your body like this," she insisted, as she pointed to the body area she believed contained the soul. She drew a picture about heaven (based on a television show she had seen about out-of-body experiences) and continued, "This is what heaven is like. First, you go down a long tunnel and all your aunts and uncles who have died wave to you. At the end of the tunnel, there is a bright light, and then there is a castle where Jesus lives. . . ."

Figure 8.7 provided a great release for Jessica as she expressed "the hurt in my heart" when she thought about her mother's death. The picture contains a lot of movement and emotional energy and, like Kellie's "sad" drawing, appears quite confused. Jessica drew "the devil" at the bottom of this drawing, whom she blamed for her mother's approaching death and for her hurt feelings. The therapist was able to relay Jessica's ideas about God and the devil to her parents and her teacher, who helped her to understand better her feelings and religious teachings.

A later drawing (see Figure 8.8), completed a few days before her mother's death at home, helped Jessica to express some of her painful emotions. The therapist asked Jessica to draw a picture about being sad, to which she responded, "Nothing." Then she questioned, "The saddest thing in my life?" and drew Figure 8.8. As she finished the drawing, Jessica said, "It's my mom's grave," and then "I'm getting ready to cry." The therapist held and comforted Jessica as she began to experience the pain of her loss.

Following her mother's death, Jessica began to write a book about her mother. Her first pages, which were illustrated with her paintings, show her attempts to understand the loss. (Note her use of both present and past tense in reference to her mother.)

> My mom was a great mom. She loved everybody. My mom had cancer. Cancer is a very terrible disease. So when my mom was 38, she died. . . . My mom was pretty. She is nice to . . . [sic]. I loved my mom. . . . Some nights my mother reads a story in the Bible.

Subsequent art therapy sessions enabled Jessica to confront and release her feelings of grief through more symbolic means. Her mother

Figure 8.7. Jessica's Expression of "The Hurt in My Heart"

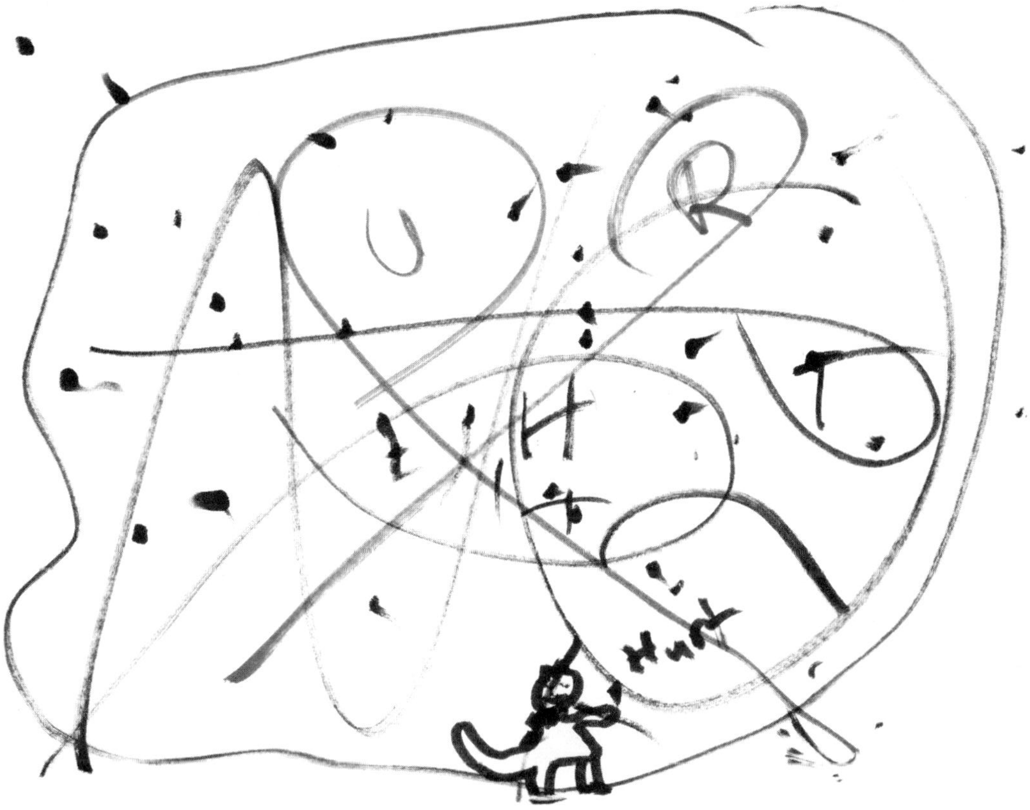

Figure 8.8. Jessica's Drawing of "The Saddest Thing in My Life"

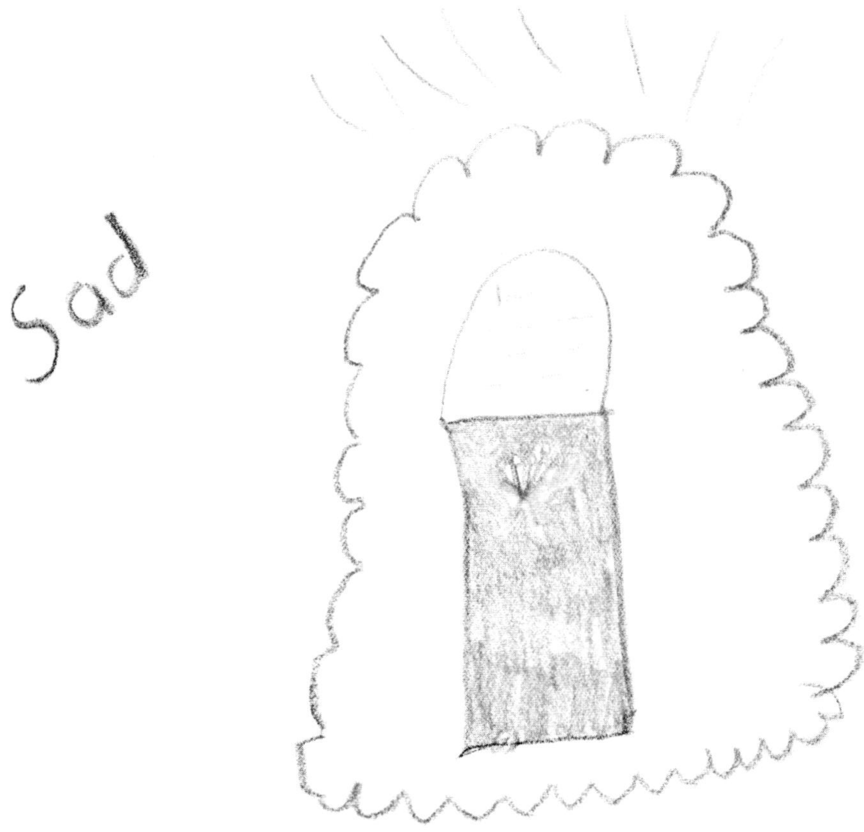

was portrayed in various images, and Jessica was able to express her grief through stories she created about those images.

Conclusion

The value of expressive therapy in general and art therapy in particular in caring for the terminally ill and grieving child lies in their ability to provide an alternate means of communication and expression for those children. Such therapy recognizes these children's needs as unique and important. It serves to strengthen the child and strives to promote the child's integrity and growth. Whether the child is confronted with his or her own terminal illness or that of a family member, he or she has particular concerns that need to be communicated and that deserve attention. By providing means through which children can share themselves with caregivers, expressive therapy improves the child's ability to cope and deal with crisis. By facilitating and encouraging children to express themselves and their worlds in their own unique ways, expressive therapy enhances a child's quality of life.

References

Bach, Susan R. von, "Spontanes Malen Schwerkranker Patienten," *Acta Psychosomatica* (Basle), 1966.

Blom, G. E., "The Reactions of Hospitalized Children to Illness," *Pediatrics*, 1958, *22*, 590–600.

Bluebond-Langner, M., *The Private Worlds of Dying Children*. Princeton, NJ: Princeton University Press, 1978.

Blumberg, M. L., "Depression in Children on a General Pediatric Service," *American Journal of Psychotherapy*, 1978, *32*, 20–32.

Burns, R. C., & Kaufman, S. H., *Actions, Styles and Symbols in Kinetic Family Drawings (K-F-D): An Interpretative Manual*. New York: Brunner/Mazel, 1972.

Furth, G. M., "The Use of Drawings Made at Significant Times in One's Life," in E. Kübler-Ross, *Living with Death and Dying*. New York: Macmillan, 1981.

Grollman, E. A. (Ed.), *Explaining Death to Children*. Boston: Beacon, 1967.

Grollman, E. A., *Talking About Death: A Dialogue Between Parent and Child* (2nd ed.). Boston: Beacon, 1976.

Grove, S. "I Am a Yellow Ship," *American Journal of Nursing*, 1978, *78*, 414.

Jewett, C. L., *Helping Children Cope with Separation and Loss*. Harvard, MA: Harvard Common Press, 1982.

Kagin, S., & Lusebring, V., "The Expressive Therapies Continuum," *Journal of Art Psychotherapy*, 1978, *5*, 171–180.

Koppitz, E. M., *Psychological Evaluation of Children's Human Figure Drawings*. New York: Grune & Stratton, 1968.

Lowenfeld, V., & Brittain, W. L., *Creative and Mental Growth*. New York: Macmillan, 1975.

McCollum, A. T., *The Chronically Ill Child: A Guide for Parents and Professionals*. New Haven, CT: Yale University Press, 1981.

Oaklander, V., *Windows to Our Children: A Gestalt Therapy Approach to Children and Adolescents*. Moab, UT: Real People Press, 1978.

Plank, E., *Working with Children in Hospitals*. Cleveland: The Press of Western Reserve University, 1962.

9

Amanda the Panda

JoAnn Zimmerman

Introduction

Amanda the Panda is a seven-foot costumed character in the form of a panda who wears a heart around her neck. Pandas are native to the bamboo forests of the Himalayan region, and have been much in the news in recent years as symbols of good will exchanges between the Chinese government and the government of the United States. Most people know pandas as large black-and-white creatures, and it is commonly assumed that they are a kind of bear. However, in fact, pandas are probably more closely related to the racoon family. But Amanda is not concerned with her own genetic heritage, for she calls herself "the Bear with a Heart." Her mission is to be a special friend to children with life-threatening illnesses, and her activities have recently expanded to encompass the operation of unusual weekend camps for siblings in their grief after the death of a brother or sister. I see these interactions with dying and bereaved children as a ministry to young people in the state of Iowa. The purpose of this chapter is to describe the work of Amanda the Panda, to identify its underlying principles, and to indicate—at least by example—how others might undertake similar activities in their own local communities.

Bear Hugs for the Dying Child

When I first created Amanda, I envisioned her to be a caring presence in the community. I thought she would go into the schools on the primary grade level and teach a unit on caring—how do we show others we care for them, especially if they are different than we are? Perhaps a child has one arm or is mentally retarded—how do we show we really care? Do we laugh at them, make fun of them, ignore them? Do we include them in our play? Unfortunately, some children on our playgrounds can be cruel and very insensitive. Sometimes when sick children wear wigs to school, other children may call them names or pull their wigs off. My hope was to use Amanda to help sensitize children to the needs of others. Also, Amanda would be a tool for teaching such things as bus safety, drug safety, pride in the neighborhood, pride in oneself. There was no limit to what Amanda could teach young children.

But all of that changed when I met and fell deeply in love with a little boy named Chris. From that moment on I knew Amanda's real mission would be to dying children. Chris was seven years old and had an inoperable brain tumor. He was referred to me by a local hospice program in January 1981. The hospice staff called and asked if I would visit this very special little boy. I said yes. When I arrived at his home, I found a boy who was very polite and incredibly bright. He had been home from the hospital barely 24 hours. In fact, he was still in his pajamas and robe. Chris was very thin and his tumor had caused partial paralysis on one side of his body, immobilizing both an arm and a leg. His hair was now beginning to grow back. His body was obviously failing but his spirit was as vibrant as any child his age. He was a very normal seven-year-old who happened to have cancer.

Amanda was a very significant "person" in Chris' life. She saw him a total of 40 times before he died. He would say to her: "You're my pal, Amanda, forever and for always." And she would reply: "That's right, Chris, forever and for always you will live in my heart." This little exchange was later to become their password.

Amanda is there to be a friend to a child at a time when other children don't come around to play much anymore. When adults receive the diagnosis of cancer, they find out rather quickly who their real friends are—which ones will fall by the wayside and which ones will stick by them. Children experience the same thing but understand it even less. Other children don't want to come and play anymore for various reasons:

(1) they—or their parents—are afraid they will "catch" cancer; (2) they are afraid their hair will fall out, too; (3) it's no fun to go to Chris' house anymore because he's "throwing up" or too weak to play, and so on. For reasons such as these children don't come to play anymore.

Life becomes very lonely for children who are sick. One day blends into the next and nothing much different happens. Then one day a giant panda named Amanda hears about them and because they have cancer and because their hair has fallen out and because they are so lonely, she travels throughout the state of Iowa to their house, goes up to their door, and rings the doorbell. You can imagine their delight when the door opens and a seven-foot Panda is there with gifts for them and for their brothers and sisters!

Amanda is there to do what the child wants to do. I try to listen carefully in order to hear what the child is really saying, and then I respond accordingly. I have no preplanned agenda as I travel to their home. If a child wants to swing, we swing. If a child wants to read a story, I hold them on my lap and we read a story. If a child wants to walk around the block, we walk around the block (and *that's* an interesting sight!). And if a child wants to talk about his or her dying, Amanda talks about dying. But it's always at the child's initiative. I don't initiate anything. I simply listen to what the child says and respond accordingly.

I am there simply to lift the child's spirits, to give lots of bear hugs, and to let the child be a child again. As the mother of a nine-year-old girl with a brain tumor put it:

> Mindy has had to grow up so fast because she's facing things that would give problems to most adults. But somewhere in the process of being with Amanda, she became a child again. I've never seen her so thrilled—even with family members—as she is when she gets a call or visit from Amanda.
>
> When kids learn to look forward to something more than a blood test or spinal tap, it's just beautiful, and Amanda provides that for Mindy. Amanda does more for her than a dose of medicine ever could. (See Figure 9.1.)

Amanda is not an authority symbol. She is not a parent or doctor or nurse. Nothing she does causes pain or discomfort. She doesn't give shots or medicines that make the child ill. She doesn't give spinal taps or bone marrows. She is simply there to give generous amounts of bear hugs. She is totally accepting of the child and will remain faithful till the end. The children know that they can call Amanda anytime they need her and she will be there. They also know that they can talk to her about their dying and she will take their concerns seriously and will always be honest with them.

Figure 9.1. Amanda and Mindy Sharing a Visit Together

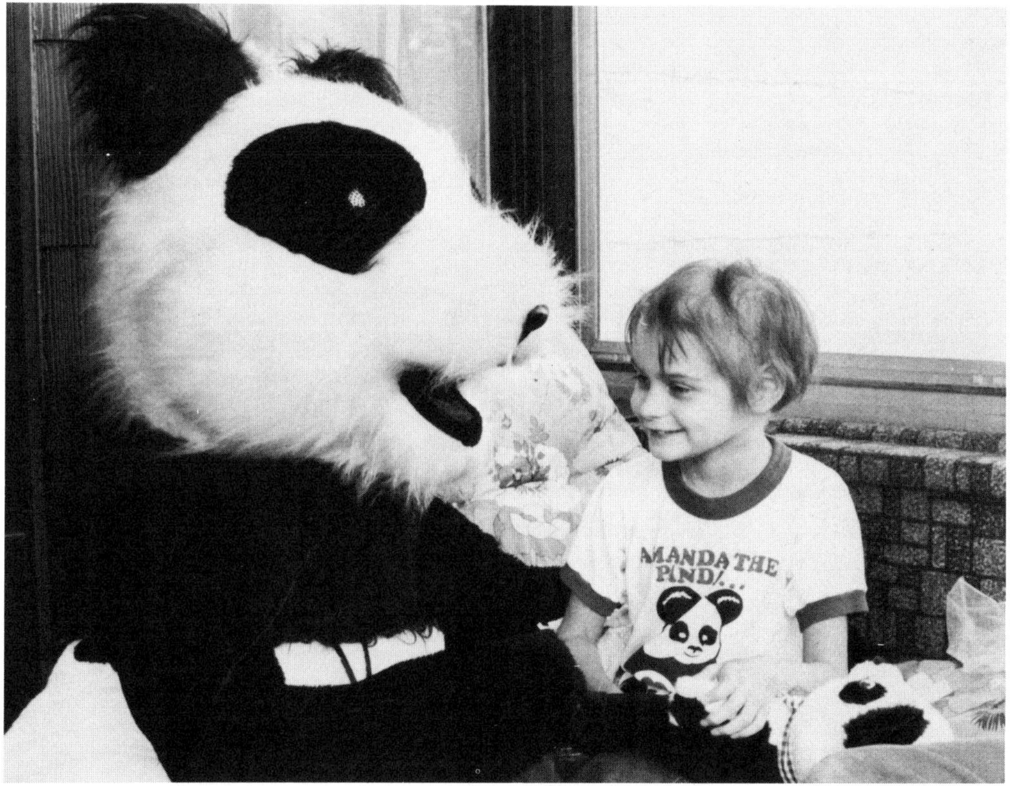

Photograph by Peter J. Dubec. Used by Permission of Photographer and *The Catholic Mirror*.

Sometimes when a child begins to talk about dying, parents or other adults will not let them continue. They will indicate either verbally or by nonverbal body language that it is not okay for the child to talk about his or her dying. In my experience I have found that if children are allowed to talk about their dying, they are not afraid. They only become afraid when they begin to talk about it and discover that it is not an acceptable topic. Adults will sometimes say to a child: "We don't want to hear any more talk like that," or, "Don't say that, you're not going to die." Or, they will physically get up and leave the child's room when he or she begins to talk of dying. It is at this point that the child discovers that it's not okay to talk about dying. The child then concludes that death must be something bad or scary. If children are allowed to talk about their fears and their feelings in an atmosphere of acceptance and honesty, then they are at peace with dying. They are not afraid. The following conversation took place between a little girl and her dad. Sara was seven years old and had leukemia. (See Figure 9.2.)

Sara:	"If I have relapse after relapse, will I die?"
Her dad:	"Yes."
Sara:	"I don't want to die."
Her dad:	"We don't want you to die, either."
Sara	*(after much thought):* "But I have Good News and Bad News. The Good News is that I will go to Heaven to be with God and Jesus, Grandpa Van and Ritchie. The Bad News is that I will have to die to get there."

As parents, we spend an awful lot of time and energy preparing our children for life. How much time do we spend preparing them to die? Is not death a part of life?

If we listen carefully to children, we will hear them talk about dying. Their language is not as concrete as ours. It is more often than not symbolic language. One day Chris was speaking to me of dying. He said: "I'm going to go on a trip, Amanda. And I want you to go with me." "Where are we going, Chris?" "We are going to go on an airplane ride. We are going to go way, high above the clouds, and the clouds are going to be soft and pillowy. And it's going to really be neat."

My role in working with dying children is simply to listen and be present. I don't feel I have to have all the answers. It is not a teacher-pupil relationship. If it were, the child would be the teacher, and I the student. It is a ministry of presence, of support, and of listening with the heart. It is also very joyful. One of the greatest fallacies among outsiders about working with dying persons is that this work is morbid and depressing

Figure 9.2. Amanda Giving Sarah a Bear Hug

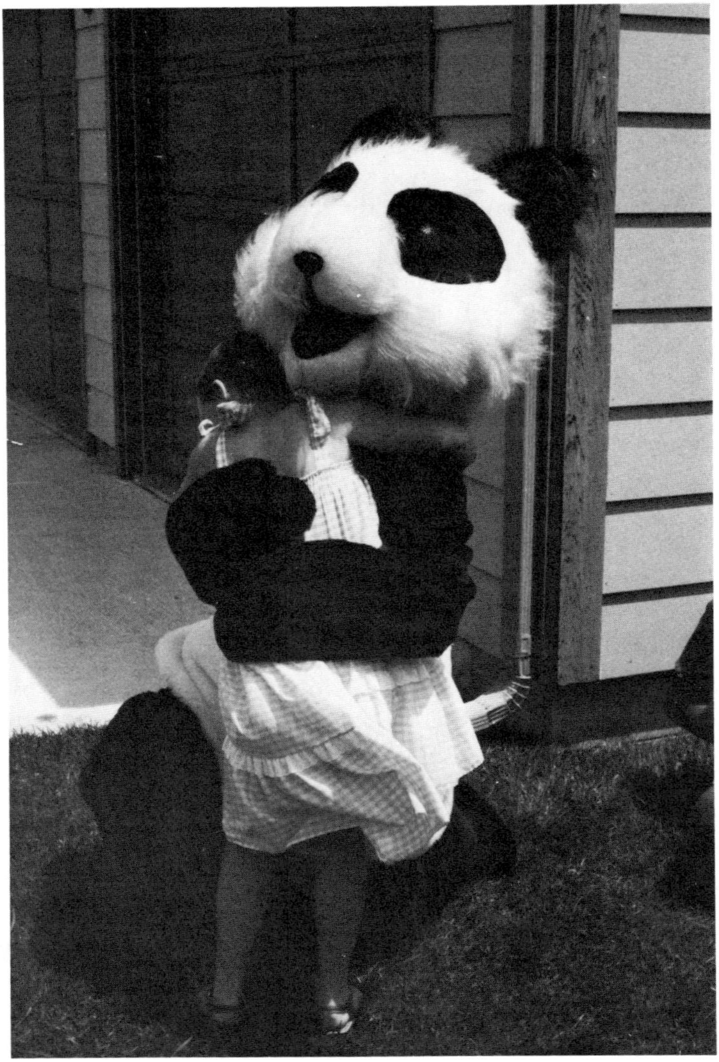

Photograph by Peter J. Dubec. Used by Permission of Photographer and *The Catholic Mirror*.

and full of pain. I am often asked: "Why in the world would anyone choose to spend their time with dying patients when they don't have to?" People who think in this way are neglecting the most important part of a dying child—his Spirit. If their focus could be that this is a child *living* with cancer instead of one dying of cancer, dying would not be so lonely.

People would continue to send their children to play with them and treat them normally.

One day Amanda was accompanied by a male newspaper photographer and a female reporter as she went to visit a child who was ill at home. After the visit was over and as we were driving home, I asked the photographer and reporter what their thoughts and feelings were during the visit. Their replies were quite interesting. The photographer spoke first. He said that when he awoke that morning he knew he was going to be accompanying me that afternoon and he started getting nervous. His main concern was whether or not he would cry. He said he is tenderhearted and he didn't know if he would be able to maintain his "macho" image. He expected the visit to be sad and he didn't know if he was up to that. He was sure he was going to "lose it."

The reporter said much the same thing. She, too, wasn't sure what to expect. She knew I went to visit children who were terminally ill, and she wasn't sure she "would be able to handle it." Both of them said they were so surprised that it was such a *joyful* visit! This little girl's joy was apparent the moment we walked in the door; her spirit was fully alive.

Oftentimes I am asked by people: "Isn't your work depressing?" The answer is an unqualified no. This work can be sad at times. It is very difficult to watch a child suffer and not be able to do anything about it. In fact, that is the hardest part of this work for me. That makes me sad. But the fact that they are going to die is not depressing. It is not depressing because of my own deep faith and the faith of the children. I know beyond any doubt that God has wonderful things in store for them, things so wonderful that we can't even begin to imagine them. I believe that after death there will be no more suffering, that they will be as free as a butterfly and will live forever in perfect love. The children themselves come from all different religious backgrounds, and their faith and trust in God is very deep and very beautiful.

The following prayer was written by Sara, five months before she died:

> Dear God,
> I don't care when you decide when it is time for me to go up to heaven with you and Jesus. I know it will be a good time.

This prayer is also written by Sara:

> Dear God,
> I know that you love us and I love you. You know I love you a lot because you are my father, my Dear Father. You have lots of people I know up there like Heather and Ritchie. I know that Heather and Ritchie are happy up there, very happy. Dear Lord, take this leukemia away, it bothers me. Lord Jesus Christ our only Son of God.

Sara died seventeen days later.

Heather was Sara's best friend. She also had cancer and died two months before Sara. Some people think that not only do children know that they are going to die; some children even know when they are going to die. Two days before Heather died she said to her mom and dad:

> I know I am going to be going to Heaven soon. But I don't want you to be sad or to cry because I'll be in Heaven with Jesus and I'll be praying for you. For the first two days when I get to Heaven, I'm just going to play. (Heather had not been able to play for a long time.) After that, I'm going to look up and hold all the babies in Heaven. And you know what, Dad? When I fall off my bike in Heaven, it won't even hurt!

That's the stuff that these kids are made of! Can you see now why this work is not depressing? Far from it. It is a tremendous privilege for me to be a part of their lives.

Camp Amanda

One of the things that we are doing in Iowa—and I believe we are unique in the nation in this endeavor—is having weekend camps for children who have experienced a death in the family: children whose mother, father, brother, sister, or grandparent has died.

In my work as Amanda the Panda, I have noticed that very little is being done, even nationally, for brothers and sisters of children so critically ill. There are support groups for almost every segment of society, but very few, if any, for siblings. And yet, siblings suffer as much as a dying child—only in a different way. They struggle with feelings of anger, resentment, jealousy, abandonment, loneliness, fear, and guilt. Most of the children that Amanda sees have been ill two years or more. Two years is a very long time for a normal, healthy sibling! Because of the total demands made on the parents, day and night, by a child who is so sick, precious little time or energy are left for the child who is well and healthy. It is not unusual for this child at some point during a two-year illness to wish that the ill brother or sister would hurry up and die so that the rest of the family "can get back to normal around here." Such siblings are not really wishing that the child would die; they are simply wishing that there was more time for them!

In our society, we place a lot of emphasis on wishes coming true. We say to a child who is very young: "Look up at the sky at night, pick the first star, and make a wish—and it will come true." Or, we tell a child to blow out the candles on a birthday cake, make a wish, and it will come true. At

Thanksgiving time we play tug of war with the turkey breastbone. The one who wins is supposed to make a wish and it will come true. Imagine the child who, at some point during a two-year illness, has wished that his or her brother or sister would die. And then that child does die. Imagine the guilt that the surviving child is left with. And the healthy brother or sister says: "My God, it's all my fault! I didn't mean it, God, honest! I really didn't mean for her to die. I take it back, God." But the dead child doesn't come back to life.

I heard a true story about a year and a half ago that touched me so deeply I resolved then and there to commit myself to doing something for this segment of society that has too long been neglected. A very warm, sensitive, intelligent, and caring woman told this story. She said that several years ago, after having been divorced, she took her two young children on a vacation. While they were vacationing, her two-year-old son drowned in a swimming accident. He had been in the care and company of his older sister who was then about eight years old. For reasons known only to her, the eight-year-old could not talk about the feelings deep inside her. Ten years later, on the anniversary of her little brother's death, she committed suicide. The story of this mother's tragedy, in large part, led to the creation of Camp Amanda.

Camp Amanda is a weekend camp experience for children who have had a death in the family. The purpose of the camp is twofold: first, for the children to run and play and laugh and make noise again—to really have a good time. Fun and laughter are extremely important and a top priority. Camp activities are geared to the age level of the campers. For six to 12-year-old children we have activities such as horseback riding, totem pole painting, games, cookouts, campfires, arts and crafts, puppets, and sing-a-longs. For teenagers we have cross-country skiing, hiking, rappelling, disco dancing, candlemaking, photography, and drama. The second purpose of the camp is for the children to meet other boys and girls their own ages who also have had a death in the family. By meeting others like themselves, the children discover that they all share the same feelings, that those feelings are normal, and that they are *okay* for having them. When one grieves alone, one doesn't realize that all the feelings which take over one's life at different times during the grief experience are very normal. It is very important to realize that what is happening to them happens to others also. Camp Amanda tries to provide the place and space for children throughout the state of Iowa to come together in an atmosphere of love and acceptance where they can meet others like themselves and have lots of fun together and where their pain is understood.

Our first Camp Amanda was held in October 1982, and was a huge success. Twenty-seven children, ages six to 12, attended from all over

Iowa. Seven children had experienced the death of a sibling; twenty had a parent who died (18 of the 20 parents who died were fathers).

The camps are held at existing campsites in central Iowa. We provide the food, the cooks, and the counselors. The camp provides the horses and two girls responsible for horseback riding. My staff members are chosen primarily on the basis of their love of children, their warmth, sensitivity, compassion, and huggability. The counselors are from all walks of life, all ages, and of both sexes.

The children are put into groups of six with two counselors, one male and one female. In this way, children whose fathers have died have a male influence and those whose mothers have died have a woman's influence. These groups of eight eat all their meals together at the same table. They are similar to a family unit and they sleep together in the same tent, boys with the male counselor and girls with the female counselor. At all other times, the children are free to relate to any of the other counselors or campers as they wish.

The staff gathers together on Friday evening beginning with supper. It is a time for all to get acquainted, be briefed on any particulars, determine which groups the children will be assigned to, take care of last-minute items, make any schedule changes, and just relax together before the children arrive.

The campers arrive on Saturday morning at 10 a.m. They bring sleeping bags, flashlights, and clothes that they can play in, as well as a few other assorted and "unusual" items. As they arrive, they are immediately introduced to their counselors who present them with a Camp Amanda T-shirt and a hand-painted name tag made of wood. The counselors take the campers to their tents and help them put their gear away. Campers are encouraged to show their parents their tents and anything else they have already discovered.

Amanda is there to greet them and to welcome them as they arrive. For some children, it is the first time they have seen Amanda. She is a big hit with all of them. She stays for the first hour or so. Then she disappears so that I can be present for the rest of the weekend. Before Amanda leaves, she promises the children she will be back. She returns at the very end of camp to give every child a bear hug and send them on their way. Throughout the weekend, the children keep asking about Amanda. They wonder where she went and when she will be back. When she does return, the children have all kinds of things to show her and tell her. Very few children discover that Amanda and I are the same person.

After the parents have had a cup of coffee, and have been shown around the camp by their children, it is time for them to leave so that Camp Amanda can officially begin.

One of the first orders of business is for everyone to get acquainted. All the children know that everyone there has had a death in the family, so we begin by having them tell something about themselves including who died in their family. This is done early so the children can quickly identify which child lost the same member of the family (mother, father, brother, or sister) as they did. During free time, they may want to go for a walk together or sit under a tree and talk. This get-acquainted session lasts approximately an hour and then it's time for a campfire cookout. The children go in search of sticks and twigs on which to roast their hot dogs. Everyone gets to roast his or her own hot dog on an open fire under the watchful guidance of the counselors. All other meals are prepared by our cooks. The children also go on a scavenger hunt in search of wildflowers and other items they deem appropriate to create the centerpiece for their table. (Some very interesting centerpieces emerge; a few even have living creatures crawling about them!)

After lunch, there are lots of games, free time, arts and crafts, and small group sharing. One of the most popular activities is totem pole painting. One of the counselors takes two or three children into the woods in search of a downed tree branch. The children do the actual sawing of the limb from the tree. Then, with great pride (they are just beaming!), they carry it out of the woods. They strip the bark and place the limb on a table in the sun to dry. After it is dry, everyone joins in to paint it every color imaginable. It is now our totem pole and is placed around the campfire where everyone can admire it. The children are very proud of the totem pole and it is one of the first things they show their parents when they come to pick them up.

Earlier in the afternoon, our cooks will have been busy baking chocolate chip cookies. These cookies come out of the oven about the same time the kids are returning from their hike. The cookie dough is made up ahead of time, but the cookies are actually baked at camp. I feel it is important to have the smells of home-baked goodies at camp. In some cases, it may have been a long time since their parents have had the time or the energy to bake home-made cookies. Also, there is nothing neater than to come home to the smell of something baking in the oven! It is a warm feeling we never outgrow.

After supper we have two guests, a doctor and a nurse. They are at camp to answer any medical questions the children might have. (See Figure 9.3.) I had a very strong feeling that the children would have many unanswered questions. In many cases, few of the children have actually had the opportunity to speak to a doctor in this manner and to receive answers to their questions in a language they could understand. Our doctor and nurse answer all questions honestly and with great sensitivity

Figure 9.3. A Camper Listening to the Doctor Explain How her Father Died

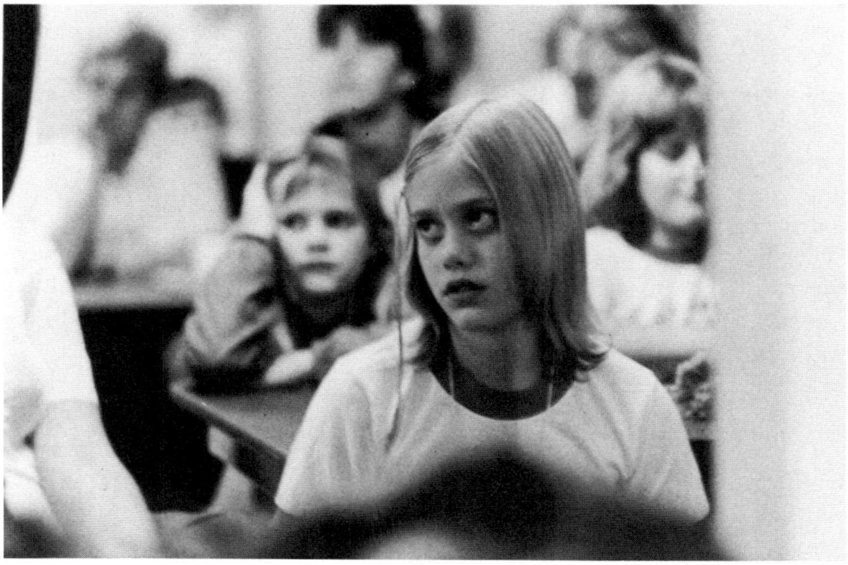

Photograph by Peter J. Dubec. Used by Permission of Photographer and *The Catholic Mirror*.

and clarity. The questions do not center solely on death. They run the full range, all the way from birth to death. All questions are taken seriously and the question-and-answer period ends only when the questions end.

At this point it is usually dark outside and time for a campfire sing-a-long.

Around 8:30 or 9:00 p.m. we have our candlelight service around the campfire. Each child is given a candle in the shape of a panda. This candle represents the person in their family who has died. We talk a little about death and about darkness and light. We talk about how there is no more darkness surrounding death because of Jesus and how He is the light of the world. How He lived and died and then rose from the dead and lives now in a whole different way. Then we talk about how their mom or dad or brother or sister also lived and died and now lives in the light of Jesus. At this point a white candle is lit. This candle represents Jesus. I light my panda candle from the Jesus candle and tell who it represents. Then the children go around the campfire lighting their candle from the person next to them, while at the same time telling who their candle represents.

As we went around the campfire one night, a little girl lit her candle and said: "This candle represents my mom and my dad and my sister." Little Beth, who was seven years old, looked up at her counselor on whose lap she was sitting and said: "Boy! That little girl lost her mom and her dad and her sister! And now she lives in a foster home! I'm lucky! I lost my sister but I still have my mom and dad!"

At the end of the candlelight service, when everyone's candle was lit, I suggested we sing, "This little candle light of mine." The little boy sitting next to me said: "Let's sing, 'When the Saints Go Marching In'." Amen!

After the candlelight service it is time for bed. The children are asked to settle in for the night in their tents. They may talk quietly for one-half hour or so. Then it is time to sleep. At that time, the staff meets to go over the day's activities and to make any changes for the next day.

Sunday morning we have a "Sunrise" service (the sun rises for weary campers at approximately 8:30 a.m.). We gather around the campfire and listen to the sounds of silence and how everything around us, in nature, praises God. The reading chosen is from "Hope for the Flowers." We may read a psalm about how the sun and the moon praise the Lord, or how the birds and the flowers praise the Lord. Then there is time for silent prayer and anyone who wants to may pray out loud. We then have a song, and we close by holding hands and praying the "Our Father" together. It is a very simple service, one intended to fit the occasion and the surroundings.

After breakfast is the activity everyone has been looking forward to—horseback riding. The children take turns by groups. While one group is riding horses for one-half hour, the other two groups are doing arts and crafts, playing table games, or working on skits for their parents.

When everyone has had their turn at riding horses, we gather together again in one large group. This time we have another guest: a puppet lady. She and her puppets spend an hour with the children talking about feelings. The children are very attentive and responsive, and she soon has them laughing and singing with her.

After the puppets, it is lunch time and then time for the children to clean out their cabins and pack up their gear in preparation for going home. Any extra time can be spent polishing up the skits each group has prepared for their parents.

I invite parents to come one-half hour early to pick up their children so we can have a cup of coffee together. As we sit together, I try to answer any questions they may have and to fill them in on some of the things we did during the weekend. After this informal session, the parents gather around the campfire with their children and the skits begin.

I leave at about this time so that Amanda can return in my place. As soon as children spot her, they immediately leave the campfire and run to the waiting arms of Amanda. They tell her all about camp and run to get their candles to show her. They tell her about the puppet lady and about horseback riding. Then Amanda gives them a great big bear hug and sends them on their way. Camp Amanda is over.

As I said earlier, most children do not know that Amanda and I are one and the same. At our first Camp Amanda, I had given all the children a bear hug and they were on their way home when, five minutes later, a car pulled up and three of the children returned. I was still in my Panda costume when the following conversation took place:

Me:	"What are you guys doing back here again?"
Them:	"We came back for one more bear hug!"
Me:	"Okay." *(Hugs given to everyone.)*
Them:	"Goodbye, JoAnn."
Me:	"Goodbye—Wait a minute! What did you call me??"
Them (with much glee):	"JoAnn! We thought we recognized your voice but we weren't quite sure. We had to come back one more time to check it out. Goodbye JoAnn."

At the end of camp each camper is given a typed list of every camper and counselor, together with their addresses and telephone numbers. New friendships are made at camp and the children want to keep in touch. Those living in different cities become pen pals. Sometimes they will call one another just to talk, thus developing their own support system. This is especially true of our teenagers who come to camp. Lasting friendships are made. Often the teenagers meet later and go to a movie together or stay overnight at one another's homes. Throughout the camp weekend, the teenagers kept saying: "It is *so* good to be here. Everyone understands where we're coming from! Kids at school just don't understand." One 15-year-old girl wrote: "When my mother brought me to camp, I wasn't sure I wanted to stay. When she came to pick me up, I didn't want to go home."

Camp-A-Panda

In addition to Camp Amanda, which we now offer four times per year to an average of 25–30 children in each session, I am happy to announce the creation of Camp-A-Panda, a week-long camp for children living with cancer. This camp was a dream in my heart for a long time before it became a reality in the summer of 1984. It took me three years to raise the money to put on such a camp, but the effort was worth every minute and more! Children with cancer have the same normal longings and desires to go to camp as other children do. Unfortunately, because of their medical histories, they are not always allowed or welcome to attend "regular" summer camps. At Camp-A-Panda, the focus is on their childhood, not on their illness.

Camp-A-Panda was a huge success; it far surpassed my hopes and expectations. I was hoping to have 25–35 children for our first effort at such a camp; instead, 68 children came to camp and had a wonderful time. They participated in everything: horseback riding, swimming, canoeing, fishing, arts and crafts, riflery, archery, miniature golf, campfires, games, and much, much more. They even got to ride in a hot-air balloon! Most of all, they made new friends and felt very much at home: no one stared at them or made them feel uncomfortable in any way. They went home more self-assured and self-confident. One father of a seven-year-old boy summed it all up in the following poem which he wrote about Camp-A-Panda:

They came to camp
To play and run
To forget about Cancer
And just have some fun

Amanda the Panda
Was there to please
She watched them ride horses
And climb in the trees

The Doctors watched over them
And the Counselors did, too
In case they got sick
Or maybe just blue

It's a chance to escape
To be well for awhile
For nothing's as rewarding
As a child with a smile!

I am deeply grateful to all counselors, staff, and special guests at all Camp Amandas and at Camp-A-Panda. These very generous, warm, loving people donate their time so that our camp costs can be kept at a minimum.

There is one last thing I would like to say about our camps: they are FREE! There is no charge to any child or family at any time. The actual cost of a weekend Camp Amanda is between $850 and $1,000. Expenses for Camp-A-Panda this year were $24,000, and next year's camp costs will be even higher because our camp rate will increase as will our attendance! These costs are absorbed through donations made by individuals, churches, civic groups, and service organizations. We are also hoping for corporate donations. All such donations are tax deductible and can be sent to Amanda Cares, Inc., a non-profit corporation, at 4116 65th Street, Des Moines, Iowa 50322.

Conclusion

In my ministry as Amanda the Panda, I specifically chose a Panda for several reasons. Pandas are in danger of becoming extinct, just as the notion of caring for others without expecting something in return is becoming extinct. Pandas also enjoy an image of playfulness and friendliness, which other bears sometimes lack. There is nothing frightening or sad about Pandas; they are lovable and fun to watch.

It is my dream to have Amandas in all parts of the country in the future, as well as Camp Amandas in every state. At the present time, we have an Amanda the Panda in the Minneapolis area. It is not necessary that future Amandas share my specific religious convictions (I am Catholic and the Minneapolis Amanda is Lutheran), but I do feel it is important to have a belief system of one's own and, for me, a prayer life is crucial to the quality of my work. I also feel very strongly that it is totally inappropriate to impose one's own religious beliefs on dying patients. I am not there to convince, convert, or convey my own religious beliefs—I am there to listen and affirm the child's belief in the goodness of God and His total and unconditional love for them. Amanda the Panda is a copyrighted name and, as such, can only be used with my permission. The name Amanda is from the Latin word *amanda* which means worthy of love. And that is Amanda's message to children.

If there were one thing that I wish could be changed regarding our attitude toward people with terminal illnesses, it would be this: to switch our focus from dying to living—to focus on the quality of life rather than on the quantity of our years. If our focus indeed changed to a positive response and attitude, we would see the problems of isolation and loneliness among dying patients become greatly diminished, if not entirely eradicated. We would not be afraid to spend time with dying patients, nor would we be judgmental. We would listen with our hearts and, in that listening, we would discover that dying patients and especially dying children, are alive and have needs and feelings that deserve acknowledgement, respect, and appropriate outlets. Most of all, we would discover the joy and the gift that such patients truly are.

IV

Caring For Bereaved Children, Family Members, and Staff

Hospice care does not end with death. The promise of hospice is that those to whom care is offered will not be abandoned. High standards for the quality of one's life should be achievable before death. But however that may develop, hospice providers pledge to maintain the gift of presence, to keep company, to listen, and to care. That pledge is offered to the dying person as well as to his or her family members. We offer the assurance to the dying person that friendship and support will continue to be available afterwards for those who live on. Hospice provides responsiveness to needs and continuity of concern to the new circumstances and problems of bereavement.

Survivors of a death may be children, parents, family members, friends, or caregivers. Their bereavement will encompass a number of shared characteristics, as well as unique qualities depending on individual coping styles and the nature of the loss experienced by different persons. For our purposes, two main forms of bereavement that require attention are the grief of children and that of parents. The former is considered here by Stephen Fleming, the latter by Charles Corr, Ida Martinson, and Kay Dyer. In both cases there is a thorough exploration of the typical patterns and dimensions in these two important sorts of grieving, a discussion of key variables which may influence the course of bereavement, and a set of practical suggestions for helpers.

On the basis of the guidelines in Chapters 10 and 11, it may be appropriate in some cases to establish new programs of follow-up care for bereaved children, parents, or other family members. But it is not always necessary to inaugurate new services, especially when existing community resources may already be meeting the need. Further, there is much to be learned from the well-established mutual- and self-help models, represented here by Candlelighters and Compassionate Friends. The careful analysis of the main features of these models by Dennis Klass in Chapter 12 is an additional source of information and insight on ways to help the bereaved cope with loss.

A final group of survivors—mentioned often throughout this book, but not always in terms of their own needs—is that composed of the staff of the caregiving program. Whether professional or lay, paid or volunteer, these individuals are human beings. As they work with ill, dying, or bereaved children and other family members, caregivers themselves must be expected to have their own feelings and needs for support. In Chapter 13 Marcia Lattanzi identifies numerous ways to respect the importance of caregiving staff by acknowledging and anticipating sources and manifestations of stress; by carefully thought-out organizational programs of staff selection, education and training, supervision, and support; by individual attention to methods of constructive coping; and by the development of an overall approach to caring that serves our requirements as caregivers in an effective manner. In this way, our last word about services for children, families, and others is essentially the same as our opening comments on hospice approaches: sensitivity to real needs, imaginative responsiveness in caring, and scrupulous attention to detail—all in the interest of supporting or improving quality of life for living persons.

10

Children's Grief: Individual and Family Dynamics

Stephen J. Fleming

Introduction

In contrast to the voluminous literature on adult grief, relatively little has been published on the topic of this chapter, namely, children's responses to the death of a parent or sibling. And, unfortunately, most of the available resource materials discussing children's grief are not based on the systematic study of unselected, recently-bereaved, normal children; rather, the research tends to be retrospective or samples of bereaved children who have already decompensated (Arthur & Kemme, 1964), are institutionalized (McConville, Boag, & Purohit, 1970), or already in analysis (Furman, 1974). Further, insight into grief at a sibling's death tends to rely almost exclusively on death from leukemia. There is some evidence that bereavement responses to other types of fatal illness, for example, cystic fibrosis, may be different (Kerner, Harvey, & Lewiston, 1979).

Acknowledging such limitations, this chapter: (1) initially considers the controversy surrounding whether children are capable of experiencing grief; (2) discusses the physiological, cognitive, behavioural, and

The author would like to thank Michelle Cohen for her assistance in the preparation of this chapter.

affective dimensions of a child's response to the death of a parent or sibling; (3) considers variables influencing or moderating the outcome of bereavement; and (4) offers suggestions for intervention.

Do Children Experience Grief?

There has been considerable debate over whether or not children have the intellectual and emotional maturity necessary to experience the full range of physical and psychological responses that follow the death of a loved one. Two quite distinct approaches to resolving this issue are evident on examination of the literature. One approach has been to stress the relationship between cognitive development and attitudes toward death; another approach, influenced by psychoanalytic theory, has focused on the intrapsychic processes and ego functions necessary for grief to occur.

Developmental psychologists claim that the child under five years of age—confronted with loss and puzzling over "where people go"—is not capable of intellectually appreciating the universality and biological irreversibility of death. Although frequently referring to "death" and "the dead," the child attributes life to the latter, feels death is reversible, and is highly vulnerable to magical thinking when considering causes of death. Such a conceptualization of death in which one appreciates and laments separation, and considers the deceased to be living under changed circumstances while maintaining hopeful expectations of their return, will markedly affect the nature and quality of the grief experienced.

Often the child from six to eight years of age personifies death as scary, frightening, disturbing, and dangerous (Nagy, 1948). If death is an external agent such as a skeleton, ghost, or bogey-man, then escape is possible. So, we are not biologically programmed to die, death is not something that will happen to all of us; instead, by calling on a number of strategies such as being exceptionally good or running exceptionally fast, one can avoid death. The nonuniversality of death might well serve to distance some of the trepidation children feel surrounding this mysterious event and permit them to actively pursue concerns regarding causality. In fact, Piaget (1966) felt these middle years of childhood brought a surge of interest in what causes death as part of the child's attempts at mastering cause-effect relationships in general.

During these early years the child also struggles with a tendency to ascribe life or living characteristics to inanimate objects. The developmental transformation of this concept, termed animism, has a number of distinct stages. Initially, the child believes anything active is alive (e.g., the stove is alive because it cooks); then movement connotes life (e.g., water and clouds are alive); followed by life being equated with spontaneous movement. Finally, during the fourth and final stage, the notion of life is similar to that of adults.

In spite of the tendency to personify death and the inherent conceptual confusion, the child from six to eight is moving from a position of little understanding of death to one of searching, questioning, and acknowledging this reality. This is a cognitive turning point in the child's understanding of death and is said to lead to the realization, between ages nine and twelve, that death is final (irrevocable) and marks the cessation of corporeal life. There is the recognition, too, that death is an internal, physiological process that happens to all of us (Childers & Wimmer, 1971; Nagy, 1948). So, the child of approximately nine years has a biologically correct concept of death and now approaches loss with the same intellectual or cognitive tools as his or her adult counterpart.

In researching the question, "Can children mourn?", psychoanalytic theorists have been guided by Freud's definition of adult "mourning." He wrote:

> Mourning occurs under the influence of reality-testing; for the latter function demands categorically from the bereaved person that he should separate himself from the object, since it no longer exists. Mourning is entrusted with the task of carrying out his retreat from the object in all those situations in which it was the recipient of a high degree of cathexis. (1926, p. 172)

In Freud's view, mourning demands that the child be capable of a number of complicated intrapsychic processes including remembering and representing an object (person) in one's mind even when the object is absent. This is not possible prior to age one (Rosenblatt, 1967). One must also be able to test reality or to distinguish the real world (external reality) from the subjective world of wish and imagination (internal reality). Whether response to loss is principally determined by fantasy or by realistic thinking is a function of the child's ability to test reality accurately. In addition, other ego functions have to be developed, among them the ability to separate oneself from the deceased (for he or she no longer exists); a tolerance of painful affect including longing, anger, and guilt; the acceptance of the loss as permanent; and a gradual shifting of emotional ties to others.

Fleming and Altschul (1963), Moriarity (1967), and Miller (1972) share the opinion that the process of mourning requires the operation of ego functions to which the child does not yet have established access. Wolfenstein (1966), observing children at the time of loss, reported curtailed feelings of sadness, little weeping, immersion in activities of everyday life, and no withdrawal into preoccupation with thoughts of the dead parent. Seemingly, the ego of the child is not sufficiently developed to tolerate the stresses that grief work entails so self-protective measures are implemented, for example, denial of the reality of the parent's absence and repression of affect. Wolfenstein concluded that the intrapsychic operations that characterize the process of mourning in *adults* are not possible prior to adolescence.

In summary, for the majority of psychoanalytic theorists, children lack the necessary ego strength and are incapable of mourning until adolescence. From a cognitive perspective, children have the developmental ability to comprehend death logically and biologically, and thus to grieve, as early as age nine.

Much of the controversy stems from Freud's conception of mourning in *adults* and the direct application of this model to *children*. The term "mourning," as Freud used it, refers to complicated mental processes emanating from inner, intrapsychic conflict and demanding considerable ego differentiation; in short, it is restricted to adolescent and adult reactions to loss. To refer to a child's response in the face of death as "mourning" is to use the term in a way that differs substantially from this original meaning.

Cognitively, the development of the concept of death seems to be a gradual process revealing pronounced differences between adult and child in appreciating the universality, causality, and irrevocability of death. So, a child does not mourn as an adult does. However, as Lampl-deGroot (1976) has argued, the *affective* responses to death for both child and adult are quite similar, being characterized by pain, sadness, protest, and guilt.

Perhaps, as Worden (1982) advocates, what is needed is the development of a model that reflects the unique aspects of a child's response to death rather than the imposition of an adult model. In any event, as a result of the inappropriateness of the term "mourning," it will not be used in this discussion. Instead, "grief" will refer to the child's physiological, cognitive, behavioural, and affective responses to death.

To the rephrased question, "Do children grieve?", the answer is an unequivocal "yes."

Exploring a Child's Grief

The following discussion is restricted to the child's reaction to the death of parent or sibling. It is beyond the scope of this chapter to consider reaction to other types of parent-sibling loss, for example, divorce, desertion, or separation.

The rupture of the incomparably rich and intense parent-child relationship deprives the child of a principal source of support and confronts him or her with a major adjustment. It was my original intention—in recognition of the uniqueness of this relationship, particularly the powerful dependency needs—to explore the physiological, cognitive, behavioural, and affective ramifications of the death of a parent and the death of a sibling separately. However, in spite of the contrast in parent-child and sibling-sibling attachments, there is a remarkable similarity in the child's response when death occurs, so they will be discussed here jointly. Where differences in either the nature or the dynamics of the grief response exist, these will be indicated.

Physiological Responses

While the physiological concomitants of adult grief have been well documented (Worden, 1982; Parkes, 1972; Lindemann, 1944), such reactions have not been shown to play a prominent role in a child's grief response. Although vague somatic complaints such as headaches and stomach discomfort may be reported, more frequently is found the distressing fear that the survivor will develop the same disease that "killed" the parent or sibling (Kerner, Harvey, & Lewiston, 1979).

Although physiological symptoms theoretically may represent unmanifested grief, one should not assume that since children are relatively symptom-free they are overtly and directly expressing the pain of their loss. For example, in the absence of obvious grief, Arthur and Kemme (1964) report a number of masking behavioural responses (restlessness, inappropriate laughter, regression to soiling and excessive eating) that reflect the trauma of experienced loss. It may well be that children struggling with loss do not respond physiologically as adults do, however, more attention will have to be paid to this dimension of grief prior to the drawing of any firm conclusions.

Cognitive Responses

The struggle to gain cognitive mastery over the concept of death reflects an attempt to turn a sudden, strange, often frightening event into something understandable and hopefully manageable. Not surprisingly, given the child's limited intellectual ability and defective reality testing, distorted concepts of illness, death, and the relationship between illness and death often result.

Finality and causality are the principal dimensions of death that present the child with a genuine intellectual problem. The verbalized uncertainties and misconceptions regarding death *per se* betray the incomprehensibility of finality. The child appreciates the absence of a parent or sibling and is convinced that the deceased *is* somewhere, that he or she *is* active, and that he or she *will* return (Arthur & Kemme, 1964). Children under six years of age (Piaget's preoperational stage) tend to translate the finality of death into known, concrete terms (Kaffman & Elizur, 1979). If mother is in heaven, then "Can she see us?", "Can she hear me?", "Does heaven have trees?", or "Daddy looks like he's sleeping, maybe we should wake him up now," or "Daddy's been gone on his trip long enough, isn't it time he came back?". Young children are particularly vulnerable to this cruel expectation of reunion, for in all likelihood previous separation from significant others has been temporary. In the relatively unusual case when separation is final, the expectation of reunion does not yield readily to reality.

In contrast, children from six to ten years of age tend to express realistic concerns about dying and death as a means of appreciating finality (Kaffman & Elizur, 1979). Such comments as, "What happens to your body when you die?", "Janet [sister] can't eat, sleep, or talk because she's dead, can she?", or "When you're dead your heart stops and your body rots," reflect a grappling with the biological irreversibility of death.

The incomplete mastery and distortion of causality is evidenced by the inability to differentiate not only between similar events but also between events occurring closely in time. Arthur and Kemme (1964) have observed when a parent dies accidentally or from illness that a child may react with exaggerated concern or panic at his or her own illness or minor mishap. These events are interpreted as portending one's own death ("bruises cause death"; "riding in cars causes death").

In conceptualizing death and specifically causality, the prominent feature is often not *what* caused the death but rather *who* caused it, *who* was responsible. Believing all world events to be purposive and largely influenced by one's own personal desires, the child may feel that his or her evil thoughts, aggressive actions, or misdeeds (real or imagined) were instrumental in causing parent or sibling death. This effect is particularly potent when the thoughts, behaviours, or feelings in question (e.g., "I wish I had another father", or "I want my brother's room") occur temporally close to the tragedy. Recollection of (innocuous) parental responses such as, "you'll be the death of me yet," uttered prior to any tragedy, affirms the child's sense of guilt and omnipotence, and further confuses psychological and physical causality.

Behavioural Responses

A number of behavioural responses have been associated with the child's reaction to death including: remembering and longing; searching for a substitute parent; identification with the dead parent or sibling; augmented dependency; and increased aggressiveness.

Remembering and Longing. If encouraged, children will verbalize memories of the deceased, look at photographs, reflect on items of clothing, and sing favorite songs. The nature and quality of these recollections tends to vary with age. Younger children, that is, those under six years of age, recall or reenact concrete events experienced with the deceased. This "remembering with action" (Furman, 1974) is exemplified by the child's demanding to go on walks he or she had taken prior to a parent's death, or the surviving sibling continuing to play the games previously enjoyed with a dead brother. Children older than six years of age speak less of the deceased but often in private look at photos, read letters, and not infrequently, ask to visit the grave (Arthur & Kemme, 1964).

Searching for a Substitute Parent. To guarantee family continuity, stability, and the fulfillment of needs following the death of a parent, bereaved children may demand attention and affection from a father or mother substitute. Other motivations for seeking a "new father" or "new mother" include a desire to provide comfort for the surviving parent and an attempt to combat pervasive, frightening feelings of helplessness by *doing* something.

Identification with the Dead Parent or Sibling. As part of a child's normal development, identification with parents is most likely to occur. With the death of a parent, however, this identification may become temporarily enhanced with the child reproducing traits, mannerisms, and behaviour patterns of the deceased. According to Furman (1974), there are both positive and negative repercussions to this; on the one hand, increased identification enhances one's sense of self and mitigates the painful process of longing for and gradually disengaging from the deceased. Unfortunately, assuming characteristics of a deceased parent has the potential of adversely affecting the development of new object relations.

Although the published literature stresses identification with a deceased parent, identification with a deceased sibling may also occur. In a case to be discussed later in this chapter, a boy of six adopted numerous mannerisms of his deceased older brother in an attempt to keep the brother alive. Through behaving "as if" he were the deceased, the survivor hoped temporarily to avoid facing his perceived culpability in the tragedy and simultaneously to bring some small measure of relief to his parents' pain.

Dependent Behaviour. Following the death of a parent or sibling there is a sharp increase in feelings of vulnerability and insecurity, along with the dread that the surviving parent(s) may also become inaccessible. Given their emotional significance, it is not surprising to witness a corresponding increase in dependency needs. In contrast to the child's behaviour prior to bereavement, there is greater clinging, difficulty in parting, and more requests for assistance in previously-mastered tasks. Augmented dependency behaviour of this sort is most frequently evident in younger bereaved children.

Furman (1974) considers an immediate post-death increment in dependency needs to be a normal, predictable response in the face of death; only when it becomes exaggerated in intensity and duration is it considered regressive. Style of parenting can affect the nature and expression of dependency needs. For example, parental overprotection, defined by excessive giving of comfort and consolation, and by extraordinary attempts to protect the child from pain, sorrow, and anxiety, tends to foster strong, prolonged dependency behaviour.

Aggressiveness. In contrast to their demeanor before suffering a loss, aggressive behaviour of a moderate nature is not uncommon among children during bereavement (Kaffman & Elizur, 1979). Included is the repeated use of force or violence in relationships with peers, quarreling and disturbing others, temper tantrums, dramatic outbursts of anger, negativism, and classroom discipline problems.

Although there may be no age-related differences in the frequency of aggressive behaviour, there are differences in how this behaviour is manifested. Kaffman and Elizur (1979) found that younger children of preschool age exhibited more temper tantrums, negativism, stubbornness, and discipline problems. In the older group, age six to ten years, there was more quarreling, cursing, rage, and irritating behaviour. Generally, anger was most frequently directed toward the surviving parent(s), but due to the strong dependency relationship, it was exceedingly difficult to tolerate and express.

In her extensive account of childhood grief experience, Furman (1974) documented a number of additional behavioural responses to the death of a parent. These included: sleep difficulties (related to guilt and characterized by thoughts of someone coming to get them, take them away, or kill them); phobic responses (also related to guilt over the death, and the underlying fear the deceased would return for revenge); academic difficulties; restlessness; enuresis or urinary incontinence; increased sibling rivalry; and eating problems.

Affective Responses

As with the other dimensions of grief expression in childhood, emotional or affective responses are multifaceted and reflect the child as an individual, the nature of predeath family relationships, circumstances surrounding the death, and the family's attempts at dealing with the trauma of parent-sibling death.

Fears of Abandonment and Death. A marked increase in fear has often been associated with reaction to loss. Although objects and situations involved may vary greatly, the prominent concerns focus on abandonment and death, and reflect a frightening sense of helplessness in the world.

Because the child feels abandoned by the deceased, his or her sense of confidence and security in the world has been shattered; in its place is apprehension, uncertainty, and a fear of recurring tragedy. For some children, such feelings of being left behind often trigger fantasies of reunion with the deceased which may take the form of: (1) wanting the deceased to return and join you in life; or (2) wanting to join the deceased in death (Arthur & Kemme, 1964). Younger children tend to blandly assert their conviction and hope of an eventual reunion "when Daddy returns from his trip" or "with my brother in heaven." By contrast, older children, with a greater understanding of death, are more apt to actively contemplate or even attempt suicide.

An example of reunion fantasy was contributed by James, age six, during an interview he and his mother participated in shortly after the accidental death of his younger sister, Tammy (age 20 months). In the six months since the accident, James' parents felt overwhelmed by their grief and largely ignored him. James was told that Tammy was in heaven, that heaven was a happy, warm place, that Tammy was with her grandparents now, and that someday they would all be together again.

Contrasted with the trauma of Tammy's death (which he witnessed) and his parents' despair and lack of interest, heaven seemed a wonderful place. It was not surprising then to find the note reproduced in Figure 10.1 on completion of the interview.

It should be stressed that James was not actively suicidal. He was relating his dual loss (sister and parents) and the uncertainty and turmoil of his current life situation to the imagined peace and tranquillity of his sister's life in heaven.

In the course of normal parent or sibling relations, the child encounters numerous frustrations which result in the expression of anger and ill will. As a function of age-related misconceptions regarding death, incomplete differentiation of self from the deceased, and an exaggerated sense of omnipotence, children fear for their own lives after the death of a parent or sibling. Absolutely convinced that their anger or ill will caused this tragedy, they expect punishment for the culpable party. Looming large are "talion fantasies," that is, the child fears he or she, too, will die at precisely the same age, or from the same cause, or under the same circumstances as the deceased (Cain, Fast, & Erickson, 1964).

Figure 10.1 James' Note

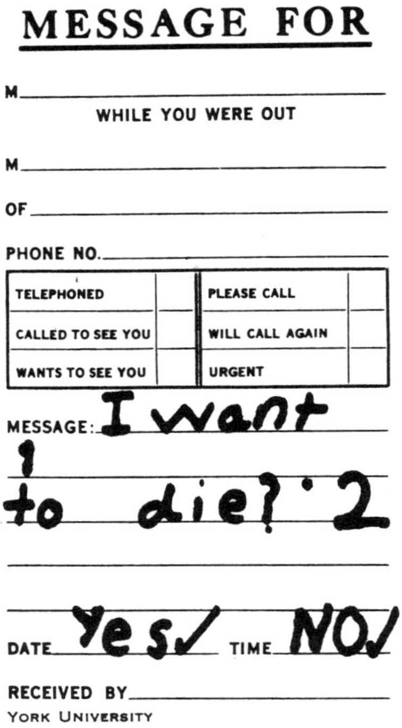

MESSAGE FOR

M

WHILE YOU WERE OUT

M

OF

PHONE NO.

TELEPHONED		PLEASE CALL	
CALLED TO SEE YOU		WILL CALL AGAIN	
WANTS TO SEE YOU		URGENT	

MESSAGE: I want to die? 2

DATE Yes✓ TIME NO✓

RECEIVED BY

YORK UNIVERSITY

Such feelings of guilt, if not consciously recognized and verbally acknowledged, may be indirectly expressed through punishment-seeking behaviours (Hare-Mustin, 1979), accident-prone behaviour (Cain, Fast, & Erickson, 1964), marked concern with blame for major tragedies and minor mishaps (Arthur & Kemme, 1964), and attempts to undo the death by assuming the identity of the deceased and thus keeping him or her alive. Consider Paul (age six) who was seen in therapy at his mother's insistence. Three months earlier, Paul and his older brother, Anthony (age nine), were returning home from school. Unfortunately, when crossing a heavily-traveled street, Anthony was fatally injured by a motor vehicle. Paul seemed to be adjusting well to the death until he began to adopt many of his brother's characteristics. He imitated Anthony's laugh, repeated many of the brother's jokes, wore his clothes, and demanded to sleep in his bed.

When I asked Paul to draw what happened at the accident scene, he drew the sketch reproduced in Figure 10.2. Paul related calling out to his brother who was some distance ahead and crossing the road. On hearing his name, Anthony stopped near the curb (in the position indicated by "B" in the figure). At that moment, Anthony was struck by a car.

Figure 10.2 Paul's Drawing

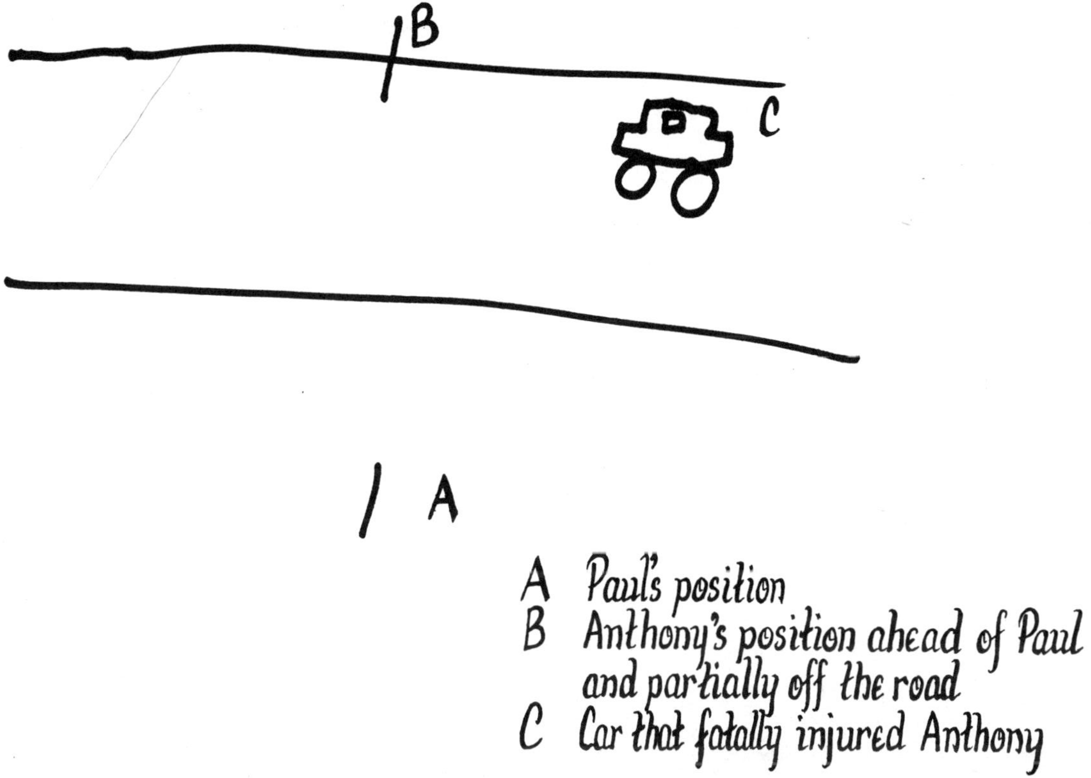

Paul's unverbalized feelings of guilt are readily evident. On gentle probing, we were able to explore the issues of blame, his perceived responsibility for his parents' hurt, and his fears of dying. Consequently, identification with Anthony stopped.

Fear of Physicians, Hospitals, and God. Some authors (Hare-Mustin, 1979; Schiff, 1977; Cain, Fast, & Erickson, 1964) have reported an increase in a child's fear of physicians and hospitals following the death of a sibling. One no longer "goes to the hospital so the doctor can make you better"; for the bereaved child, hospitals are now associated with death. Physicians are seen as impotent in the face of illness and closely aligned with illness and death. Such fears are given added credibility when parents are openly critical of the care and treatment provided by physicians and nurses.

At this time, too, children are frightened and confused about God, His nature, and His role in the death of a parent or sibling. There may be anger and hostility directed at God who is perceived as responsible, some puzzlement over His portrayal as benevolent, a reluctance to pray or place one's trust in Him. "I hate God for taking my Daddy!", and "If God is so good, why does He kill children?", are common responses in the face of death. At the same time, the child is also in awe of this "God person" and fearful that his or her hostile reactions will meet with punishment.

Denial of Death. Cognitive and affective factors combine to make denial of death, particularly for younger children, a common response in bereavement. With insufficient cognitive maturity, confusion over causality and finality, suffering in the pain of separation, and a need for protection from the danger of further deprivation, most preschool children speak of the deceased as if they are still alive. Repeatedly asking about a sibling's return, or the convincing announcement that "Daddy *is* coming home tomorrow," are other examples of the intense need to preserve emotional attachments to the deceased (Kaffman & Elizur, 1979; McConville, Boag, & Purohit, 1970).

Although denial may be implemented, older children tend to use more elaborate and sophisticated defenses like isolation and intellectualization after the death of a parent or sibling.

Anger. Another prominent response to the death of a parent or sibling is anger and rage (Hare-Mustin, 1979). Common objects of resentment include: (1) the surviving parent(s) for not adequately protecting and sensitively caring for the deceased, and for not parenting well since the death; (2) the deceased parent or sibling for "leaving"; (3) a malevolent God; and (4) physicians and nurses who could not defeat death. Anger toward one's surviving parent(s) is often combined with an idealization of the deceased.

Factors Moderating Outcome

The death of a parent or sibling has an extensive, disruptive impact on virtually all aspects of the child's functioning. To this point, it has been stressed that a child's response to death is largely a function of his or her developmental capacity to understand its meaning. The nature and quality of grief is also affected by the environmental climate surrounding the child, for example, the reaction of the parent(s) to the death and the availability or unavailability of support and comfort to the child. This section will focus on factors that affect adjustment and, in so doing, suggest ways of successfully intervening to facilitate the expression of grief.

Communication During the Dying Process

Intervention with bereaved children ought not to be conceptualized as beginning after parent or sibling death. There is evidence implicating family response to illness, particularly predeath communication about the disease, in helping both patient and family cope with the disease process and in facilitating postdeath family adjustment.

Share (1972) has succinctly reviewed the two opposing perspectives on communication with the life-threatened child.[1] The *"protective" approach* maintains that the ill child and often his or her siblings should be shielded from diagnostic and prognostic information. Three arguments are made in support of this position. First, the hospitalized, life-threatened child often responds to his or her condition with passive silence, seldom verbalizing any concerns about fate and the future. It is concluded that this reflects the child's wish not to know about the illness or the child's fears of discussing it openly. Second, since younger children fear separation from parents and injury from medical procedures, it is thought that they are not concerned with death. Finally, it is asserted that awareness of the nature of one's disease would create overwhelming anxiety. Thus, advocates of the protective strategy maintain that the only humane, constructive approach is to bolster denial and otherwise assist the child in repressing cues as to the prognosis of the disease. This results in the presentation of an optimistic demeanor, an emphasis on "getting well again," and pressure to make life appear as normal as possible.

Proponents of a more *"open" approach* respond that the child as young as age six, if not aware of impending death at a conceptual level, is at least

[1]Although this section deals mainly with the dying child (sibling), there is evidence that the dynamics are similar when an adult (parent) is dying (Mount, 1974; Glaser & Strauss, 1965 & 1968).

aware something is seriously wrong (Spinetta, 1974; Binger et al., 1969) and is willing to talk about it. In addition, far from being a humane approach, attempts at denying the seriousness of the disease are said to increase anxiety and foster a pervasive sense of isolation, loneliness, and abandonment. The passive, unquestioning demeanor of fatally-ill children is seen as a response to the inability or unwillingness of parents and staff to deal with the child's awareness (Bluebond-Langner, 1978; Vernick & Karon, 1965). There is some evidence that younger leukemic children use the symbolic language of play and art to communicate their awareness, while older children withdraw so as to "protect" the adult (Binger et al., 1969; Morrissey, 1965). Finally, advocates of open communication maintain, a "closed awareness" situation (Glaser & Strauss, 1965) where the disease is not discussed may ultimately end in failure as Bluebond-Langner (1978) found in her study of leukemic children.

> The leukemic children acquired a great deal of information about the hospital, staff, rules and procedures; about the disease, its treatment, process and prognosis, before they died. The fact that they managed to acquire so much information was even more remarkable because they learned in a situation in which the parents and the staff unconsciously conspired to keep them in painless ignorance. (p. 165)

It is important to appreciate what the open approach does *not* encourage, namely the provision of diagnostic and prognostic information to the young child. The focus is on conveying a willingness to deal with the child's fears—whatever they may be.

> The question of whether a child should be told that his illness is fatal is meaningless; rather the questions and concerns which are conscious to the child threatened with death should be dealt with in such a way that the child does not feel further isolated and alienated from his parents and other meaningful adults. There should be no curtain of silence around his most intense fears. (Waechter, 1971, p. 1172)

Research evidence of the outcome of this open approach has not been extensive. Vernick and Karon (1965) held group meetings for children hospitalized with leukemia, their parents, and hospital staff. These were designed to "develop an environment in which [children] feel perfectly safe to ask any question, and completely confident of receiving an honest answer" (p. 393). Results revealed no significant adjustment problems; when withdrawal and depression occurred, they were always transient. Karon and Vernick (1968) noted that when given the opportunity, children would ask technical and highly searching questions about their illness and its implications. Spinetta, Swarner, and Sheposh (1981) found that the child with higher adaptation levels to illness tended to have parents who provided the information and emotional support needed during the course of the illness (at a level consistent with age and level of development). Furthermore, parents who were successful in the provision of an environment in which the child felt supported and comfortable enough to discuss his or her illness were better adjusted after the child's death.

Intervention designed to foster an atmosphere that effectively "gives permission" to the child and family to explore their fears and concerns should be mounted early in the course of a life-threatening disease. Whether professionals (e.g., physicians, counselors, clergy) or self-help groups (e.g., parents of leukemic children) are involved, the purpose is identical, namely to support, not supplant, the family. An atmosphere of acceptance and assurance allows each family to manage their own lives and to arrive at a solution most adequate for them.

With the patient-and-family as the unit of care, and intervention directed at "total pain" (physical, psychological, social, and spiritual), the child often needs assistance in verbalizing his or her anxieties and assurance, in an atmosphere of hope, that he or she will not be alone and that pain will be controlled. Particular attention to magical notions of causality and the interpretation of medical procedures as punishment for real or imagined wrongdoings is indicated. Struggling with the pain of watching a child die, parents must also deal with anger, self-blame, depression, and fatigue. Unfortunately, fathers have frequently been unable to tolerate this stress and often restrict their contact with the child to routine, brief visits (Lansky, 1974; Binger et al., 1969). If this situation develops, fathers may need professional assistance in verbalizing their anguish and in gaining insight into the impact of such avoidance behaviour. In addition, dying children may present child-rearing challenges such as excessive dependency, and parents may experience anxiety over disciplining.

Sensitivity to the plight of siblings is also necessary, for they, too, may be plagued by misconceptions and magical thinking regarding causality; they may be fearful of their own death, jealous of the preferential treatment accorded the ill child, and guilty for such evil thoughts. Wilson (1982) has suggested that support be extended to include grandparents, aunts, cousins, even schoolmates, where necessary.

Finally, staff who work with a dying child need support in dealing with feelings of inadequacy, failure, sadness, and often anger at parental behavior. Bluebond-Langner (1978) found that staff openly ostracized and were highly critical of parents whom they considered cruel and uncaring because they encouraged open, sensitive communication about their child's disease and treatment. Physicians and nurses who were too closely involved with "curing" the disease were unable and unwilling to recognize openly the child's concerns about dying. Perhaps, as Martinson and her colleagues (1977) and Wilson (1982) have urged, the most desirable location for the terminally-ill child is the home. When the child is more secure in familiar surroundings, family members are nearby exercising some control, and the hospice home care staff can teach and support, the family's ability to handle the disease and subsequent bereavement will be enhanced.

We are a long way from prospectively identifying those effective coping strategies that will help families deal adaptively with the stresses imposed by disease and its treatment. However, the encouragement of open communication by the family during the period of illness and anticipation of grief before death itself is a good first step.

The Period of Bereavement

Following parent or sibling death some children respond with appropriate sobbing, crying, and moodiness (Kaffman & Elizur, 1979), while others exhibit only minimally visible affective responses. Parents may interpret the latter as a sign of adjustment or feel relieved that the child is not posing "painful" questions. Others may express some concern that "the child never cries" or "he only cried the day of the funeral."

When a child possesses the intellectual sophistication needed to understand death, yet confuses physical and moral causality and believes death is reversible, it is evident that the emotional implications of examining the loss are profoundly threatening and inhibit grieving. According to Furman (1974), there are two factors that may interfere with the ability to deal with the tasks of grieving: the assurance that one's needs will be met consistently, and the continuation of other relationships.

At the time of death, to the extent that the deceased did fulfill a child's physical and psychological needs, death represents a danger. For one who invests a great deal of love in the members of his or her immediate family, the death of a parent is the elimination of a major source of need gratification. The surviving parent is ideally suited to provide the sense of continuity and emotional gratification that "helps to establish a position of internal and external safety from which, under favourable circumstances, the work of mourning can begin" (Furman, 1974, p. 114). Although ideally suited, the death of a spouse often renders the surviving parent incapable of understanding and supporting a grief-stricken child. Surviving spouses tend to "protect" both themselves and their children by avoiding or curtailing discussion of death and the feelings related to it (Becker & Margolin, 1967).

With the death of a parent, the child faces the physical loss of one parent; at the death of a sibling, the child is confronted with the functional loss of *both* parents. We are currently in the process of documenting the extensive family disruption the death of a child creates (Fleming, 1984; Trowhill & Fleming, 1980). At one and two year postdeath assessments, bereaved parents[2] completed a self-report Social Adjustment Scale (Weissman et al., 1978) evaluating instrumental performances, interpersonal relations, and satisfactions in five major roles (work, social and leisure activities, extended family, marriage, and parenting).

Up to and including two years postdeath, bereaved parents report significantly greater maladjustment in all areas of functioning than a group of nonbereaved controls. Responses on the marital and parental subscales indicate poor adjustment. The marital subscale reflects such issues as a reported lack of affection, disinterest in sex (and feelings of dissatisfaction and guilt when it occurs), domineering behaviour, dependency, and submissiveness.

In a personal account following the death of a child, Schiff (1977) elaborates on the other crises stressing the marriage. There is a "loss of illusion" about each other (that is, the expectation of comforting one another dissolves in the midst of overwhelming pain), a blaming of one another in the incessant struggle to answer "Why?", and a helplessness that the marriage is doomed endlessly to face defeat and despair. In addition to financial stress and religious differences (even among those of the same faith), parents indulge in what I call a "dance of grief." The expectation that one can effectively support a spouse in grief, a simultaneous desire to protect, along with resentment if, on an "up" day, you are confronted with your mate's grief, all combine to create parental disharmony. Not surprisingly, considering the accompanying sentiments, this "dance" leaves many bruised partners in its wake.

The parenting subscale of the Social Adjustment Scale reflects a lack of affection (or at least a lack of energy to show affection), lack of involvement, and impaired communication. Communication, particularly surrounding the dying and death of a child, is an extremely touchy issue. Parental distress is great and parents may be understandably reluctant to discuss difficult topics with surviving children. The latter, in turn, are well aware of the trauma their parents experience and often conceal expressions of anguish and fear (Hare-Mustin, 1979; Cain, Fast, and Erickson, 1964). Schiff (1977) acknowledges this formidable barrier to open communication:

> It would be a rare child that could face his tear-stained bereaved mother and tell her "I hated my brother sometimes. I even used to wish he was dead. Is that why he died?" (p. 90)

[2]Members of the Bereaved Families of Ontario, a self-help group offering formal and informal programmes for bereaved parents and siblings following the death of a child.

If parents get a glimpse of a child's grief from a very normal response, such as, "I'm glad my sister is dead, now I can have her room," they may be enraged. An understanding and appreciation of the child's inability to conceptualize death, its causality, and its finality, is completely overshadowed by the seeming callousness of the remark. The child is left with increased feelings of guilt and inadequacy, and is now isolated and alone in grief.

Krell and Rabkin (1979) have explored communication problems that result from family defensive manoeuvres to create a new equilibrium out of feelings of guilt, sorrow, anger, and despair. If certain parenting styles become the predominant method of handling stress, the child and family are predisposed to develop complications in grieving. The first maladaptive style focuses on how the child died. If parents believe the child's death was preventable, that they could and should have intervened, then discussion of the circumstances surrounding death is impossible. Parents and child(ren) share a "conspiratorial distribution of guilt"; their only protection is not to discuss the event for to do so risks exposing the guilty party. Suppression of facts related to causality creates an atmosphere of tension in which the surviving child is "haunted by something mysterious and uncertain, knowing and yet not knowing, and afraid to ask for clarification" (p. 474).

A second parental protective device which impedes communication and impairs healthy adjustment to loss is the according of special status to a surviving child. The death of one's child is a poignant illustration of parental powerlessness and vulnerability. One response to this intolerable situation is a futile attempt at controlling fate by obsessively guarding against all real or imagined dangers. Although a certain degree of overprotectiveness with a surviving child is a common occurrence, extreme shielding and protecting denies autonomous functioning and leads to an immature, unstable personality with heightened fears for one's own physical well-being.

Finally, parents may want to replace a deceased child. The most common method of substitution is to designate one of the surviving children to play this role. Cain, Fast, and Erickson (1964) report parents actually changing the name of a living child to that of the deceased. Other methods of substitution include biological reproduction, where mothers are of childbearing age, and adoption. Where the new offspring is intended to fill a family void, individual identity is denied as he or she is forced to live a dual identity, one's own and that of the dead child. Parents often utter consistently unfavorable comparisons, based on the idealized image of the dead child, between the surviving child and the deceased.

With the nature and expression of grief so intimately tied to how one's parent(s) grieves, the child is in a vulnerable position. Marital and parenting dysfunction and the destructiveness of Krell and Rabkin's (1979) "family protective manoeuvres," have the potential to create extensive pathology. It must be recognized, however, that most families are not at risk to develop complications such as these following the death of a parent or sibling. Grief is a very normal response, in effect, the emotional price we pay for loving. And as a normal response to loss, formal intervention may only be necessary where the parent(s) and/or child exhibit maladaptive responses.

In most instances, since grieving tends to be done in private or with supportive family and friends, professional contact will be intermittent. However sporadic, professional assistance and/or participation in a mutual- or self-help bereavement group can represent a potent force in the prevention of bereavement complications. Both these modes of intervention offer a supportive atmosphere which encourage the exploration and expression of grief. Equally important, they help the parent more adequately help the surviving child by stripping much of the mystery from this unknown, often uncontrollable and frightening, human experience called grief. To quote Erikson, "healthy children will not fear life if their parents have integrity enough not to fear death" (1963, p. 233).

For a parent, then, befriending one's own grief is crucial for resolution; it is also imperative that the parent(s) befriend the child's grief. To enter this seemingly unintelligible and bizarre world, one must have some appreciation of the uniqueness of the child's struggles with such factors as reality testing, the universality and finality of death, animistic thinking, causality, and the relationship between illness and death, vulnerability, guilt, feelings of omnipotence, and acute fears of abandonment, mutilation, and death. Thus armed, the physiological, cognitive, behavioural, and affective dimensions of a child's response to loss are less puzzling and the probability of gentle, sensitive mediation is enhanced.

Even though familiarity and foresight may be overshadowed by sorrow, Schiff (1977), nevertheless, offers other suggestions to facilitate or guide a child through grief. These include:

Labor to maintain a focus on the surviving children and their hurt.
Try to spend time with each child individually.
Remind them that it is natural during a quarrel to wish ill of a sibling, but this does not cause death.
Reflect on the good things children did for the dead sibling.
Do not condemn children for laughing and playing during early stages of grief.

Appropriately share your grief; do not avoid talking about the deceased but don't idealize the dead child and make unfavorable comparisons.

Maintain discipline and a sense of continuity and caregiving as much as possible.

Conclusion

In examining physiological, cognitive, behavioural, and affective responses to the death of a parent or sibling, no "loss" syndrome that might be considered typical of childhood bereavement is clearly evident. The particular pattern or combination of symptoms is largely a function of such variables as age, developmental level, and family response to death. For children and adults, the potential for maladjustment is markedly reduced when loving, supportive family and friends have the courage to stand with the bereaved through the pain and helplessness of grief.

References

Arthur, B., & Kemme, M. L., "Bereavement in Childhood," *Journal of Child Psychology and Psychiatry*, 1964, *5*, 37–49.

Becker, D., & Margolin, M. S., "How Surviving Parents Handled Their Young Children's Adaptation to the Crisis of Loss," *American Journal of Orthopsychiatry*, 1967, *37*, 753–757.

Binger, C. M., Ablin, A. R., Feuerstein, R. C., Kushner, J. H., Zoger, S., & Mikkelsen, C., "Childhood Leukemia: Emotional Impact on Patient and Family," *New England Journal of Medicine*, 1969, *80*, 414–418.

Bluebond-Langner, M., *The Private Worlds of Dying Children*. Princeton, NJ: Princeton University Press, 1978.

Cain, A. C., Fast, I., & Erickson, M. E., "Children's Disturbed Reactions to the Death of a Sibling," *American Journal of Orthopsychiatry*, 1964, *34*, 741–752.

Childers, P., & Wimmer, M., "The Concept of Death in Early Childhood," *Child Development*, 1971, *42*, 705–712.

Erikson, E., *Childhood and Society*, 2nd ed. New York: Norton, 1963.

Fleming J., & Altschul, S., "Activation of Mourning and Growth by Psychoanalysis," *International Journal of Psychoanalysis*, 1963, *44*, 419–432.

Fleming, S. J., "Parental Social Adjustment After the Death of a Child." In preparation, 1984.

Freud, S., "Inhibitions, Symptoms and Anxiety" (1926), in *The Standard Edition of the Complete Psychological Works of Sigmund Freud*, translated by J. Strachey, 24 vols. London: Hogarth Press, 1959, Vol. 20, pp. 87–172.

Furman, E., *A Child's Parent Dies*. New Haven, CT: Yale University Press, 1974.

Glaser, B. G., & Strauss, A. L., *Awareness of Dying*. Chicago: Aldine, 1965.

Glaser, B. G., & Strauss, A. L., *Time for Dying*. Chicago: Aldine, 1968.
Hare-Mustin, R. T., "Family Therapy Following the Death of a Child," *Journal of Marital and Family Therapy*, 1979, *5*, 51–59.
Kaffman, M., & Elizur, E., "Children's Bereavement Reactions Following Death of the Father," *International Journal of Family Therapy*, 1979, *1*, 203–229.
Karon, M., & Vernick, J., "Approach to Emotional Support of Fatally-Ill Children," *Clinical Pediatrics*, 1968, *7*, 274–280.
Kerner, J., Harvey, B., & Lewiston, N., "The Impact of Grief: A Retrospective Study of Family Function Following Loss of a Child with Cystic Fibrosis," *Journal of Chronic Disease*, 1979, *32*, 221–225.
Krell, R., & Rabkin, L., "The Effects of Sibling Death on the Surviving Child: A Family Perspective," *Family Process*, 1979, *18*, 471–477.
Lampl-de Groot, J., "Mourning in a Six-Year-Old Girl," *Psychoanalytic Study of the Child*, 1976, *31*, 273–281.
Lansky, S. B., "Childhood Leukemia: The Child Psychiatrist as a Member of the Oncology Team," *Journal of Child Psychiatry*, 1974, *13*, 499–508.
Lindemann, E., "Symptomatology and Management of Acute Grief," *American Journal of Psychiatry*, 1944, *101*, 141–148.
Martinson, I. M., Geis, D., Anglim, M. A., Peterson, E., Nesbit, M., & Kersey, J., "When the Patient is Dying: Home Care for the Child," *American Journal of Nursing*, 1977, *77*, 1815–1817. [See also Chapter 2.]
McConville, B. J., Boag, L. C., & Purohit, A. P., "Mourning Processes in Children of Varying Ages," *Canadian Psychiatric Association Journal*, 1970, *15*, 253–255.
Miller, J. B. M., "Children's Reactions to the Death of a Parent: A Review of the Psychoanalytic Literature," in S. Chess & A. Thomas (Eds.), *Annual Progress in Child Psychiatry and Child Development*, 1972, *5*, 487–506.
Moriarity, D. M. (Ed.), *The Loss of Loved Ones*. Springfield, IL: Charles C Thomas, 1967.
Morrissey, J. R., "Death Anxiety in Children with a Fatal Illness," in H. J. Parad (Ed.), *Crisis Intervention: Selected Readings*. New York: Family Service Association of America, 1965, 324–338.
Mount, B. M., Jones, A., & Patterson, A., "Death and Dying: Attitudes in a Teaching Hospital," *Urology*, 1974, *4*, 741–747.
Nagy, M., "The Child's Theories Concerning Death," *Journal of Genetic Psychology*, 1948, *73*, 3–27.
Parkes, C. M., *Bereavement: Studies of Grief in Adult Life*. New York: International Universities Press, 1972.
Piaget, J., *The Child's Conception of Physical Causality*. London: Routledge & Kegan Paul, 1966.
Rosenblatt, B., "Reactions of Children to the Death of Loved Ones—Some Notes Based on Psychoanalytic Theory," in D. M. Moriarity (Ed.), *The Loss of Loved Ones*. Springfield, IL: Charles C Thomas, 1967, 135–145.
Schiff, H. S., *The Bereaved Parent*. New York: Crown, 1977.
Share, L., "Family Communication in the Crisis of a Child's Fatal Illness," *Omega*, 1972, *3*, 187–201.
Spinetta, J. J., "The Dying Child's Awareness of Death: A Review," *Psychological Bulletin*, 1974, *81*, 256–260.

Spinetta, J. J., Swarner, J. A., & Sheposh, J. P., "Effective Parental Coping Following the Death of a Child from Cancer," *Journal of Pediatric Psychology*, 1981, *6*, 251–263.

Trowhill, A., & Fleming, S. J., "Parental Bereavement: The First Ten Months." Paper presented at the Annual Meeting, Canadian Psychological Association, Calgary, June, 1980.

Vernick, J., & Karon, M., "Who's Afraid of Death on a Leukemia Ward?" *American Journal of Diseases of Children*, 1965, *109*, 393–397.

Waechter, E. H., "Children's Awareness of Fatal Illness," *American Journal of Nursing*, 1971, *71*, 1168–1172.

Weissman, M. M., Prusoff, B. A., Thompson, D., Harding, P. S., & Myers, J. K., "Social Adjustment by Self-Report in a Community Sample and in Psychiatric Out Patients," *Journal of Nervous and Mental Disease*, 1978, *166*, 317–326.

Wilson, D. C., "The Viability of Pediatric Hospices: A Case Study," *Death Education*, 1982, *6*, 205–212. [See also Chapter 1.]

Wolfenstein, M., "How is Mourning Possible?" *Psychoanalytic Study of the Child*, 1966, *21*, 93–123.

Worden, J. W., *Grief Counseling and Grief Therapy*. New York: Springer, 1982.

11

Parental Bereavement

Charles A. Corr, Ida M. Martinson, and Kay L. Dyer

Introduction

We have heard many bereaved parents share the following statement with each other and with those who have not walked in their footsteps. They say: "The death of a parent is the death of my past, the death of a spouse is the death of my present, the death of a child is the death of my future." This statement is intended to drive home the differing impacts of three of the most prominent and typical encounters with death that may occur in a lifetime, and to draw special attention to the situation of the bereaved parent.

In this chapter, we will explore the experience of parental bereavement, especially as it is related to hospice approaches for the care of dying children and their families. In order to place this subject in context, we begin with a brief account of some typical features of grief, bereavement, and mourning. After that, we turn to our specific topic of parental grief and bereavement. This is highlighted by a series of issues that are distinctive of this particular form of bereavement and by data from extensive interviews with bereaved parents as much as two years after the death of their child. Finally, we suggest some principles to guide those who may be in a position to give help and assistance to bereaved parents.

We recognize from the outset that parental bereavement is a sensitive and complex topic. It is a very personal and individual experience, one that touches the whole of a person's life and one that is affected by many variables. Some bereaved parents may find this chapter hurtful insofar as it reopens old wounds. To them we can only offer our deep sympathy and concern. Our apology for proceeding nevertheless is that other bereaved parents may benefit from this discussion and that our society very much needs to learn more about the situation of bereaved parents and about ways to offer constructive assistance.

Grief and Bereavement

A basic premise of all hospice care is that death is a psychosocial and spiritual event, not merely a physical or biological one. All of these dimensions must be recognized and given attention, not just in the dying child but equally in his or her family and friends. Further, while death puts an end to the problems faced by the child who is dying, it raises a new set of issues for those who live on. This is what Toynbee (1968, p. 267) has called the "two-sidedness" of death. Thus, recognition of what is involved in grieving prior to a death and in bereavement thereafter is an essential prerequisite for any effective giving of care.

It is the ties of past relationships that define the character of our losses. Where there has been no relationship, there will be no sense of loss. Similarly, *grief*—the emotional reaction to loss—will be proportioned to the kind of loss experienced and to other relevant variables (Jackson, 1979 & 1957). Thus, a mother who is involved in a difficult labor and delivery that culminates in a dead infant may grieve not only for the loss of her child but also for the death of a part of her very self. By contrast, her husband will also grieve the death of the child, but he will be grateful that his wife is alive and safe. Sometimes it is in the intensity of our grief that we first begin to fully appreciate the depth of our loss and how much the relationship had really meant to us.

Grief is sad, but it is also a natural, healthy, and altogether proper reaction to loss. "To grieve," as Edwin Shneidman has said (1983, p. 29), "is to pay ransom to love." Only those who never love, who live a life of loneliness, estrangement, and isolation, need not grieve. By reaching out in love everyone else is made vulnerable to *bereavement,* that difficult condition of survivors who are forced to go on with their own lives after the death of someone precious. Death, as it were, is a thief who steals the person we love and leaves us sad, forlorn, and bereft.

More precisely, as Parkes (1972) has suggested, bereavement seems to have three components: (1) the initial loss or taking away of the loved person or object; (2) its ongoing deprivation or absence; and quite often (3) a certain stigma or change in social attitudes of the sort experienced by some bereaved parents who are shunned by other young couples who find their presence too painful a reminder that their own children could also die.

Mourning

If grief is the reaction and bereavement the situation consequent upon a death, then *mourning* is the process of management, adaptation, and resolution. Mourning is, as Parkes (1972) has argued, a kind of *realization,* whereby our psyche adapts to or makes real in its own inner universe that which is already real in the outer world. Mourning is the way in which we channel or express our grief—usually in familiar personal and social patterns. Thus, mourning is often ritualistic as in cries of lamentation or customary funeral practices. It is in having the ability to mourn, as Imara (1983) reminds us, that we are blessed or touched by God and can hold on to the promise or expectation of finding comfort. Our hope is in the resources within us and in those that surround us as we move from what has been in the past, and through our grief that now is, to what will be in the future. With this in mind, we will consider in this section common or ordinary patterns in mourning, abnormal grief, the basic tasks of mourning, and its goals.

Dynamics of Grieving

The dynamics of grieving have been conceptualized in many ways (e.g., Westberg, 1962), but the most impressive and widely accepted account is that developed by John Bowlby (1980) and Colin Murray Parkes (1972). This account postulates four phases or dominant dimensions in the mourning process. The first is *shock and numbness,* a common initial reaction when we are confronted by trauma and tragedy, though one which may also recur. This phase is marked by a feeling of being stunned or overwhelmed. Even when a child's death is anticipated, it may be difficult to believe it actually has happened. Life appears as a bad dream from which we expect to awaken. Overall functioning is impeded and it is difficult to make judgments or to maintain concentration. There may be outbursts of intense panic, distress, or anger, but the fundamental characteristic is resistance to stimuli. What Lifton (1967) termed "psychic numbing" in the Japanese survivors of the atomic bombing of

Hiroshima is thus essentially a familiar defense of a besieged and overloaded psyche.

We are told that burn victims most feel pain some time after the initial searing of skin tissue when nerve endings begin to regenerate and function again. So, too, as the shock of a death fades and numbness thaws there is an acute awareness of stimuli. This is called *yearning and searching*. The quite understandable desire to experience once again the presence of the loved child and the search for familiar sights, sounds, and smells associated with the deceased are marked by restlessness, anger, and ambiguity. Like a probe in a raw wound, reexamination of the full scope and impact of the loss is extremely painful. This testing of reality confirms the magnitude and permanence of our loss.

As testing is transformed into awareness of reality, mourners find themselves in the midst of *disorientation and disorganization*. Feelings of depression and loneliness are common. Basic functioning is diminished: with energies depleted one lives in a kind of "slow-motion" universe where sighing, loss of appetite, insomnia, or inability to find restful sleep, and similar somatic disorders are common. Especially during the first year of bereavement there is ample reinforcement for sadness and disorientation as the survivor lives through all of the "first times"—birthdays, holidays, and special times, culminating in the anniversary of the death itself—without the child.

For the vast majority of bereaved people mourning leads in its own time to healthy *reorganization*. This is signaled by the more or less gradual resolution of conflicts. It appears in a growing sense of confidence and an increased ability to function in the tasks of life. One's perspectives become more and more congruent with reality itself. Life can once again be accepted and affirmed, and new challenges undertaken. Drawing on lessons that "came not from schooling but from suffering," Harriet Schiff (1977, pp. xiii & 7) offers a very hard-won truth: "It was only when I could think 'Robby is dead' that I could also think 'but I am alive.' " This is not an abandonment or betrayal of the dead child; rather it is a precondition for realistic respect of the present situation of both parent and child.

Mourning, or "grief work" as it is sometimes called, is a demanding occupation. It is likely to dominate our lives for some time, typically a longer period of time than most people expect (Davidson, 1979). In the disequilibrium of mourning, many people think they are "losing their minds"; that is almost never actually the case. The strength and power of our grief and the truly hard work of mourning are unusual and hard to believe. But they are rarely abnormal. We surprise ourselves both by our capacity to grieve and eventually by our ability to overcome our burdens and to survive.

Abnormal Grief

Abnormal grieving or pathological mourning is difficult to define in any simple way, but it usually centers on excessive, fixated, or dysfunctional behavior. An inability to mourn or conduct that is in some serious way harmful to self or others are more significant indicators of difficulty than tears, tiredness, or paranormal experiences in which one senses the presence of the deceased. Properly speaking, abnormal or complicated grief goes beyond mere prolonged or chronic grief, and this must especially be kept in mind as we learn more and more about the lengthy time that may be involved in resolving unexceptional parental grief (see the forthcoming section titled "Two Years After a Child's Death").

Perhaps more common than frank pathological grieving, but still generally undesirable strategies in bereavement are: either the prompt and complete removal of all traces of the deceased as if she or he never existed in the first place; or the long-term enshrinement of his or her things in an unaltered memorial as if time had stopped and might again go forward when he or she steps back into life. Erasing the deceased or suspending the death indefinitely are techniques to avoid the need to mourn. They do not accord with reality or with the underlying need to come to terms with the loss of a loved child.

Tasks of Mourning

It may be helpful to think of mourning or grief work not only in terms of the broad patterns displayed, but also as a process which involves four interrelated tasks. These four tasks of mourning are (Worden, 1982):

1. To accept the reality of the loss. Effective living deals with realities, not distortions. When death has altered my world and its familiar relationships, both the facts and the meaning of the loss must be faced, acknowledged, and accepted. This is, of course, a task to be undertaken in striving; it is not something accomplished lightly or all at once.
2. To experience the pain of grief. The pain of grief is excruciating. It is one of the most disabling acute pains that humans can experience. Most people are surprised at how hurtful grief really is until they experience it for themselves. It is intense, pervasive, and enduring. In the long run, one surmounts this pain by working with it rather than against it. Our rash tendency to sedate or protect against this pain is often counterproductive. Suppression and avoidance, for example, through drugs or alcohol which mask our true feelings, usually only prolong the course of mourning. After all, death *is* painful for survivors. We cannot wish that

away. By experiencing our pain in tolerable amounts we find that it becomes less fearful.

3. To adjust to an environment in which the deceased is missing. Accepting loss and enduring pain can lead to stagnation. This is seen in a withdrawal from social contacts, a failure to try to develop skills that are needed to cope, and a general tendency to be helpless. Instead, the task is to adapt one's life to the new realities. In support of this task, well-meaning friends often rightly invoke what would have been the intention of the deceased, namely that the beloved survivor should not withdraw from living but continue to go forward and thrive. But adjustment after a rupture, a tearing of the familiar fabric of existence, is difficult. One is never one's old self again. This is aptly symbolized in the Jewish ritual of *keriah,* the rending or tearing asunder of a garment which ought not and in truth cannot ever be completely mended (Gordon, 1974). The task is to become a new self, to achieve a mode of living in which the good days at least outbalance the bad. This work cannot be rushed, as if loss and pain could somehow be bypassed.

4. To withdraw emotional energy and reinvest it in other relationships. There is a tendency to want to cling to a familiar and satisfying relationship that may have been established over many years. The task here, in part, is to loosen the grip or as some say to engage in a "letting go" of the relationship. More precisely, this is to realize that the relationship itself is now a part of our past, fixed in history but no longer actual as it once was in our present. In positive terms, this involves a reexamination and honoring of the lived relationship with the child by identifying and retaining in our memory its good qualities. Though the past is gone, such good memories can never be taken away from us even as we move forward and find meaningfulness and purpose in our new condition.

Goals of Mourning

It is wrong to think of these tasks as defining a process that leads to "forgetting" the deceased loved one or that is likely to come to completion once and for all. Significant relationships like parenthood and events like parental bereavement permanently alter our lives. A child who has died is never forgotten or simply obliterated from our being. The goal of mourning is not forgetfulness but enriched remembrance (Cantor, 1978). The loved one becomes an inner presence with human dimensions, neither an idealized hero nor a maligned villain. There is sadness when we recall the deceased, but not the continuous wrenching pain of mourning. And this sadness is compatible with warmth, tenderness, and good feelings.

The mourning process cannot be artificially accelerated or concluded; it must be given the freedom to find its own rhythms and depth. Time is a necessary, though not a sufficient, condition both for mourning and for the healing of tissue after a physical wound. Resolution is found in our ability to go on with living. But this is a tenuous balance which may be disturbed by some thought or event that recalls our loss to the forefront and evokes new grief. For example, one mother whose son had died five years earlier received in the mail a letter to her son from the Selective Service System wanting to know why he had not registered for the draft. Suddenly, she found herself flooded with tears and unexpected sadness. Even simple questions like, "How many children do you have?", can be the occasion of renewed distress for a bereaved parent. Oftentimes, such people ask: "Why can't I get over this?" In fact, one never really "gets over" a major loss. Rather, one works continuously at accepting and living with its aftermath. What we "get over" is the intensity of mourning. Normally, successive outbreaks of grief become less intense and shorter in duration. That is, as we come to terms with our bereavement more effectively, its pain tends to lessen. As one mother said, if that did not happen we simply could not survive.

The Death of a Child

In the past, the death of an infant or child was a relatively common experience. Though certainly not welcomed, it was an inescapable feature of life to which parents must have been resigned. In our time, things are so different that it is hard for us to imagine the feelings of parents who would conceive ten or 12 offspring only to see most die at birth, in infancy, or in childhood, so that only two or three would live to adulthood (Rosenblatt, 1983). Now parents on the average have only one or two children and many delay parenting for several years in the confident expectation that it is rare for a child to die. Only in an era when mortality rates for children had been drastically reduced could there be so much talk of "unfairness" when a child does die. This language betrays our unspoken assumption that the death of children is an unusual event which "ought" not to happen, as if they were born with a guarantee of long life.

But children do die, and their deaths are perhaps the most difficult events that their parents will ever have to endure (Sanders, 1980). Their deaths undercut so much of what children offer to parents: the preciousness of new life, an opportunity for giving love, a source of status and personal satisfaction, hope for the future, and a symbol of their own immortality and continuity with life. Moreover, while children do die from acute and chronic illnesses, it may be an additional burden for their parents that a relatively high proportion of childhood deaths in our society involve inexplicable origins (like Sudden Infant Death Syndrome), unnatural causes (accidents, homicide, and suicide—the three leading causes of death in adolescence), and congenital disabilities. It is particularly significant, in our judgment, that attention has recently been paid to the full spectrum of parental bereavement from miscarriage, stillbirth, and infant death (DeFrain, Taylor, & Ernst, 1982; Jimenez, 1982; Borg & Lasker, 1981; Peppers & Knapp, 1980; see also pp. 142–144 above) right through childhood and adolescence (Raphael, 1983), though we suggest two relatively new and as yet unexplored phenomena, that of adolescents who themselves become bereaved parents and cases of the adult child in which an elderly parent buries a mature son or daughter.

The death of any child is an individual and highly personal experience for his or her parents. We can only speak of general patterns here, but we recognize that the contours of bereavement will be unique for each case and for each parent. Some of the most significant variables affecting parental bereavement appear to be: the age of the child; whether the death is unexpected or anticipated; its suddenness; the pattern of the child's dying trajectory and whether or not it involved distress from illness or treatment; the individual parent's own personal resources and developed ways of coping with trauma; and the community or social resources available to assist the bereaved parent. Many experienced caregivers believe that the most influential determinants of parental bereavement are the presence or absence of an opportunity for preparation and the intermingling of guilt with grief. These deserve separate attention.

Anticipatory Grief

It is often suggested that sudden, unexpected deaths impose a more difficult coping burden upon survivors than those for which we have advance warning and time to adjust. This depends upon a claim that *anticipatory grief* eases postdeath grief. In fact, the two appear to be different in both form and duration and, in general, anticipatory grief is not a very well-understood clinical or theoretical concept (Fulton & Gottesman, 1980). Perhaps it is enough for us to say here that where time, circumstances, personal coping styles, and social context permit, preparatory grief and adjustment to prospective loss do appear to mitigate postdeath grieving at least in some qualitative respects. And death can be a relief for survivors when it is perceived as a release from the child's long period of suffering and distress. But anticipatory grief is not always possible for many of the very rapid trajectories that characterize childhood death today, and even when it does occur the finality of death is always a shock for which anticipation never wholly prepares us. In some cases, anticipatory grieving can itself become dysfunctional; though what Davidson (1975) has called the "waiting vulture syndrome" can often be avoided by meaningful involvement of parents in the care of their dying child.

Guilt

A related claim is that bereavement is eased when potential survivors have been included in the unit of treatment, that is, have had their own needs attended to while their loved one is dying, and when they have been enabled insofar as possible to help in caring for the dying person. The latter of these points particularly concerns the place of *guilt* in bereavement. Grief and guilt are separate though often intertwined phenomena. Usually, guilt exacerbates grieving. This is true whether the guilt is legitimate or, as is so often the case, unwarranted. In our grief and mourning, we often manufacture unrealistic occasions for guilt. "If I had only thought or done . . .," we say, when no reasonable person could have been expected to think or do such.

Parents find guilt an especially easy burden to assume, and Miles (1984) has identified four prominent forms: causation guilt—something the parents did or failed to do which might have contributed to the cause of their child's death; cultural role guilt—feelings of inadequacy as caregivers, nurturers, and protectors; moral guilt—failings or transgressions which are thought to have led to death as punishment; and survival guilt—whereby, as Frances Gunther (1949) says:

> I think every parent must have a sense of failure, even of sin, merely in remaining alive after the death of a child. One feels that it is not right to live when one's child has died, that one should somehow have found the way to give one's life to save his life. (p. 160)

Late in the mourning process a parent can experience guilt over his or her renewed enjoyment of life. Feelings of guilt can easily be intensified by unthinking comments or accusations from others. Such feelings will be diminished only when they can be disentangled from grief, perceived as the irrational expressions of helplessness and pain which they most often are, and relieved by being expressed and shared. Even when there is legitimate basis for guilt, parents need to learn not to forget but to forgive and have patience with themselves and to come to terms with their own human fallibility and limitations.

A Model of Parental Grieving

A useful model of the broad contours of parental grieving has been developed by Miles (1984; see Figure 11.1). Because this model is based on the general theories outlined above, many of its basic features will already be familiar. Thus, it is not surprising for Miles to speak of the following as experienced by bereaved parents: numbness, shock, disbelief, denial, and unreality; loneliness, emptiness, yearning, and searching; preoc-

Figure 11.1. A Model of Parental Grief

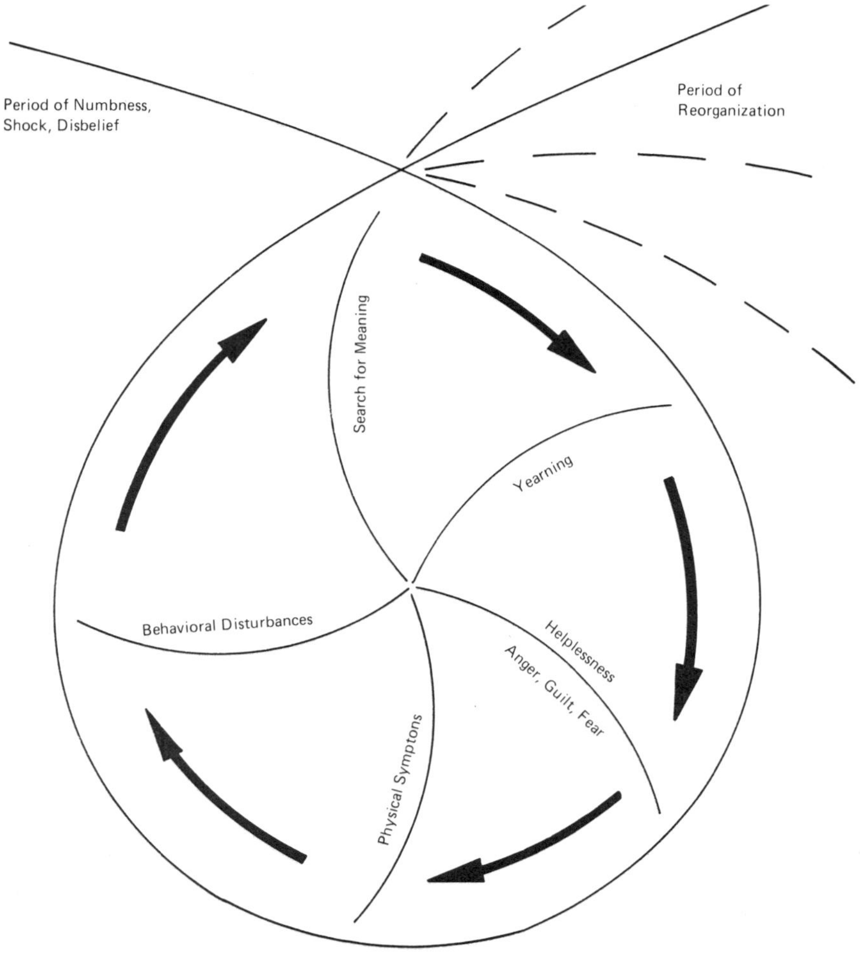

From Margaret S. Miles, "Helping Adults Mourn the Death of a Child." In Hannelore Wass and Charles A. Corr, eds., *Childhood and Death.* Copyright © 1984 by Hemisphere Publishing Corporation. Used by Permission.

cupation with thoughts of the deceased child; helplessness, anger, frustration, guilt, and fear; hostility towards God or individuals with healthy children; a wide variety of physical symptoms, such as poor appetite, insomnia, fatigue, sighing, irritability, headaches, and digestive disturbances; behavioral changes, such as inability to concentrate, disorganization, restlessness, confusion of thought processes, and a tendency either to withdraw or to become hyperactive; fear of going crazy; and an overriding search for some purpose or meaning in the child's death.

Nevertheless, this model does have several important advantages. First, it only postulates three phases in mourning: a period of numbness and shock; a period of intense grief (incorporating both what have previously been called dimensions of yearning and searching, and of disorganization and disorientation); and a period of reorganization and recovery. A tripartite division of this sort rightly tends to focus attention on the dominant central period here termed "active" or "intense" grief in which one may easily become stuck and remain spinning around without purpose for a relatively long time. Second, this model attempts to avoid "staging" grief or dividing it into a progressive linear order by emphasizing the shading of expression into one another both within and between periods. Especially in the period of intense grief, the model explicitly acknowledges that feelings, symptoms, and behaviors may occur and recur at any time either separately or simultaneously. The image chosen to represent this is a wheel or kaleidoscope of tumbling manifestations. And third, the model indicates that when and as it occurs reorganization may have several outcomes. In resolution, most parents, according to Miles, find themselves at roughly the same level of growth and development as before their loss, though some may grow while others deteriorate in their status.

Some Ramifications of Parental Bereavement

Thus far, we have mostly discussed parental bereavement as an individual or intrapsychic phenomenon. It is, of course, also an interpersonal and social experience, one which may have ramifications for marital relationships, for relations between parents and surviving siblings, for grandparents, and for others. Some discussion of each of these will be helpful.

Marital Relationships

In many family crises, including other sorts of deaths, only one partner is primarily involved emotionally while the spouse is available as a significant source of support. After a child dies, however, both parents are bereaved. Their loss is both shared and unique. To the degree that it is shared, both are wounded and bereft. To the degree that it is unique, each will grieve in his or her own personal way. One may become withdrawn while the other acts out strong feelings, one may be angry and the other depressed, one may cry while the other turns away from tears. If they are tolerant of each other's differing rhythms in mourning, each may be a source of strength and support to the other at different times. However, it often happens that the pain of each is so great that neither can help the other very much. Those experiencing intense grief may lack the resources to be available to a mate and may even find that the needs and behavior of a spouse only add to their own pain and isolation. Synchronicity is jeopardized in what would otherwise be a balanced dyadic relationship.

In other words, stress can have diverse effects both on individuals and on social relationships. A good deal has been said about high rates of separation and divorce among bereaved parents; some claim an incidence of 70 to 80 percent. We think these figures are not very reliable and we believe it fair to question in many cases whether the parting can be traced directly or solely to the child's death. In our view, the death of a child may drive the surviving parents together or it may push them apart. Much depends on the quality of the relationship prior to the death. The key is how, individually and jointly, they handle their feelings and communicate with each other. Anger and guilt are two dominant issues that must be faced and worked through.

It is also popularly asserted that fathers grieve differently than mothers. That is, in our society men are said to be socially conditioned not to express their feelings, while women are granted freer disclosure. Further, husbands are often encouraged to "be brave" or "be strong" for their wives. No doubt there is truth in these observations. But it is wise not to rely too heavily upon stereotypes nor to construct them too simply. Our concern is for individual bereaved parents with all of their personal characteristics and variations, not for gender models. And the pregnant mother mentioned above who is engaged in a difficult delivery that ends in a dead infant was at risk in fact and in her husband's eyes in a way that he never was in her view. Both will grieve the dead child, but the full panorama of their feelings will inevitably be different. Husbands are often compelled by force of circumstance to return promptly to work with its diversions and pressures that repress mourning, while nonworking wives may well find themselves at home with more occasion to dwell on and express their feelings. Single and divorced parents who are bereaved will face special difficulties and complexities that cannot be addressed here.

Siblings

Intensely-felt grief over the death of a child may render a bereaved parent incapable of offering much help to a surviving sibling. Even parents who are able to support and comfort each other may neglect other members of the family. This is often reinforced by adult assumptions that children are too young to understand death or to feel the sadness of grief. The grief of children is considered elsewhere in this book (see Chapter 10), but it is surely nonsense to think that a surviving child is not affected by the death of a brother or sister, as well as by the nonavailability or withdrawal of one or both parents. Children keenly sense the emotional currents with in a family, they have a right to share in its sadness as well as in its happiness, and their needs deserve full attention. Sometimes relatives and friends other than the parents can help to fill in here, but often only a parent will do despite his or her own grief. Further, an understandable preoccupation with the child who has died—especially when that follows upon a lengthy process of dying that demanded much in parental time and energy—may lead surviving children to conclude that by comparison they are of little worth.

Just as no one can replace or become the dead child, a surviving sibling has a right to live his or her own life and to have legitimate needs satisfied. Parents should be encouraged neither to neglect surviving siblings nor to smother them with what is all-too-often a guilt-driven overintensity. By attempting to maintain an honest and responsive relationship with surviving children, bereaved parents will benefit themselves in the end. It may seem burdensome to require a bereaved parent to be available to his or her surviving child. But children call us back to life in a wholesome fashion. And a child can often be a significant source of comfort and support to a grieving parent. Needs and manifestations of grief may differ in parents and in children, but it is foolish to assume that life-giving love and consolation only flow from the elder to the younger generation.

Grandparents and Others

Grandparents, a favorite aunt or uncle, a teacher, the mother for whom a young girl used to babysit, a high school boy's former employer—these and others too varied to mention may all be affected by the death of a child (Gyulay, 1975). It will be enough here to concentrate on grandparents as perhaps the most visible and noteworthy of these oft-forgotten grievers. Our point for any of the members of this group is simply to note that they may form attachments to the child for which death also brings loss, grief, and mourning.

In particular for grandparents, grandchildren are special and precious. This is true whether the grandparents are involved in the child's daily care or are free to take delight without the burdens previously incurred in raising their own children. Relationships are inevitably a bit complicated since they jump across an intervening generation and involve a son- or daughter-in-law, and because a grandparent is usually not the child's primary caregiver and guardian. So grandparents are at once entangled and removed. They will grieve the loss of the child through death, as well as the "unnaturalness" of surviving their own offspring's children. And they will bear a kind of double grief for the ache being experienced by the child's parents and siblings.

Like other grievers, grandparents can help or hinder parental bereavement. Thoughtless comments, questions, or accusations which spring from the grandparent's own pain, helplessness, and frustration can deeply wound a vulnerable parent. Equally, grandparents can be an abundant source of support, encouragement, and practical assistance. Often there are few outlets through which grandparents and significant others can share or express their grief. The death of the grandchild may reactivate an unresolved loss from the past or may add to the bereavement overload experienced by some elderly people in the present. We encourage bereaved parents and grandparents to be sensitive to each other's needs and feelings, and to draw upon the mutual aid which each has to offer the other. We remind helpers to take note of the grief of grandparents and significant others in the larger circle of bereavement that emanates from a child's death, and to include them where possible in the creation of a healing community.

Two Years After a Child's Death

In the Home Care Project described in Chapter 2, interviews were conducted with parents 24 months after the death of their child (Martinson, Nesbit, & Kersey, in press; Martinson, Moldow, & Henry, 1980). The parents interviewed represented 54 of the 58 families served by the Project in its initial two-year period. Selected results from these interviews may further our appreciation of parental bereavement, especially as it follows upon a hospice-type service of the sort discussed in this book. For example, when asked about conversation concerning the dead child almost 60 percent of these parents reported either that they talk about the child "all the time" or that they had talked about the child within the preceeding 24 hours. Further, while only 28 percent reported that the deceased child is mentioned within the family or by others daily or practically every day, another 32 percent reported that the child naturally occurs in conversation within the family. Clearly, for many the name and memory of the dead child is a familiar presence in their lives, even though others are still having difficulty talking about their child two years after his or her death.

Two particularly revealing questions offer insight into the duration of these parents' bereavement. The first asked parents if they felt they had returned to their normal life style. Of the 88 parents responding, 74 (84 percent) replied that they had returned to their normal life style. Comments made by the 14 (16 percent) parents who replied in the negative included the following:

> We're back to the routine but not the normal, because your life is never the same. You're not the same person because so much has happened.

> No, I don't think so. It's too deep in my soul and myself. He had changed my whole life and my perspective in life.

> I don't think you ever do. There's always kind of something missing. I think you live more in the past than you ever did because you want to think of things you did in the past.

The second question asked parents to identify when the most intense time of their bereavement was over. Responses shown in Table 11.1 indicate wide variability across parents. Over one-fifth reported that the most intense time of their bereavement was not yet over at 24 months after the child's death. Another one-fourth indicated that the most intense time of their bereavement was not over until 12 to 18 months after the child's death. It would appear also from responses to this question that there is some difference between mothers and fathers on this point. That is, fathers were more than twice as likely as mothers to report that the most intense part of their bereavement was over within a few weeks

Table 11.1. Parents' Responses 24 Months After Child's Death to Question: When Was the Most Intense Time of Your Bereavement Over? (Mothers versus Fathers)

	Mothers		Fathers		Total	
	Number	Percent	Number	Percent	Number	Percent
First few weeks	5	9.4	4	12.9	9	10.7
One month	2	3.8	5	16.1	7	8.3
Three months	6	11.3	5	16.1	11	13.1
Six months	8	15.1	1	3.2	9	10.7
1–1½ years	14	26.4	7	22.6	21	25.0
Not yet over	12	22.6	5	16.1	17	20.2
Unsure	6	11.3	4	12.9	10	11.9
Total	53	99.9	31	99.9	84	99.9

to one month after the child's death. Clearly, for a substantial portion of these home care parents, intense bereavement is a long-term process which includes some disruption of the family's normal routine.

When asked 24 months after their child's death how they felt they had adjusted, 73 (86 percent) of the 85 parents responding said they had adjusted fairly well, that they had accepted their child's death. The remaining 12 parents (14 percent) felt they had not adjusted well. Some of the comments from this latter group are:

> We have a lot of trouble making decisions about anything. We listen to our friends and end up doing something we don't like to do.

> It just seemed like it was never going to end and it's never going to get better, so I don't care. It's like you want to give into it and the heck with the whole world.

> I feel kind of an apathy for a lot of things that I used to have more spirit for.

Self-ratings of present level of coping with grief on a 1–10 scale roughly accord with these responses, with 71 percent of the parents rating their coping at the three highest or best levels of coping.

Parents were also asked whether there was anything they could not do 24 months after the child's death. Of the 87 parents responding to this question, 59 (69 percent) reported there was nothing they couldn't do. Four parents said they could not go to the hospital where their child had been treated, three others said they couldn't attend funerals (one of these specifically mentioned funerals of children), three said they could not prepare or eat some foods that their deceased child had enjoyed, and three parents said they could not look at pictures of the child. One mother related that her husband cannot watch television shows which deal with cancer, and another mother said it was difficult to visit the child's grave. Still another said she could not decide whether to have another baby. Two couples referred to difficulties in going out with other couples. One of these couples said they could not go out with other couples because of conversations about children, while the other said they could only go out when other couples were present. Five other parents each said they could not do specific things that were closely related to the deceased child. These ranged from caring for the child's horse to reading the diary kept during the child's illness. Again, these data leave the impression of adequate coping by a large proportion of the parents and wide variability among the group who express some difficulties.

During the interviews 24 months after the child's death, parents were asked whether their grief had interfered with their ability to function in their daily activities (i.e., their job or their management of the home) in the 12 months preceding the interview. A sizable proportion—84 percent of the 86 parents responding—answered that their grief had not interfered in the past 12 months, but there was wide variation among the minority responses from the parents who answered affirmatively. These included the following comments:

> I don't have an interest in anything anymore. Everything seems like it's such a hassle.
>
> We had trouble making decisions in our daily life. It was hard to manage our house or to work.
>
> I'm not as good a mother or a housekeeper because I don't feel like getting things done. I have all these feelings inside me.

Several questions during this interview related to the effect of the parents' grief on their employment. Only six (7 percent) of the 86 parents responding said there had been days in the 12 months preceding the interview when they could not go to work. Even among these six, only one parent indicated he had missed more than one or two days in the preceding 12 months because of his grief. However, one-third (34 percent) of the parents said there had been days when they went to work but did not get much done because of their grief. Finally, parents were asked whether they had had a change in employment in the preceding 12 months. While 23 of the 100 parents on whom data are available changed employment, there were no cases where anyone had to stop working as a consequence of his or her grief. Except for one father who retired and one mother who quit work because she had a baby, all other changes were the result of changing jobs or of entering the labor market. In particular, ten mothers had begun new part- or full-time jobs in the previous 12 months.

It is important to note that all of these data derive from parents who had chosen to be involved in the Home Care Project. From that and with the support of the Project, one might have judged them to be a favored group better disposed to a positive mourning process and satisfactory bereavement outcome than many other groups of bereaved parents. For most the outcome does seem good. But it clearly took a good deal of time and, even for the majority, was not without significant difficulty. And there is a sizeable minority that reports additional difficulties and a mourning process that is not yet complete at two years after their child's death.

Some Suggestions for Helping

In our experience, no intervention is more helpful for bereaved parents than a caring human presence. This may be the presence of a spouse, a surviving child, the deceased child's grandparent, a friend, another previously-bereaved parent, a hospice caregiver, a clergyperson, or a concerned funeral director. Rarely are professional counselors or therapists required, and, if so, their involvement is usually of short duration. This is so, as we have stressed throughout this chapter, because despite the great pain entailed in parental bereavement, productive mourning is a normal human process well within the capacities of most of us.

Many potential helpers are paralyzed by not knowing what to do or say. They worry that they might make a mistake, and as a result they do the worst thing of all by withdrawing and neither doing nor saying anything. In fact, it is mostly superficiality and thoughtlessness that lead us astray. Sincere caring is never misplaced, almost always welcomed, and usually manages to find something constructive to offer to a bereaved parent. This is well recognized by Arthur Smith (1974), himself an Episcopal priest and a bereaved parent, who sets the tone for helpers in the following way:

> Death is not a private affair. Except for rare instances, every death affects many people in varying ways. The entire community is, or should be, involved in helping those affected most to resume a normal life. This should never take the form of trying to erase the memories or the hurt, rather it should enable those hurt most to accept death as a normal, inevitable, and necessary part of our humanity. (p. 55)

We encourage helpers of all sorts to make a gift of their presence to bereaved parents, to practice "active listening," and not to offer facile "answers" intended to wipe away the parent's grief. What is required is much more a matter of general attitude or outlook, than a set of formulae to be memorized, quick tricks to be learned, or definable skills. Thus, active listening is essentially a posture of attentive receptivity, a readiness to affirm the legitimacy of the grief being felt, and a concern for the deep feelings that underlie spoken words or other surface manifestations. Almost always, less talking is required of helpers than listening. Frequently, helpers who are not themselves also actively grieving can find the patience more easily than other bereaved persons to listen to the constant reiteration of events and feelings that are part of healthy realization and adaptation. If one wishes to do something helpful, then take a specific action—bake cookies, run an errand, babysit with surviving children—rather than vaguely request the bereaved parents to "call me, if you need anything."

For many, grieving is a process of anguish and questioning, a time of fluid emotions and rapid changes of focus. Personal values and faith commitments are often thrown into doubt (e.g., Claypool, 1974). Helpers need to be sufficiently secure in their own fundamental convictions so as not to be threatened by this and to see it for what it really is. The cry of an aching heart is often only the quest of a bereaved person for a return to a reaffirmation of hope, trust, and belief. In this vein, helpers encountering grieving people whose anger is projected onto God are wisely advised not to rise in defense since God can take care of Himself.

One mother in the film, "When a Child Dies" (1980) mentions the comfort she derived from a neighbor whom she sees only about once a month. She says that this neighbor invariably mentions her deceased son—not because the neighbor read in a book to do that, but because it is a normal thing to mention a parent's child. It is appropriate for helpers to mention the deceased child naturally in conversation, and thereby to affirm the meaningfulness of his or her life. We are usually wrong to maintain an unnatural silence about the child and the death, as if bereaved parents would forget their pain if we did not refer to its source. Many bereaved parents have reported that in death they lost their child and in the silence of their friends they felt threatened by the erasure of his or her public memory. For similar reasons, presence at or shortly after the death, an opportunity to hold or have time with the dead child, and perhaps permission to wash or dress the body for the funeral can all be significant factors in confirming the reality of loss. Down through the ages the rituals of funeral practice have marked death as an event to which attention must be paid and they have affirmed a closure to life which is important for survivors in their mourning process.

While positive suggestions for helpers are more in the form of a general orientation or approach, negative advice can be much more specific. Don't say, "I know how you feel," unless you really have walked in the very same path. Don't try to give answers to unanswerable questions. "He died because God wanted him," or "She is in heaven because God loves her," are all-too-facile and potentially misleading. Don't say, "Well, you have other children," for no surviving child or new baby, however loved, replaces the deceased child. When we discount grieving we unwittingly trivialize the death. Don't alter basic patterns of behavior; act normally and honestly in dealing with bereaved parents. Don't overprotect. Well-meaning but misguided protectionism is at the root of a good deal of foolishness in dealing with grieving people. When in doubt, ask the mourners. Let them guide you as to how to help. Give them options from which to choose, but let them select their own course. Don't suppress or sedate tears and mourning—especially not because they make nonmourners uncomfortable. That merely drives grief into a closet of further loneliness and isolation. "Look how well she's taking it," when said in front of the bereaved parent may actually overlook deep hurt inside and tacitly encourage further repression. Of course, one should also advise not forcing words or tears when they are not needed. Perhaps all of this is summed up in the title of a book by Doug Manning (1979), *Don't Take My Grief Away From Me.* Helpers should respect the legitimate needs of bereaved parents, act as their touchstone for reality, and simply be available as mourning discovers its own route to healing. As Stephens (1973) has said: "Grief only becomes a tolerable and creative experience when love enables it to be shared with somebody who really understands" (p. 53).

Self-help groups like The Compassionate Friends (TCF) and Candlelighters (see Chapter 12), together with other community resources, can be of great value for many bereaved parents. As Ronnie Peterson (1983, p. 9) has written, "the most important things that TCF offers are the endless capacity to listen with true empathy, and the reassurance that one is not 'going crazy.' " We heartily commend such sources of assistance and their great good work, even though we realize that no single resource is universally appropriate for such an individualized experience as parental bereavement. Many people have written about their own bereavement or the bereavement of others, both as therapy for themselves and as assistance for others (e.g., Donnelly, 1982). Helpful literature is also available both for bereaved parents (e.g., Tengbom, 1981; Miles, 1978) and for those who wish to help children deal with death (e.g., Wass & Corr, 1984; Jackson, 1965). At the proper time, such literature can be very useful, as can a constructive project into which energies can be directed.

Conclusion

Those who are not themselves bereaved parents cannot claim to know what the experience feels like from the inside. They can only seek to understand as much as is possible from the outside, and to reach out in tenderness and concern to fellow human beings. In so doing, their efforts may not appear to have much result or, perhaps, even to be appreciated. But they can at least learn to try not to add unwittingly to the hurt of a bereaved parent. They may also find ways to listen and to just be present in a time of trial. Those who aid bereaved parents in these ways may make living a little less onerous by recreating a caring human community. At the same time, helpers are likely to encounter their own limitations and vulnerability. This is difficult, but it is not undesirable. For it is in knowing our own finitude and capacity for pain that we take the measure of our humanity. And it is in helping others that we make it possible for them to help us; it is in giving freely to others that we receive back the most precious of all rewards.

References

Borg, S., & Lasker, J., *When Pregnancy Fails: Families Coping with Miscarriage, Stillbirth, and Infant Death.* Boston: Beacon Press, 1981.

Bowlby, J., *Loss: Sadness and Depression.* Vol. 3 in *Attachment and Loss.* London: Hogarth Press, 1980.

Cantor, R. C., *And a Time to Live: Toward Emotional Well Being During the Crisis of Cancer.* New York: Harper & Row, 1978.

Claypool, J., *Tracks of a Fellow Struggler: How to Handle Grief.* Waco, TX: Word Books, 1974.

Davidson, G. W., "Hospice Care for the Dying," in H. Wass (Ed.), *Dying: Facing the Facts.* New York: McGraw-Hill/Hemisphere, 1979, pp. 158–181.

Davidson, G. W., "The Waiting Vulture Syndrome," in B. Schoenberg, I. Gerber, A. Wiener, A. H. Kutscher, D. Peretz, & A. C. Carr (Eds.)., *Bereavement: Its Psychosocial Aspects.* New York: Columbia University Press, 1975, pp. 357–361.

DeFrain, J. D., Taylor, J., & Ernst, L., *Coping with Sudden Infant Death.* Lexington, MA: Lexington Books, Health, 1982.

Donnelly, K. F., *Recovering From the Loss of a Child.* New York: Macmillan, 1982.

Fulton, R., & Gottesman, D. J., "Anticipatory Grief: A Psychosocial Concept Reconsidered," *British Journal of Psychiatry,* 1980, *137,* 45–54.

Gordon, A., "The Psychological Wisdom of the Law," in J. Riemer (Ed.), *Jewish Reflections on Death.* New York: Schocken Books, 1974, pp. 95–104.

Gunther, F., "A Word From Frances," in J. Gunther, *Death Be Not Proud: A Memoir.* New York: Harper & Row, 1949, pp. 155–161.

Gyulay, J., "The Forgotten Grievers," *American Journal of Nursing,* 1975, *75,* 1476–1479.

Imara, M., "Growing Through Grief," in C. A. Corr & D. M. Corr (Eds.), *Hospice Care: Principles and Practice.* New York: Springer; London: Faber and Faber, 1983, pp. 249–265.

Jackson, E. N., "Bereavement and Grief," in H. Wass (Ed.), *Dying: Facing the Facts.* New York: McGraw-Hill/Hemisphere, 1979, pp. 256–281.

Jackson, E. N., *Telling a Child About Death.* New York: Hawthorn, 1965.

Jackson, E. N., *Understanding Grief: Its Roots, Dynamics, and Treatment.* Nashville, TN: Abingdon, 1957.

Jimenez, S. L. M., *The Other Side of Pregnancy: Coping with Miscarriage and Stillbirth.* Englewood Cliffs, NJ: Prentice-Hall, 1982.

Lifton, R. J., *Death in Life: Survivors of Hiroshima.* New York: Random House, 1967.

Manning, D., *Don't Take My Grief Away From Me.* Hereford, TX: In-Sight Books, Inc., 1979.

Martinson, I. M., Nesbit, M. E., & Kersey, J. H., "Parents at 24 Months After Death of a Child From Cancer," *Cancer Nursing,* in press.

Martinson, I. M., Moldow, D. G., & Henry, W. F., *Home Care of the Child with Cancer*. Final Report: Grant CA 19490, HHS, National Cancer Institute. Minneapolis, MN: School of Nursing, University of Minnesota, 1980.

Miles, M. S., *The Grief of Parents When a Child Dies*. 1978; 1980: The Compassionate Friends, Inc., P.O. Box 1347, Oak Brook, IL 60521.

Miles, M. S., "Helping Adults Mourn the Death of a Child," in H. Wass & C. A. Corr (Eds.), *Childhood and Death*. New York: McGraw-Hill/Hemisphere, 1984, pp. 219–241.

Parkes, C. M., *Bereavement: Studies of Grief in Adult Life*. London: Tavistock, 1972.

Peppers, L. G., & Knapp, R. J., *Motherhood and Mourning: Perinatal Death*. New York: Praeger, 1980.

Peterson, R., "The Compassionate Friends," *Forum for Death Education and Counseling Newsletter*, 1983, *6* (8), pp. 9–10.

Raphael, B., *The Anatomy of Bereavement*. New York: Basic Books, 1983.

Rosenblatt, P. C., *Bitter, Bitter Tears: Nineteenth-Century Diarists and Twentieth-Century Grief Theories*. Minneapolis, MN: University of Minnesota Press, 1983.

Sanders, C. M., "A Comparison of Adult Bereavement in the Death of a Spouse, Child and Parent," *Omega*, 1980, *10*, 303–321.

Schiff, H. S., *The Bereaved Parent*. New York: Crown, 1977.

Schneidman, E. S., "Reflections on Contemporary Death," in C. A. Corr, J. M. Stillion, & M. C. Ribar (Eds.), *Creativity in Death Education and Counseling*. Lakewood, OH: Forum for Death Education and Counseling, 1983, pp. 27–34.

Smith, A. A., *Rachel*. Wilton, CT: Morehouse-Barlow, 1974.

Stephens, S., *Death Comes Home*. Wilton, CT: Morehouse-Barlow, 1973.

Tengbom, M., *Help for Bereaved Parents*. St. Louis, MO: Concordia Publishing House, 1981.

Toynbee, A., "The Relation Between Life and Death, Living and Dying," in A. Toynbee, A. K. Mant, N. Smart, J. Hinton, S. Yudkin, E. Rhode, R. Heywood, & H. H. Price, *Man's Concern with Death*. New York: McGraw-Hill, 1968, pp. 259–271.

Wass, H., & Corr, C. A. (Eds.), *Helping Children Cope with Death: Guidelines and Resources* (2nd ed.). New York: Hemisphere, 1984.

Westberg, G. E., *Good Grief: A Constructive Approach to the Problem of Loss*. Philadelphia, PA: Fortress Press, 1962.

"When a Child Dies." (Film) Color, 23 minutes, 1980. Distributed by the National Funeral Directors Association.

Worden, J. W., *Grief Counseling and Grief Therapy: A Handbook for the Mental Health Practitioner*. New York: Springer, 1982.

12

Self-Help Groups: Grieving Parents and Community Resources

Dennis Klass

The Making of Community

Care of the dying and grieving has always been an occasion for mobilizing communities. Whether it is the neighborhood casserole brigade during the crisis of illness or the roomful of family and friends at the *shiva* or wake, one of the few constants in the way all cultures deal with death and dying is that the responsibilities are assumed to be broader than just for the immediate family. Indeed, hospice—though it is now becoming a more professionalized affair—has its roots in the old custom of giving hospitality to those outside of one's immediate kin group. Death is the maker of community, for in sharing the suffering of dying or the healing of grief individuals find the common bonds that unite them and call them to the shared meanings which become the reason for living itself.

The death of children is a special occasion for the mobilization of the community. In the past—and in some places today—the death of a child may have meanings different than it does in our contemporary culture. In our grandparents' generation, the young child was as much at risk as a retired person is today. With terrifying regularity epidemics carried away the very young. Some people have asked if the reason families have fewer children today is because of their lack of fear of losing a child. When a child dies today it seems as an intrusion on normal reality. We do not look on children today as fragile vessels of life. When, therefore, we turn our attention to the death of children, it is not surprising that we find a community mobilized to care for the tragedy of childhood death and for the spiritual and emotional pilgrimage that is the resolution of this most difficult of griefs.

But communities mobilize in different ways and at diverse levels. Thus, professional health care tends to be organized around patterns that reflect sufficient demand for services to sustain provider organizations. Even in hospice programs that specialize in care for the dying, the "normal" model for death has most often been that of a relatively slow trajectory caused by cancer at a fairly advanced age. So, too, grief has frequently been understood primarily as an experience of widowhood or the feelings of an adult child. Parental grief seems different and calls for different community responses.

For the most part, help offered to dying children and to their survivors tends to take the form of peer-to-peer rather than professional-to-client relationships. The reasons for this are partly because families have been thrown back on their own resources in a society which does not accept the death of a child as normal. Thus few formal services have been available. In their isolation, the dying and the bereaved have turned to each other and have found ways of helping each other to live and to grow. At the same time, these services also tend to be peer-to-peer because in many cases families have found that professional help has not been of much assistance to them.

There are, then, several themes that underlie the work of this chapter. Those who are concerned with care for the dying and the bereaved need not begin wholly from scratch. In every community, they will find already existing patterns of formal and informal networks. And in many places there will be groups and organizations, often with by-laws, well-developed styles of service, and national or international affiliations. Our obligations are to learn from the strengths of these groups and organizations, to give them our assistance in their work, and to build upon a whole supportive series of networks within the society at large. We will not do that if we limit our attention only to the "normal" death, if we ignore situations involving children, or if we attempt to co-opt successful lay volunteer organizations. In particular, for childhood death and parental bereavement, the opportunity is for us to join a movement to make this most unacceptable of events an occasion for growth and for building ties between people, rather than the source of bitter isolation and a withering of the inner self.

Self-Help Groups

This chapter will discuss self-help groups for the parents of dying and dead children. "Self-help" may be defined as groups composed of individuals sharing a common condition, symptom, or experience. The groups are self-governing and use consensus rather than hierarchical decision making. Distinctions within the organization of helpers and helpees are a matter of degree. The groups tend to engage in a wide variety of activities, including newsletters, resource libraries, informal subgroupings, outreach, community education, and meetings for sharing and helping each other (Lieberman, et al., 1979). The "grandfather" of self-help is Alcoholics Anonymous and the subgroups it has spun off. It is the addiction to the drug and the attempt to overcome dependence that is the requisite for AA membership. It is the insight based on the personal fight against addiction that forms the knowledge base which helps others fight their addiction. In self-help, the professional role, especially when compared to counseling or psychotherapy, is radically deemphasized. Self-help groups primarily value the experience of those who have successfully completed the process.

Self-help is different from the "support groups" which have become popular in various kinds of grief, for example, widow support groups. Two important distinctions can be made between support groups and self-help groups. First, in the support group, predetermined outcomes are established and the leader attempts to achieve those outcomes with a minimum of obvious coercion. If the leader does not claim superior status by his or her professional credentials, superior status is supplied by a specific training. Second, the support group defines the members as victims or in some other way as being in a dependent position. The client may graduate from that status, and graduation may be to leadership status, but there is always a distinction between those being helped and those helping. Usually the support group is offered as a service of an agency, whereas the self-help group is self-sustaining and relies on donations of friends and members. Some self-help groups also raise funds for the health care facility in which children of members are treated.

Two groups will be used as examples in this discussion: the Candlelighters, parents of children with cancer, and The Compassionate Friends (TCF), parents of children who have died. Many of the families who find their way to Candlelighters do not have a child die, for remissions and cures are increasingly common. But death may be a possibility, and as the hope of cure fades the group has found ways of supporting the child and family through the death of the child. The Compassionate Friends welcomes parents no matter the age or cause of death, so many in that group will have suffered the sudden death of someone close to them. These are two outstanding organizations with which we need to be familiar. There are, however, in each community many other formal and informal networks, so each "catchment area" must be investigated to find those local networks.

How Self-Help Works and How Others Can Help

The Self-Help Trajectory

While it may seem more logical to begin with the process of dying and then turn to issues in bereavement, the ambivalent place dying and bereavement play in the lives of parents of children with cancer creates some dynamics which complicate our account of that process. We will therefore first look at The Compassionate Friends and then turn our attention to Candlelighters.

Perhaps the best way to introduce The Compassionate Friends is to let a member describe her experience. Fran Cooper has completed the Compassionate Friends trajectory. That is, she has moved through the spectrum of possible relationships a member can have to the group. She began as a reluctant new attender and is now one of the leaders in the organization. She has, through her participation, found a positive resolution to the issues presented in her grief.

> I have five children; Cory, my youngest, was twelve when he was killed. He was hit by a truck. At the time I had three children still living at home and my husband and I were back together after a separation. We began divorce proceedings a year later. Cory had been just standing at the corner straddling his bike waiting for the traffic to pass when the truck swung out too far for a turn and hit him. I know I am not the only parent to say this, but Cory was a very special child. He charmed everyone with his outgoing personality, big glasses, and golden blond hair.
>
> A policeman came to tell us. I can't describe the impact of that moment, the pain and total chaos. When I came back from identifying Cory, all the kids were home within an hour. Each of them was close to Cory, so they were all bouncing off the walls in their agony.
>
> Through the visitation and funeral I was in a state of shock and probably remained that way for the next six months. I've always been considered a strong person and I managed to make plans and keep functioning, but I've never been so totally vulnerable and helpless in my life. In my struggle to continue to appear "strong," I remember saying to the Boy Scout honor guards, "Stop crying and put your head up! We are going to get through this." And we did. But each day I would

wake up thinking it was all a nightmare and then reality would hit me and absolutely overwhelm me. You don't want to hurt like that and you don't want every waking moment consumed with painful remembrances, but you are totally helpless and consumed by your grief. It was a time when our family began to get disrupted anyhow due to the kids' ages and leaving home. This was the straw that caused the ultimate disruption. There has never been a sense of unity or organization here since. I quit my job but my boss begged me not to quit but to take off as long as I wanted. My husband went back to work after three days, worked for two days and quit. We tried being home for two weeks and then I decided to go back to work. I was a zombie and it was a couple of weeks before I could get through a set of orders without having to walk out because I was crying. It wasn't until about six months that the reality hit me that Cory was *never* coming back. In some ways it was harder and the painful memories were still daily, but by then I had also made the decision that I was going to get through this.

I went to a Compassionate Friends meeting two months after Cory died. I think someone had sent me a sympathy card with a notice of the group inside. At the time though, I didn't want any association with a whole group of bereaved parents. I wasn't one of them! Someday I would wake up and this would all be gone. They sent me a newsletter that dealt with "Getting Through the Holidays." I was so angry that I tore it up! How could anyone think about "getting through" the holidays, let alone write about it? There were not going to be any holidays for me! Finally out of sheer desperation I had to try something. I couldn't survive the way I was going. I had lost 15 to 20 pounds and the doctor was angry with me that I wouldn't take any tranquilizers. But I couldn't function when I took his pills.

I don't remember too much about the first meeting except that I decided I wasn't going back—but I did. People talked about how it gets better and how there are good days and the memories become good ones, but obviously they didn't love their children as much as I loved Cory. That's really what I thought. There was no way to convince me at the time that things might get better.

For the first three or four meetings, I just stored their words of hope and advice for later, because I wasn't ready to accept them at the time. Then I noticed that Joyce, whose child was killed a month before mine, was beginning to heal. I wanted desperately to be like her. I didn't know what to do to make it any better, but decided I was going to try.

Compassionate Friends helps because it is the only place you can go and talk about your grief and your child as openly as you want. No one is going to make any judgments on you about how you are handling the situation. They reassure you that there is no "right way or wrong way." Whatever helps *you* the most is the right way. You take all the information and sift through it for what you need. Also, where else can you go to discuss what become major issues such as "When someone asks how many children you have, what do you say?"

> Between six months and a year, my motive for going to TCF changed from "taking" to "giving back"—not that I ever quit getting something from the group. Often old issues come up that aren't totally resolved or could be handled better. It seems to make the healing complete. You know, it seems when you feel like you are drowning in grief you reach out frantically and grab to whatever you can. Some grab hold of something, TCF for instance, and learn to swim. Some sink and some just float. It is hard to know who will do what. The people that just float learn to glide over the top of their pain and are not willing to go down and dredge up old wounds. You wonder what the long term consequences are though. Then some people are just takers. They go as long as they can take, but aren't willing to give back. I find that giving to others in the group is a healing in itself. It helps to give some purpose to Cory's death. At one point, I decided that he couldn't be completely happy in heaven while he knew I was so unhappy.
>
> My husband went to the group simply to please me and he went after the divorce probably as a way of holding on to me. That was so uncomfortable that I stopped going for awhile, but then went back. I don't attend now because my work schedule makes it impossible. The people in Compassionate Friends mean a lot to me. We are a tight knit group. We don't send Christmas cards and socialize outside of the group. But there is a strong bond. It is a level of understanding and caring that you don't get elsewhere.
>
> I've changed since my son died. I was strong before, but in some ways I'm even stronger now. Nothing will ever hurt me as much as Cory's death, so there is less to fear and more worth risking. I'm still a giving person and there are many people I care about, but I'll never give as much of myself or care as much about others as I did before Cory's death. I've learned to protect and take care of myself. My faith is stronger. Fortunately, I didn't go through questioning my faith like many parents do. I can now see that Cory was only meant to live 12 years. I couldn't accept that at first, but now I believe strongly that there is a reason for everything that happens. We usually receive signs we don't understand. After Cory died I found the present he was going to give me for Christmas. It was a bell with a golden-haired angel on top.

Fran Cooper has experienced the full self-help trajectory in that she went from the shock of the death and rejection of the group to learning how she could accept the help of the group. She then began finding models in the group for her own healing. Later, she discovered that she could be of help to others and that in helping others she found help for herself. Finally, she became one of the leaders in the group who stay to help others and in so doing give their child's death positive meaning through service to others.

Helping Bereaved Parents

Obviously not everyone who attends a self-help group completes the trajectory. Some never learn to accept help and others drop out when they feel a lowering of their own stress. Those of us who are not bereaved parents can increase the probability that a parent will benefit from the group by supporting the bereaved parent through different relationships to the group. It is helpful, for example, for someone to take the newly bereaved parent to the first few meetings. Often, especially if the father and mother do not come together, a friend or older child can bring the parent. It feels safer to have a familiar face at the meeting. It also helps to have someone in the car to debrief with during the ride home. It is hard to go to a meeting, for as Fran said, that constitutes an admission that the child is not going to come back. It is also frightening to think about sharing this deepest and most personal of emotions. Several times parents have reported at their first meeting that the month before they had gotten into the car and then turned back. Some even get to the door and then go back to the car and drive home. Sometimes, as for Fran, the first meeting is full of negative experiences. The parent wants to stop crying and instead the parent finds other people who are crying—sometimes even a year after the death. One person sat for three meetings with his coat on and his hat in his hand, seemingly ready to leave at any moment if it got too hard for him. In the early part of parents' relationship to the group we can be with them as they come to terms with themselves as bereaved parents.

To understand the self-help process, we must see that people move through it as their grief changes. As parents change through the group process, those of us who are not bereaved parents can be ready to change the nature of our support for those parents. There is no easy cure for the emotional and spiritual dilemmas presented by the death of a child. The Compassionate Friends and Candlelighters do work major changes in many people's lives, but it takes time. We have had professionals listen to parents who have just attended their first meeting and after just one report, the professionals decided that self-help doesn't "work" because people don't "get over it." Rather than encouraging the parent to go through their grief, the professionals identified with the parent fearfully standing at the beginning of that long lonely road through the valley of the shadow of death. It is difficult for outsiders to understand that these parents have no choice. Their child is dead. Either they come to terms with that fact or they must cut off that part of themselves which is attached to their child. Trying to protect bereaved parents from any more pain retards the cure. Those who are not bereaved parents are sometimes like the physicians, who, when their own powers to cure have been so radically threatened by childhood death, prescribe tranquilizers and antidepressants for long periods after the death. They are trying to "protect" the parents from further pain. But such intervention only postpones the grief work, and in the interim family dysfunction often increases. We do not need to worry about hurting these parents. As one said, "I lost my child; how could you hurt me more than that?"

If others want to help bereaved parents, they can support them on the long road through grief. One of the most difficult realizations those of us who are not bereaved have to make is that we have little we can say for comfort, even though we can "be there" and show we care. We may be the objects of anger—especially if we still have our healthy children. When we reach into our past for an experience by which to empathize, we are met with, "But you don't understand." They are right.

I have worked closely with bereaved parents for several years and I still cannot comprehend losing a child. Parents of dead or dying children regularly share the resentment they feel toward the ways people try to find meaning in a situation that parents find meaningless. "You are lucky to still have other children," or "At least she died young so you don't have so much to miss," are comments bereaved parents get all the time. Unless we have lost a child, we must realize that we do not understand what they are experiencing. We can love and care for these parents. We can be with them, listen to them, and hurt with them, but we cannot bear their burden. They must find their own path through the grief. But it is easier to travel that path when the parents find others on the same journey. Self-help groups are about communication with others who are traveling on the same strange and frightening road.

Help From Bereaved Parents

There is a wide range of help that parents can give each other. Information is shared. For example, a parent at his or her first meeting may timidly ask, "Is it normal to be tired all the time?" or "Do other people find themselves worried about their other kids?" Solutions to practical problems are shared, for example, how to include the dead child in a holiday celebration. (Readers may go to a cemetery the day after Christmas to see the trees and toys on new child graves.) Usually at some point a new member finds someone in the group who is further along and uses the "veteran" as a model to emulate. Sometimes simply being able to share the child with others is helpful as, like parents everywhere, the members tell stories about and show pictures of their children. Some Compassionate Friends chapters have a photo album in which members place pictures of their children—symbolically sharing the child with the group. As parents mature in the group, helping others becomes a way of helping the self, for now the love which was formerly given to the child is available to be shared with others like the self. Soon that love will be available for any reinvestment the parent chooses.

The help that comes from others on the same path is not possible from someone whose child is not dying or dead. But professionals and friends can help bereaved parents by supporting them on the long road through death and grief. They can be especially supported in their Compassionate Friends membership. Parents can be encouraged at the beginning of their experiences with a self-help group by taking them to meetings or by listening to the accounts of the meetings or to their response to items in the newsletter. As parents begin to find techniques for dealing with problems such as how to celebrate holidays, others can cooperate in those solutions. As parents begin to make positive identification with a model within the group, others can note the changes and be patient as the bad days still sometimes come. Finally, as parents take leadership in the group, passing their experience on to those who are new in death and grief, those of us who are not bereaved parents can give the positive regard which is rightfully due to one who has triumphed in one of the most difficult personal challenges life can offer.

Parents of Dying Children

While the majority of childhood deaths are sudden, the long process associated with various childhood cancers and other diseases calls for some additional help from others in the same predicament. We find that parents feel the sense of isolation from natural support systems, and that they have banded together to aid themselves in this most difficult parenting. The Candlelighters vary from chapter to chapter, but all have as their aim the support of parents whose children have cancer. Because cancer no longer means automatic death—and to these parents it cannot mean death, at least until late in the child's illness—the Candlelighters are not concerned primarily with death and bereavement. Their emphasis is on support and cure. They work hard at making sure their children have opportunities to experience life through fishing trips, summer camps, Christmas parties, ball games, and the like. They work very hard at fund raising, much of which is devoted to research into the cause and cure of cancers in children. Thus the parents understand that they are contributing to the effort to save their children's lives and that they are not simply passive victims of an overwhelming force called cancer. Hope based in realistic assessment of their situation is the centerpiece of the Candlelighters' message. In the newsletter are reports of children's normal progress in school or scouts, and reports of children now off chemotherapy.

But there are also reports of the children that have died and personal remembrances of each of those who lost the fight against cancer. The group understands its role as parents supporting other parents in *all* the phases of childhood cancer. Special parties for the children, Mom's night out, information on various treatments, and sharing family dynamics—as well as bereavement support—are all part of the same process for this group. That means that we cannot completely separate activities which are pointed toward recovery from those which prepare for or cope with death. Both remission and death are possible at most points along the road Candlelighters must walk. Unlike cancer in older people, where death may be understood as "natural," and where the surviving children have already cut the primary emotional dependence on the dying parent, when young children are in danger, their parents cannot cut those bonds, and death is not regarded as "natural" even though it may be recognized as possible.

The trajectory through the Candlelighters' process is somewhat more complex than the trajectory through the Compassionate Friends. We find the basic self-help set of changes: from parents looking for help, to parents defining models in other members of the group, to parents learning that helping others is a way to help the self. As in Compassionate Friends, at each of those changes, people outside the group can support the Candlelighter. Intertwined with the trajectory of the relationship of the self to the group, however, is the trajectory of the illness itself. Candlelighters serve parents of children with life-threatening illness, parents of children who have recovered from life-threatening illness, parents of terminally ill children, and parents of children who have died. The parents' relationship to the self-help process is within the changing course of the child's illness.

It seems, then, that there are two primary roads through Candlelighters—one ending in recovery and one in death. But the parents do not know which road they are on until late in their Candlelighter membership. Those parents for whom the outcome is still unknown may not want any hint that death may be the end for their child. They must hope not just for their child to live fully the life he or she now has. They must hope that the child will be given a long enough life that the parent will die before the child. The Candlelighters want clearly to be associated with the acute care facility, because recovery and life are their goals. We cannot take that away from them. But some of these children do die and those concerned with care of the dying and bereaved might find ways to support the work of Candlelighters without being the overeager grim reaper that these parents hate so.

Virginia Hitchcock, whose child has been dead for five months, described her relationship with the Candlelighters this way:

> It's not something you really choose to join, but when Daniel was diagnosed with cancer, I desperately needed to talk to someone who knew what I was going through. I started calling other mothers just to talk and got a lot of support. When Daniel relapsed, it's amazing how many others came to my aid—they came to relieve me and encourage me to get out for a while; came to clean my house once a week. They were there whenever I needed them, but they don't bug you when you don't want to be bugged.
>
> None of the parents want to face their child dying, but at some point you need to be told what to expect and what you will have to cope with. The problem is that the time for being able to hear is different for each family. You certainly don't want to hear it when your child is first diagnosed. One mother wanted to bring in a hospice worker to talk on death and dying. Most of the parents wanted nothing to do with it.
>
> I still turn to Candlelighters for support. Right now I'm getting so upset with people for telling me how I should be. They think I should be getting over my grief by now, but it's really getting harder. The reality is setting in. I'm learning to put on a mask for most people, but I still desperately need someone to talk to. Before Daniel's death I didn't allow myself to get to know Donna Morgan. Her daughter had already died and I would think, "You're threatening me. I don't want to see you." Now I call Donna at any time and she will let me talk about Daniel for hours. That's also true of a lot of Candlelighters whose children are still living. They don't know exactly what I'm going through, but they listen to me and don't expect me to "get over it."

In the Candlelighters, as in the Compassionate Friends, parents first join because they need help, but at some point they begin reaching out to others and discover the great secret of the self-help process—in helping others, the helper is healed as much as those who are helped. Volunteer parents staff the clinic to be there when new parents come in and that process develops the contacts that lead to participation in other group activities. Unlike the Compassionate Friends, the Candlelighters tend not to have meetings aimed at emotional sharing, that important task is done in the hours together in the clinic and in the relationships that develop between parents and between children. Meetings are informational, and to some extent are aimed at education in the community. After the death of the child, however, more formal sessions of sharing and support—such as the Compassionate Friends uses—are available in many Candlelighter chapters. In others, some of the bereaved parents tend to move to the Compassionate Friends.

What Works with Whom

Not everyone seems to take to the self-help process, though we have no way of predicting at this time who will find it useful. We also find that some parents find other support systems are useful to them in addition to the self-help group.

Of all the parents in a community, we do not know which are likely to join a self-help group. Children die in such decentralized settings that only a large-scale research project would show patterns. In a rather small way we tried to answer the question of who stays with Compassionate Friends by telephoning parents who had been to one or two meetings, but did not come back. We found two kinds of responses. One set of people seems to have found a more informal group which performed some of the same functions as Compassionate Friends does formally. They had an extended family or friends, some of whom might have also lost children, with whom they could share, cry, offer support, and be supported. Many of those people spontaneously reported that they read the monthly newsletter from cover to cover, and some passed the newsletter on to friends. In one case the informal support network was two women who had met at what was for each their first TCF meeting. As we listened to those parents talk, we found that several subgroups of members form for periods of time spontaneously, especially among people whose losses are similar.

The other kind of response we got from those who came once or twice and had not returned was characterized by attempts to control or hold down the strong negative feelings brought on by the death of the child. These people reported that they were trying not to feel so bad and that going to the Compassionate Friends meeting only made them feel worse. A few of these parents cut short the phone conversation, saying "I don't like to talk about it because it depresses me." One person suggested that we call Compassionate Friends because "they like to talk about it there." In describing themselves, several of these parents used phrases such as "Well, I'm not much of a talker" and described rather strong implicit agreements in the family not to discuss the death.

After we had completed that research project, we tried to predict who at that first meeting would be back and who would not. We failed so often that we stopped trying. Often we have on first impression assumed that the newly bereaved family was strong with excellent natural support networks. After several months, however, it became clear that stresses which had been put aside during the dying process had now reemerged. Sometimes, though both parents would not stay with the group, one did. By contrast, we have occasionally observed people tightly clenching their jaws during three or four meetings. We thought they were trying to repress the strong feelings and would not return. But suddenly they started talking and clearly they had been assimilating everything they heard.

For a few other people we interviewed, the first meeting of Compassionate Friends was not relevant to the situation—for example, a person who had lost her only child had come to a meeting in which there was a presentation on helping siblings. Yet others who came to an inappropriate first meeting have returned and later became central members of the group. We need not try to predict who will benefit from the self-help process. At this time, it appears that the bereaved parents, not others, should make that decision.

Clearly, the crisis that the death of a child presents reaches deep into the psyches of each member of the family and affects the most hidden aspects of the relationships between family members. There is no such thing as an acute grief response which is tied to a particular loss. Eric Lindemann (1944), who first claimed the existence of acute grief as a definable psychological syndrome, said that the predictive factors he found for the syndrome were a previous history of psychological problems or a major disturbance in the social relationship. So the death of a child, as upsetting as it may be, is not sufficient reason to recommend professional help. Yet we do find that some of the parents report that therapy or marriage counseling is useful. Others observe that they have tried professional help and have been very disappointed. Except for an almost universal rejection of the drugs offered by physicians, in our research with parents for whom The Compassionate Friends process has been, by their own reports, successful, we have found no consistent pattern of the relationship between self-help and professional help. A very common comment is, "Dr. ______ is really good in helping me understand a lot of things about myself, but he just doesn't understand my grief. Only the people here understand that." So it would appear at this time that receiving professional help before, at the same time as, or after being in a self-help group is in no way contradictory. Just as we do not hesitate to recommend multiple interventions for other afflictions, it seems that we should think in terms of several options for the bereaved, and let them choose for themselves what is helpful.

Helping Self-Help Groups

The realization that we cannot comprehend the experience of a parent of a dying or dead child and that we cannot help them in ways we would like to is difficult. That realization is, however, balanced by a realization that we can help the groups that help the parents. This is the "good news/bad news" which is at the center of the relationship of the professional to the self-help process. The strength of the self-help process is that it provides something the professional by definition cannot: the experiential knowledge that comes from having "been there." The initial step in affiliation with both Candlelighters and The Compassionate Friends is in the realization that others share the experience and that "I am not alone." As parents move into the group, they begin to own it, taking responsibility for both the group needs and the needs of those who are newer to the process.

The question for the helping professional is how people who do not share the experience can support that process without diminishing its strengths. The Compassionate Friends has given some thought to the role of the professional and has issued the following policy statement:

> Chapters of Compassionate Friends are and should be organized with bereaved parents responsible for programs and activities and with members of the helping professions serving in consulting roles. . . .
>
> Someone who has not lost a child should not attempt to play a central role in this [self-help] process.
>
> However, Compassionate Friends can benefit from maintaining a cooperative and friendly relationship with members of the helping professions. . . .
>
> The selection of the individuals themselves is of paramount importance. They should have demonstrated commitment to the self-help principle, and be comfortable in a consultative capacity. . . .
>
> Chapters may want to invite a professional to attend meetings. This person could serve as an invited speaker, a facilitator, or may simply be present as a resource to be called upon if the group feels the need. The professional should be there to react, not to initiate (The Compassionate Friends).

Patricia Codden, a clinical specialist nurse who works with the St. Louis Candlelighters at Cardinal Glennon Memorial Hospital for Children, says her role with the group is simply being liaison and facilitator. "The fine line for professionals is to provide enough support to keep them moving along, but not enough to take away their autonomy and power. The group is its own vitality. What the professionals can do is to provide a home base—a person to identify with and to provide some consistency to the group since many parents come and go."

There is clearly a difference between the roles the professional might take with the Candlelighters by contrast with The Compassionate Friends. In Candlelighters the professional is in the clinic playing an active facilitator and referral role. There are also parents volunteering their time in the clinic. Thus, there is a more steady ongoing interaction between the members and the professional, as parents come in on the child's medication days and spend long sessions at the hospital when their child is an inpatient. The professional is also a part of the treatment team, in contact with the physicians regarding medical orders. In The Compassionate Friends members are more isolated because there is no central institution that binds them together and they have no place but the graveyard where they can go to be with their children. Meetings are usually held only once a month. When a child is dying, the parents' activity level may be higher than usual, for the crisis spurs attempts which are aimed at saving the child. Their down days result as much from exhaustion as depression. By contrast, the bereaved parent has little energy and may find it an effort even to come to a meeting at first. It would seem, therefore, that the professional working with the families of dying children might be more active and direct—without interfering with any group processes—than can the professional working with groups for the bereaved. Thus, the professional is probably a more significant source of information in Candlelighters than in The Compassionate Friends.

In either case, any help given the self-help group should grow from an understanding of the range of activities and relationships within the group. There is a misunderstanding among professionals that self-help is an amateur form of psychological intervention. On the contrary, self-help should be seen more like a community with communications, shared understandings, ongoing leadership development processes, traditions, and business matters. It is a process different than professional intervention, but one that has its own integrity which must be maintained (Klass & Shinners, 1983). In the long run, for example, it may be a better use of a professional's time to recommend that a service organization donate $500 for newsletter mailing costs than to try to speak in a helpful way to a single parent. At one point one TCF chapter was having problems because people said the meeting depressed them. The solution turned out to be lending our professional prestige to convince a church board with a more cheerful room to let the group use the church even though the meeting would last long after the custodian left. It probably did not require a Ph.D. to accomplish that task, but those few phone calls and the letter were one of the best things we ever did for the group. A group for parents of dying or dead children always needs publicity because it is the kind of group many people would rather not know about. It costs a lot of money to produce and mail newsletters, so institutions with mimeograph and folding machines might just add that to their schedules. Professionals often come into contact with other professionals who seem to have a good style and new material. Self-help groups are always on the lookout for good programs and speakers, so a phone call or note about new resource persons may be enough to establish a useful contact. The leaders of any group have their problems and frustrations. It helps them to have someone who can listen while they think through what they should do. Sometimes a suggestion helps, but just as often a well-asked question is better. Needs may be greater at one time than another. The professional can be there when he or she is needed.

Professional Intervention and Self-Help Compared

The key to the success of self-help is that there are a variety of communication channels and modes of communication which are appropriate to the situation. The professional model of helping usually narrows the modes of communication since each use of the professional's time must pass the test of cost-effectiveness. The self-help group expands its therapeutic effectiveness with each expanded communication mode. Thus, a professional cannot spend hours on the telephone going over the details of the treatment or death again and again with a client. But two parents who are going through the same process will both be helped by those same hours on the phone to each other. The professional may write for a newsletter and help the readers, but if a group member is encouraged to write, the writing itself helps the writer and the feedback from readers will reinforce the growth brought about by the writing. Someone once humorously defined psychotherapy as a relationship between two people in which both of them change, hopefully one more than the other. In self-help, all the participants in the relationship change and that is precisely the point. For every communication we can foster in self-help we double the benefits.

We might best understand the processes of Candlelighters and The Compassionate Friends by a concept which Thomasina Borkman (1976) has introduced, "experiential knowledge." Experiential knowledge is knowledge acquired by direct acquaintance with an affliction or condition. It is based in immediate experience and in the multiple ways the individual must respond in order to meet and overcome the affliction or condition. Because experiential knowledge is from the point of view of the experiencer rather than from the outside point of view typical of professional knowledge, experiential knowledge is always wholistic whereas professional knowledge is fragmented and based only on the professional's expertise.

For example, an issue which is problematic for bereaved parents is what to say when people ask how many children they have. On first glance, it seems to be such a practical question that no psychological or sociological attention need be paid. But the question reaches deep into the nature of the parental bond; what does it mean when people say they "have" a child? After all, only under specific conditions do children understand that they "have" their parents. Even if we were to "work through" the nature of that bond in therapy so that the bereaved parents realize that they "have" the child in a different way, the parent is still left with the practical problem of what to say in the social situation. For when people ask how many children someone has, it is a casual question for the inquirer, while to the bereaved parent an appropriate response depends on the degree of intimacy there is in a relationship before one's loss is shared. The issue of degree of intimacy is related to factors in the culture having to do with uncomfortable responses people make when they hear about the death of a child. So the question raises the social role of a bereaved parent in a death-denying society. Clearly, such role issues are beyond the professional ken of psychology or psychiatry, and really not in the province of social work either, for the problem is with the society, not with the parent. But all that theory still leaves the parent not knowing what to do or say.

In the group there will be other parents who have found answers to the question of how many children they have. Not all the answers are the same. One parent may say, "I have four," and then if the questioner goes on to ask the ages will report the ages of the three living children and add, "and one would have been 17." Another parent might subtract the dead child from the total before giving the first answer; while a third might say, "I used to have three, now just two." Each answer positions the parent differently toward the underlying issue of "having" a child and toward the problematic social role of being a bereaved parent. The parent facing this difficulty can thus choose a position from among several available models in the group. At the point of choice, the underlying issues are understood clearly in a way that is both concrete to the social situation and congruent with other existential positions that person takes in life.

The problem was not that parents needed to learn what it means to "have" a child; they understood that all too well. They also understood all too well the marginal nature of their social role. What the experiential knowledge has given them are options for existential action. To change the metaphor a bit, scientific professional knowledge can analyze body movement, eye-hand coordination, and the effects of air pressure differential on moving objects. But the batter in a baseball game must integrate all of these into one experience of responding to a pitch. Like bereaved parents at a meeting, ball players work on their "stance" during practice; during the game they just do the best they can. If they go into a slump, they may want to try a different stance for a while. A good coach is usually someone who played the game, but who had to work at being good. Superstars do not make the best coaches. Ordinary parents further down the path are the people who make the best coaches for parents whose children are dying or dead. It is easiest for these parents to follow the lead of those they know have played the game a little longer than they have.

The self-help group thus provides a resource which cannot be duplicated. If we were to begin "support groups" as opposed to self-help groups, in effect we would make the claim that the power to change is limited and we would perpetuate a view that these parents are victims. It is in taking charge of their own lives by helping others and then owning the group that the parents move from being passive to active. The existential stance which is given in experiential knowledge is an active interaction with the world. Within that stance, meaning-making, relationship-building, and self-imaging are a product of action. A support group, with its passive role for the participant, can ease the pain, and it can provide measures of change, but it cannot provide the sense of autonomy and agency that the self-help group can. Part of that sense of agency comes from the full ownership of the group and the processes within the group. Most Compassionate Friends chapters begin their meetings and every newsletter with a statement that the group is of, by, and for bereaved parents. The social isolation in the marginal social role which bereaved parents feel is thus not denied, nor is the attempt made, as would have to be done in a support group, to break down that isolation. Rather the social isolation is used positively, to form *a community of the isolated.*

Conclusion

We who are not parents of dying or dead children can, if we wish, learn to give all the support to these parents that we can. We can break some of the social isolation by being willing to talk about the child and about the death. We can provide help for daily tasks when the parents' energy is low. We can be their friend as they struggle to heal the part of themselves that has been torn out and as they learn to reinvest themselves in the world in new ways. But there is a distance between their world and ours. We cannot fully share their experience. By supporting parents as they join groups such as The Compassionate Friends or Candlelighters, we can put parents of dead or dying children in touch with a strong potential source of help. By assisting the groups themselves in ways which do not co-opt their strengths, we can encourage a community of understanding which is available to people when their child dies.

Care of the dying and the grieving has always been an occasion for mobilizing communities. The death of a child in this culture at this time in history is a very special kind of grief, and in response to that special grief the community has been mobilized in a special way in self-help groups.

We can be part of that mobilized community as we encourage parents of dying and dead children in their membership. As we find ways to help the groups themselves without diminishing the strengths of such groups, we become helpers in the process of mobilizing the community. In so doing, we may even discover the self-help secret that in helping others we ourselves are helped even more.

References

Borkman, T., "Experiential Knowledge: A New Concept for the Analysis of Self-Help Groups," *Social Service Review*, 1976, *50*, 445–456.

The Compassionate Friends, "Policy Statement Regarding Relationships to Professionals."

Klass, D., & Shinners, B., "Professional Roles in a Self-Help Group for the Bereaved," *Omega*, 1983, *13*, 361–375.

Lieberman, M. A., Borman, L. D., & Associates, *Self-Help Groups for Coping with Crisis*. San Francisco: Jossey-Bass, 1979.

Lindemann, E., "Symptomatology and Management of Acute Grief," *American Journal of Psychiatry*, 1944, *101*, 141–148.

Bibliography

In the spirit of self-help, I asked some of The Compassionate Friends members and some Candlelighter members to suggest some books which they thought were particularly helpful to people in their situation. I added newsletters to the list because I often hear how helpful they are for these parents. The list is by no means exhaustive, but it may show the kind of communication these people use in healing.

Claypool, J., *Tracks of a Fellow Struggler*. Waco, TX: Word Books, 1974. A bereaved father and well-known pastor uses autobiography to describe his journey of the soul. He shares in a most moving and human way.

Grollman, E., *Living—When a Loved One Has Died*. Boston: Beacon, 1977. This book is about death at any age, but many parents report that it is helpful to them. Grollman is an experienced counselor with practical advice.

Hewett, J. H., *After Suicide*. Philadelphia: Westminster Press, 1980. Compassionate dealing with one of the more difficult types of deaths. Because teenage suicide is on the rise, every TCF chapter has a significant group of suicide survivors.

Peppers, L. G., & Knapp, R. J., *Motherhood and Mourning: Perinatal Death*. New York: Praeger, 1980. The authors are social scientists who interviewed parents who had experienced fetal or neonatal death. They report findings, offer interpretations, and give some practical advice, especially on the relationship between spouses.

Schiff, H., *The Bereaved Parent.* New York: Crown Publishers, 1977. This seems to be the first book given most often to newly bereaved parents. Writing from her own experience and with great compassion, Schiff lays out the territory and offers many clues for healing. If anyone were to read only one book on the subject, it should be this one.

Stephens, S., *Death Comes Home.* New York: Morehouse-Barlow, 1973. Stephens is the founder of TCF. His book is the story of the early TCF in England, but along the way Stephens gives some pointed insights about parental grief and healing.

Newsletters: Most chapters of TCF and Candlelighters put out a regular newsletter which includes chapter news, meeting notes, and articles by members. Those writings are part of the healing process for members as they write to define and vent their feelings. Many times the poems and letters are quite moving; at all times they are informative to those of us who have not shared the experience. When you ask to be put on the mailing list be sure to send a contribution to pay your fair share.

13

An Approach to Caring: Caregiver Concerns

Marcia E. Lattanzi

Something we were withholding made us
weak until we found it was ourselves.

—*Robert Frost*

Introduction

In contagious or radiating ways, caregivers experience stresses similar to those of the families with whom they work. The care of critically ill, dying, or bereaved children and their families creates major sources of distress. Parents and caregivers struggle with feelings of helplessness and role conflicts. While the stresses are situational and relational, the most significant impact is intrapersonal.

In the course of normal childhood growth and development, there are numerous causes for the pressure, strain, and disruption that define stress. Children are on rapid trajectories of change and growth that make adaptation a constant process. In his pioneering work, Selye (1956) reminds us that stress plays a role in such diverse manifestations of life as aging, the development of individuality, the need for self-expression, and the formulation of an individual's ultimate aims. Clearly, stress cannot be avoided, and stress in and of itself is almost essential for creativity. In the context of working with dying or grieving children and their families, caregivers can attempt to channel stress in creative directions and to keep its damaging effects to a minimum.

It is important to recognize that other occupations also contain inherent stresses. For example, it would be difficult for those outside this daily work to imagine the functional demands and challenges of a junior high school teacher. Nevertheless, medical caregivers are generally seen as individuals who are at high risk. With constant exposure to disease, pain, and trauma, and with ongoing personal and consumer expectations of treatment successes, a consistent level of role-related tension exists. This chapter will discuss some of the unique situational concerns and elements of support related to care of dying and grieving children and their families. It will address an overall approach to caregiving and caring from this particular perspective that has potential for generalization to other settings and circumstances.

Situational Stresses

Hospice approaches to caregiving center around offering families *choices*. When choices are available, human beings are usually able to maintain enhanced feelings of participation and control. For example, the option of home care inherent in hospice services becomes a key factor in managing parental stress. With the ill child at home, parents and other siblings seem to achieve a sense of relief. Ida Martinson (1976) has pointed out two primary interventions for the family that a home care service offers: (1) parental control; and (2) limiting uncertainty. Active involvement and participation in care increases one's ability to deal with the situation. When parents are allowed to set schedules and routines, and to deliver care to their child, there is heightened opportunity for positive interaction. Information and explanations to the parents about difficulties that might occur limit not only the uncertainty, but also the stress that fear of the unknown creates.

In a time when support persons to the family may, because of their own distress, be avoiding or distancing themselves from what they perceive as an uncomfortable situation, hospice caregivers become increasingly important. The family's functional patterns are disturbed prior to and following the death of a child. Changes in routine, increase in caregiving demands, and shifts in usual patterns of communication and roles involve constant adjustment at a time when physical resources are strained and diminished. Many of the stresses and difficulties experienced by caregivers are related to attempts to assist and protect the family.

In general, when a child is involved most caregivers experience an intensification of all the usual stresses experienced in terminal care. Hospice challenges caregivers to experience their own limitations. A situation with such inherent human conflicts can lead individuals to question their own professional adequacy.

Caregiver Concerns

When asked, nurses and other hospice caregivers are usually readily able to identify the elements that are most difficult in providing care for a dying child (Lattanzi, 1982). All of these elements are related to: (1) role ambiguity; and (2) emotional responses experienced by the caregiver. Typical examples of stressors in each category are outlined below. Note that the stress which results is based upon conflicts that are within the caregiver during and following his or her involvement with the child and family.

Role-Related Stresses

Ambiguity. The philosophy of hospice entails that the professional function as an advocate for the child and family. Delivering care in the context of the family's wishes and under their control can create significant role uncertainty for caregivers. There may also be certain needs that a nurse may feel uncomfortable addressing, for example, spiritual concerns. And, care must be maximized in the home setting in the context of periodic and limited contact.

Protection. Medical and nursing practitioners often are cast in the roles of "protector" or "guardian." In the situation surrounding the death of a child, however, there are few ways that we can protect the family and child from the distress they are experiencing. When we are unable to restore health, our goals become comfort-related, reflecting the realities of the situation and the limitations of our interventions.

Mediation. Caregivers often act as buffers in a tense and trying situation. Conflicting family views or goals must be worked with in a collaborative way. Parents may develop an alliance with a particular caregiver, making attempts to include the other partner necessary. The role of balancing different needs entails that the professional act as a buffer and mediator in a situation where stress can force parents to focus anger on medical personnel.

Functional Conflicts. Terminal care has become an increasingly accepted practice. The more typical gratifications and definitions of medical success must be reframed in this new context of care (Lattanzi, 1981). Caregivers face a challenging task in maintaining levels of optimism, idealism, or altruism. Caregiving that is associated with significant human experiences of grief and loss demands greater levels of adaptation. Responding to tensions, frustration, and insecurities surrounding the death of a child becomes a complex process where ongoing adaptation is difficult.

Emotional Stresses

Powerlessness. Health care professionals are prone to an emphasis upon and a belief in curative interventions. By our efforts, we attempt to improve health status and functioning. In terminal care situations involving children, our desire would be to perform the miraculous. Instead, the situation creates feelings of frustration and helplessness. In spite of all our best efforts and advancing technology, we are unable to save the life of a dying child or to eliminate the pain of bereavement.

Witnessing Suffering. Adults in general, and caregivers in particular, find it difficult to see a child experience the distress associated with a critical illness and related treatment, or with bereavement. Caring adults experience the reflection of the pain that the child and the parents experience. Kollar (1982) points out that we are reminded of our own vulnerability, insignificance, and transience, and are transformed as a consequence of our own suffering and that of others.

Identification. As parents and members of families, the concern that we feel for others mirrors fears for our own children. In our own ways, we recognize and take part in the anguish that parents experience during or following the terminal illness of a child. In so doing, we may come to participate in and identify too closely with the family's experience. This identification can take place with one specific parent or with the child. It is possible in this way to lose one's objectivity, especially when there are family conflicts and differences.

Overinvolvement. In working with a dying or bereaved child and family, caregivers can try to supply all the support for all the need. It is not difficult to feel engulfed by the intensity of the need. Nurses and other caregivers can react to the level of need by offering to be of greater support to the family than would be desirable or optimal.

Grief. A significant part of the stress involved with care of a dying child is related to the loss of a special being who never had the opportunity to develop his or her full potential. Another issue relates to the loss of the person who was the object of a great expenditure of effort and energy. There is also a cumulative effect of grief, particularly when there is no specific opportunity for its expression. Because one loss evokes a realization and fear of other losses, it may become difficult to remember that not all children are dying.

Understanding the nature of the stresses caregivers experience can generate new insights and possibilities for coping. Knowledge has an empowering, even a curative value. Beyond understanding the stresses involved in working with dying or grieving children and their families, the greatest challenge lies in developing the potential for meaning that the experience can hold for living beings.

Manifestations of Stress

For families and for caregivers, indicators of stress are barometers that can be used to determine the amount or type of intervention and support that may be desirable. Coping styles and patterns are important, but there are times when the concerns are so consuming and longstanding that resources become worn and depleted. A threatening situation evokes stress responses throughout one's entire being.

Perhaps the most apparent demonstrations of distress occur in *physical health:* headaches, fatigue, sleep disturbances, eating disturbances, injuries, muscular pain, especially back and neck pain, complications or recurrences of preexisting conditions, and lowered resistance to infectious processes (e.g., colds, flu, etc.) are all common experiences. Grieving persons are not unfamiliar with these symptoms or illnesses.

Emotionally, people in high levels of distress can experience distancing, depression, fearfulness, guilt over one's healthy state, paranoia, difficulty in concentrating, and nervous tics. Most parents feel that they could endure personal pain more easily than the pain of watching their child suffer.

Behaviorally, high levels of stress and distress interfere with one's sense of well-being. Rapid mood changes are not infrequent. At one moment the child or parents may feel hopeful and optimistic, and at another feel scattered and frantic in their actions. Hyperactivity can become a manifestation of the stress that parents experience in caring for their terminally ill child. Caregivers often marvel at the energy and efforts of parents during the time of the child's illness. Another typical way of responding to stressful situations involves dependency-related behaviors, such as increased consumption of food, alcohol, and medications. These responses are largely avoidance. They have the potential to bring about temporary anesthesia, and sometimes transient relief, but they do not relate to high levels of well being or optimal functioning.

In a *spiritual* or *values* context, a crisis that centers around the questioning and even the possible loss of faith can occur. Occasionally, there may be a dramatic or sudden shift in one's values or beliefs. These spiritual or value-related responses influence one's outlook and attitude. An air of frustration or hopelessness, and possibly even cynicism, can be experienced. Another response that could occur is an attitude involving an overly critical approach to caregivers as well as to one's friends and acquaintances.

Perhaps the most significant strain during times of distress is experienced in *relationships.* The occasion of a significant crisis can lead individuals to feel either a sense of isolation or a need to be overly dependent. Alternatively, responses to things or people around them may become mechanical. Successes in the treatment and care of a terminally ill child require us to address the issues of increasing anger and isolation with the child who is ill. Work-related stresses often lead to conflict with friends and nuclear family members. Finally, these conflicts create a sense of social isolation, limiting the support that is available to the individual and the family (White, 1981).

There are a number of ways that human beings express and demonstrate their distress. Basically, these ranges of responses and experiences generate the observation that there are ways that stress can be manifested which can limit or exclude available support.

Preventive Measures

Professionals and volunteers involved in the care of critically ill or dying children are involved in a situation with inherent distress. The image that corresponds best to this work is that of standing near a fire. The challenge is to stand near enough to feel the warmth, and yet to maintain a suitable distance that will prevent one from getting burned. Harper (1977) believes that caregivers are challenged to accept the responsibility of learning to know in a deep and significant way the children and families with whom we work. Against this, it is not unusual for some caregivers to use professional demeanor as a defense against emotional involvement with patients and families (Quint, 1967). Since health essentially involves adaptation and balance, it seems necessary for caregivers to develop and maintain their own personal resources. Both organizational and individual approaches are essential in this process.

Organizational Approaches

Staff Selection. A primary consideration related to *staff selection* involves an assessment of the individual's coping abilities based on previous work and personal experiences, along with the availability of support outside the work setting. Individuals who have had successful work or life experiences bring not only a sense of their personal gifts and talents, but also a knowledge of their boundaries and limitations. The balance that this work demands can only be achieved if one possesses insight based on one's own life experiences, a hopeful outlook, and the personal experiences of love, friendship, and good moments in one's life. People who are operating at a deficit or who are in times of deprivation in their own lives will find it extremely difficult to balance the demands of this work. Even caregivers with good coping skills and excellent support will, at times, find working with dying or bereaved children and their families challenging to integrate into their lives.

Education and Training. These are key elements that significantly influence the ability of staff and volunteers to manage stress, and do the caregiving work. The initial team training in a hospice program is an important team-building effort. It also serves to set the tone and to present models that will encourage individuals to function as effectively and comfortably as possible in their roles (Lattanzi, 1983a). Training programs need to include information on self-care and options for support. Ongoing as well as initial education and training efforts optimally include consideration of one's own resources. Modeling of this sort and reflection upon one's personal resources help to clarify deficiencies and strengths prior to the time when one will be in significant need.

Supervision. This is another aspect of ongoing staff development and maintenance. Individual consultation is an important part of the supervisory process. The relationship between the caregiver and the supervisor is one of the primary variables thought to be beneficial to the adjustment process of professionals working with dying or bereaved children and their families (Harper, 1977). Supervision may be exercised in a wide range of formal and informal interactions, and is of central importance in establishing the overall environment and administrative tone which underlies the individual's ability to cope with stress.

Mutual Support. Support within the hospice team or the clinical context is also essential. In particular, the support available from a caregiver's primary functional unit, for example, the miniteam of those involved with a given family in the home, or one's identified peer group, is an invaluable and sustaining element. The functioning of the interdisciplinary team encourages examination of current concerns and patterns of involvement and interaction. Team members challenge each other in an effort to ensure the highest possible quality of care. In addition, the shared perspectives and knowledge base of many professionals and lay volunteers add to the understanding and the diverse assets available to individuals on the team. The interdisciplinary team lets caregivers confront biases and difficulties encountered by individual caregivers, and encourages the extension of perspectives as well as the broadening of an individual's knowledge base. The significant stresses inherent in hospice care are balanced by the remarkable potential for professional and personal expansion.

Individual Considerations

Support is neither a simple nor a constant source of energy in individual attempts to manage stress. Much of the support human beings experience comes from within themselves (Lattanzi, 1983b). One's personal orientation and ability to sustain oneself during both difficult and pleasant times is the foundation upon which other sources of support exist. Workshop participants are able to identify a range of patterns of support and coping styles (Walker & Lattanzi, 1982). Mechanisms of coping fall into the following general categories:

Activities. Individuals can find comfort through the distraction and pleasure of enjoyable activities. The range of possible options includes physical exercise, meditation, reading, writing, playing a musical instrument, hobbies, and so on.

Time Alone. In addition to, or as a part of one's activities, there is a need for solitary, reflective time. Privacy allows for the examination and clarification of one's experiences. Individuals who are engaged in constant activity or involvement with other people have little opportunity to integrate their processes and progress.

Outlets for Emotional Expression. It is necessary to have opportunities for emotional release available to us on a daily basis. People to cry with, people to laugh with, people with whom it is safe to express anger, and people who will listen to any emotional reaction without judgment or censure are essential in maintaining health.

Rituals. Personal or group-related rituals involve social acknowledgement of experiences. They offer individuals permission to publicly give and receive support related to significant events. As society becomes more sophisticated, there are no apparent replacements for traditional rituals and their potential for meaning in our lives.

Personal Philosophy. There are moments when all internal and external ways of coping seem inadequate. Many caregivers experience times of crises when the only sustaining element is one's personal life view, or the meaning one finds created out of one's work and relationships. This element of support takes on a very important role in the struggle to continue to adapt. When all other available support is inadequate to address the depth of the distress, one turns to an inner reservoir maintained for the most difficult times. This reservoir includes one's commitment to ongoing life. Caregivers need a level of maturity to face and to go beyond their fears. In its purest sense, compassion begins in the acknowledgement of and surrender to one's own pain. This personal philosophy is essentially the quality of open-heartedness.

Clinical Experiences

Various approaches to support can be seen clearly in clinical experiences. The two cases that follow illustrate diverse ways in which families and caregivers respond to difficult situations. No one dimension of support is adequate in and of itself. Rather, these situations demonstrate the need for each individual involved to create a collage or composite picture of support that includes a variety of elements as well as persons.

Judith and Rick

Judith, a nurse involved with hospice home care for only four months, began her relationship with the Holter family in early May. The middle child, Rick, 16, had been ill for less than six months with widespread metastatic carcinoma. Rick's older brother, Don, 19, and his younger sister, Barbara, 14, were very active and involved in Rick's treatment and care. In response to their high levels of distress, Rick's parents often withdrew into their jobs or into household activities. Nevertheless, with continuing attention and encouragement from his friends, Rick was able to spend short periods of time at the high school up to three weeks before his death.

Hospice involvement in Rick's care was concurrent with even greater levels of anxiety for the parents. Preexisting family conflicts emerged. Mr. and Mrs. Holter often disagreed about treatment options and directions. Judith's role with the family emerged as one supporting the two siblings, Don and Barbara, and of encouraging Mr. and Mrs. Holter to involve Rick in choices and decisions. Over the seven weeks of hospice services, the siblings began to become more and more active as caregivers. As is typical in families with adolescents, there was some evident separation from the parents. Judith's main task was to act as an intermediary and advocate for Rick. She worked to improve patterns of direct communication, especially in regard to treatment and care considerations. Judith experienced a great deal of warmth in her relationship with Rick. Many of their important interactions occurred over the telephone.

Because she respected the family's boundaries, Judith felt frustrated in her desire for optimal care for Rick. She also felt that there was little that she could do to satisfy Mrs. Holter. In a most appropriate way, Judith expressed her emotional responses to involvement with the Holter family at interdisciplinary team meetings. She continued her aerobics classes, her yoga practice, and spent time alone in her mountain home. Nearer to the time of Rick's death, Judith asked for more opportunity for emotional expression. Seeking out specialized time for supervision and direction allowed her to clarify her role. Judith's role was limited by the family. She spent approximately two to three hours per week talking with nursing coworkers in an attempt to clarify directions and to receive support. As a newer member of the hospice team, Judith was defining her own boundaries, as well as seeking feedback on the appropriateness of her involvement and interventions. Judith had a desire to be more active in the family. She did, however, respect the family's wishes and needs. At team meetings, Judith mentioned her feelings of inadequacy and uncertainty in working with the Holter family. In addition to receiving significant support, Judith realized that it was the family that had identified her role within the work setting.

Marilyn and Jeffrey

Following a referral from the hospital social worker, Marilyn became involved with the Stiltner family. Jack and Sandra are parents in their late twenties, with three sons aged five, three, and 18 months. Their fourth son, Jeffrey, was born with untreatable congenital cardiac anomalies. The Stiltner family decided to take Jeffrey home to spend with them the two to three weeks that he was expected to live. Marilyn met the parents prior to Jeffrey's discharge from the hospital four days after his birth. The Stiltners had a positive relationship with open communication and helpful exchanges with the other sons. Jeffrey appeared to be a normal infant, and presented few care problems in the home. The concerns of the parents centered around the time of death. They were concerned about how the other children might react to Jeffrey's death, especially if he should struggle for breath or experience pain.

Marilyn focused all her energy on supporting the parents. She arranged for a visit to the local hospital for a trial run in the event the decision was made to bring Jeffrey there near the time of his death. Marilyn made numerous home visits to reassure the family and to offer ongoing assessment of Jeffrey. Her relationship developed with the other boys, and she was helpful in discussing Jeffrey's illness and "sick heart" with them. One of the most difficult concerns for the family was the seeming unreality of the situation. The visible signs of Jeffrey's apparent health created more questions for the parents and other children. Jeffrey lived 26 days and died at home in his mother's arms. Marilyn was very pleased with the eventual outcome of the involvement, and developed a great respect and affection for this young family.

The stress that Marilyn experienced was related to the unusual and poignant dimensions of the involvement. Marilyn based her coping strategy upon her own spiritual beliefs. The Stiltner family was active in the church that Marilyn attended. Marilyn was supported, as were the Stiltners, by their minister. Marilyn also sought additional support and consultation regarding ways to best respond to the other siblings. At interdisciplinary team meetings, in private and often spontaneous conversations, and with her husband, Marilyn talked about the emotions and concerns that she was experiencing in working with this young family. Marilyn also continued her twice-weekly hikes in the mountains. While the pain of the Stiltner family was great, Marilyn felt that the stress for all involved was minimized by the act of focusing on Jeffrey's comfort and presence in the home.

These caregiving experiences demonstrate some ways that stresses can be addressed both within and outside the context of a hospice approach. The fact that the care was of children is an inherent dimension of the stress experienced. LaGrand (1980) points out that elements on the job that make one feel inadequate generate stress. While the hospice caregivers were unable to change the circumstances or the situation they were able to manage the stresses by defining standards for quality internally. More importantly, they brought comfort and special moments to the parents and surviving siblings.

Management of Stress

At certain points in the caregiving process, there is an escalation of anxiety and stress levels. Harper (1977) outlined the helping behaviors necessary in the face of the trauma of terminal illness, death, and bereavement. She believes that the professional person needs to:

1. Understand the behavioral dynamics and emotional responses of patients who will not recover.
2. Relate to responses and reactions of family members.
3. Offer emotional support and strength to the patients and family members.
4. Understand and deal with his or her own anxieties and feelings.

There is an intensity about work with dying or bereaved children and their families that can create significant levels of anxiety. The fact that children are involved and especially that it may be a child who dies adds to the already considerable demands placed upon caregivers who work with dying persons and their families. In these situations it becomes more probable for caregivers to experience excessive degrees of anxiety that can be disorganizing and can deter healthy adaptation.

One of the most effective ways to manage anxiety lies in the ability to focus on positive and possible actions that can be helpful to the child and family.

Within the framework of Harper's identified helping behaviors, there are certain things that caregivers can do to increase their functional and personal levels of comfort. In the context of understanding the responses of dying children, there are significant data that suggest that children are very aware of their situations (Bluebond-Langner, 1978). Beyond that, children's reactions to an experience or threat of death are greatly influenced by the ways their parents and other significant adults or authority figures respond.

Kalish (1969) suggests that children's fears would be allayed if adults were able to speak more factually and freely. Children's responses parallel adult responses to death. In many situations, caregivers have marveled at a child's calm and his or her level of understanding.

The major focus of our efforts can be in determining from the family what information the child has been given, and discovering from the child what he or she knows about the situation. Also, caregivers can do much to manage the emotional responses associated with physical pain and procedures. The fact that a child is dying or grieving cannot be changed, but one can attend to individual needs and responses.

Perhaps the primary area of intervention with a dying or bereaved child lies in the support of his or her parents. The negative psychological consequences of helplessness (Seligman, 1975) are a critical factor for parents. The possible psychological benefits to parents of providing care for their own children are obvious. The efforts of caregivers need to be directed not only toward the responses and reactions of family members, but also to the active and primary involvement of parents in the care of their children.

Hospice care attempts to recognize the needs of the person who is ill or grieving, as well as those of the family. Nurses spend a large portion of their professional time providing emotional support (Martinson, et al., 1978). Very often other family members are more in need of support than the child. When they receive adequate emotional support, parents are then able to face the task of caring for their child. A relationship with a caregiver should never supplant or interfere with a parent's role. Rather, caregivers need to be available for the roles that the family cannot fulfill. The involvement of a caregiver should make it more feasible for a parent to care for his or her child.

Caregivers have a responsibility to manage their own reactions and feelings. Work in an interdisciplinary context offers a number of opportunities for expressing and managing reactions. The task is to seek out the support that is available. It is important to keep their caregiver anxieties and fears out of the family situation where there is already an overload of emotional responses. Hospice workers must put into perspective their past experiences and their present and future fears. The goal is not to eliminate all anxiety, but rather to manage it constructively and to deal with it outside of the context of the family situation.

An Approach to Caring

> A candle loses nothing of its light by lighting another candle.
>
> —*Cort R. Flint*

Caregivers often experience a great deal of ambiguity over appropriate interventions and ways to support family members and each other. It is a very basic and yet difficult task to define what is involved in caring for others. Nouwen (1974) reminds us that *caring* as a word originates from the Greek "Kara," which means "to lament," "to grieve," "to cry out," and "to experience sorrow with." The process of caring for those who are suffering and grieving involves a journey that Imara (1983) believes could be made easier. He suggests that caring involves (1) clarifying reality frames by asking appropriate questions related to our actions; (2) supporting the need to express pain; and (3) standing by while there is an attempt to make meaning out of apparent madness or abnormality. On the surface, these goals seem simple enough. Experienced caregivers know that it is very difficult to tolerate the uncertainty and lack of control that these efforts involve. Once the needed elements of support have been identified, there is an ongoing challenge to channel our efforts in constructive directions.

Developing a Meaning Framework

Beyond exploration of the causative factors for distress—the reasons why some individuals are affected more deeply by work with dying or bereaved children and their families—and the ways caregivers cope, the relationship of this work to one's own life experience and beliefs is an important dimension.

Care of critically ill, dying, or bereaved children and their families demands an approach wherein caregivers learn to practice and to live their own advice. There are no simple "how to" lists for dealing with the personal impact of such work. The central focus is the relationship with the family, together with the supportive relationship with an interdisciplinary team. Individual caregivers are challenged to face and acknowledge the limitations of their efforts, and yet to continue to expend efforts and energy toward providing the child and the family members with whatever care and comfort may be possible. Standards for determining whether or not a good job has been done or quality care has been provided are appropriately different in the hospice context. Feedback from other members of the interdisciplinary team is extremely helpful. More than that, caregivers need to operate out of an internally-defined meaning framework within which this work can be examined and integrated.

Helping persons can have difficulty asking for support. Usually the act of asking for support involves considerable growth beyond the traditional need to be the person who is giving, rather than the one who will receive. Frankl (1959) points out that the power is in our response to difficult circumstances. In the act of witnessing grief, our personal values and beliefs are challenged. Caregivers involved with dying and bereaved persons find themselves forced to face the discrepancies and inconsistencies between their values and the tangible way they are living them in their own lives. This unsettling process of reexamination demands evaluation of one's own life and one's relationships. Caregivers who work in terminal care settings are pushed beyond the borders of their previous experiences and beliefs. An emerging and deepening philosophy of life is the key to reestablishment of homeostasis and to any eventual levels of personal meaning and comfort related to work with dying and grieving persons.

Emotional survival depends upon the establishment of internal norms. Caregivers must feel a level of comfort and satisfaction related to their activities and interventions. A critical factor for caregivers has to do with their sources of internal strength and hopefulness. Just as the persons with whom we are involved need a will to live, our ability to function is related to our ability to experience vitality in our own lives. In truth, we often gain our sense of strength and hope from the children and families with whom we work. One of the major rewards in caring for children who are dying involves the challenge to maximize the intimacy and meaningful contact with people for whom we care. Another significant reward is related to continued involvement with the family during the time of bereavement. Families who experience the death of a child grieve intensely. Many, out of their understanding of suffering, become very generous and more deeply caring people. Just as grief can be a transformative process for individuals with whom we work, it is also an opportunity for personal transformation for involved caregivers. Health involves not the *avoidance* of stresses, but rather *attention* to our experiences. The stress of facing pain is somehow less than the costs of avoiding or repressing it. We are most aware of the rewards involved in hospice care when we experience the richness of our own lives. The most effective way to minimize and manage work-related stress is to maximize enjoyable moments in our own lives.

Selye (1956) proposed that most of our tensions and frustrations come from our compulsive needs to act the role of someone we are not. He quotes the wisdom of Matthew Arnold: "Resolve to be thyself: and know that he who finds himself, loses his misery." The principle born out of psychoanalysis is that knowing what hurts one has an inherent curative value. Our failure to adapt and adjust to life situations is the source of disease-producing conflicts. Psychotherapy is a helpful example in that it encourages us to adapt ourselves to our life circumstances.

Beyond adaptation, there is a challenge associated with addressing and being close to the mysteriousness of death. Involvement with death, an experience larger than our conscious mind can contain, puts other daily life concerns in a different perspective. Selye (1956) suggested that contact with something infinitely greater than ourselves could lead to a sense of equanimity and a peace of mind.

Being in Relationships

Individuals who choose to work in hospice settings tend to value relationships. Because of their close contact with children and families at critical moments, often a deep intimacy is experienced. This closeness is both satisfying and difficult. Relationships do not generally operate at the level of intimacy that hospice caregivers experience. There can be the desire on the part of caregivers to experience that intimacy in all their meaningful relationships. It is no coincidence that there is little boredom experienced by hospice caregivers.

Finally, the challenge is to develop our caregiving skills and our human potential to the degree that our presence in a situation where a child is dying or grieving is made perhaps a bit more easy. The process of personal development is a continuing one. A hospice nurse for the past five years remarked about the constant impact of the work upon her being. Many stressful work settings do not encourage seasoned workers to stay. By contrast, in a hospice program of care an experienced worker is increasingly able to operate and react from a functional base of sensitivity and compassion. Just as growing older demands a certain degree of grace and courage, continued involvement in hospice care can allow us to become more and more ourselves.

The process of clarifying, transcending, and deepening of our experience of life is related to what we learn in relationship to the people for whom we care.

In her lovely book, *The Velveteen Rabbit,* Margery Williams (1981) gives us some idea of what the outcome of stress can be. The Rabbit asks the wise old Skin Horse what it means to be "real." Here is the response and the ensuing dialogue.

> "Real isn't how you are made," said the Skin Horse. "It's a thing that happens to you. When a child loves you for a long, long time, not just to play with, but REALLY loves you, then you become Real."
>
> "Does it hurt?" asked the Rabbit.
>
> "Sometimes," said the Skin Horse, for he was always truthful. "When you are Real you don't mind being hurt."
>
> "Does it happen all at once, like being wound up," he asked, "or bit by bit?"
>
> "It doesn't happen all at once," said the Skin Horse. "You become. It takes a long time. That's why it doesn't often happen to people who break easily, or have sharp edges, or who have to be carefully kept. Generally, by the time you are Real, most of your hair has been loved off, and your eyes drop out and you get loose in the joints and very shabby. But these things don't matter at all, because once you are Real you can't be ugly, except to people who don't understand."
>
> "I suppose you are Real?" said the Rabbit. And then he wished he had not said it, for he thought the Skin Horse might be sensitive. But the Skin Horse only smiled.
>
> "The Boy's Uncle made me Real," he said. "That was a great many years ago; but once you are Real you can't become unreal again. It lasts for always."*

References

Bluebond-Langner, M., *The Private Worlds of Dying Children.* Princeton, NJ: Princeton University Press, 1978.

Frankl, V. E., *Man's Search for Meaning.* New York: Pocket Books, 1959.

Harper, B. C., *Death: The Coping Mechanism of the Health Professional.* Greenville, SC: Southeastern University Press, 1977.

Imara, M., "Growing Through Grief," in C. A. Corr & D. M. Corr (Eds.), *Hospice Care: Principles and Practice.* New York: Springer; London: Faber and Faber, 1983, pp. 249–265.

*From Margery Williams, *The Velveteen Rabbit.* Philadelphia, PA, Running Press, Copyright © 1981. Used by Permission.

Kalish, R. A., "The Effects of Death Upon the Family," in L. Pearson (Ed.), *Death and Dying: Current Issues in the Treatment of the Dying Person.* Cleveland, OH: Case Western Reserve University Press, 1969, pp. 79–107.

Kollar, N., *Songs of Suffering.* Minneapolis, MN: Winston Press, 1982.

LaGrand, L. E., "Reducing Burnout in the Hospice and the Death Education Movement," *Death Education,* 1980, *4,* 61–76.

Lattanzi, M. E., "Coping with Work-Related Losses," *Personnel and Guidance Journal,* 1981, *59,* 350–351.

Lattanzi, M. E., "Learning and Caring: Education and Training Concerns," in C. A. Corr & D. M. Corr (Eds.), *Hospice Care: Principles and Practice.* New York: Springer; London: Faber and Faber, 1983a, pp. 223–236.

Lattanzi, M. E., Group exercises conducted in workshops and seminars taught in 1982.

Lattanzi, M. E., "Professional Stress: Adaptation, Coping, and Meaning," in J. C. Hanson & T. T. Frantz (Eds.), *Death and Grief in the Family.* Rockville, MD: Aspen Systems Corp., 1983b, pp. 95–106.

Martinson, I. M., "Introduction to the Home Care Project," in *Home Care for the Dying Child: Professional and Family Perspectives.* New York: Appleton-Century-Crofts, 1976, pp. 3–14.

Martinson, I. M., Armstrong, G. D., Geis, D. P., Anglim, M. A., Gronseth, E. C., MacInnis, H., Kersey, J. H., & Nesbit, M. E., "Home Care for Children Dying of Cancer," *Pediatrics,* 1978, *62,* 106–113.

Nouwen, H. J. M., *Out of Solitude.* Notre Dame, IN: Ave Maria Press, 1974.

Quint, J. C., *The Nurse and the Dying Patient.* New York: Macmillan, 1967.

Seligman, M. E. P., *Helplessness: On Depression, Development and Death.* San Francisco, CA: W. H. Freeman & Co., 1975.

Selye, H., *The Stress of Life.* New York: McGraw-Hill, 1956.

Walker, J. R., & Lattanzi, M. E., *Understanding Loss and Grief.* Boulder, CO: Boulder County Hospice, Inc., 1982.

White, W. L., "Managing Personal and Organizational Stress in Care of the Dying," in *Hospice Education Program for Nurses.* Hyattsville, MD: Health Manpower References, DHHS Publication No. HRA 81-27, 1981, pp. 291–337.

Williams, M., *The Velveteen Rabbit.* Philadelphia, PA: Running Press, 1981.

Index

Index

Abdellah, F. S., 49
Acting out by terminally ill children, 160–161
  by grieving children, 167, 204
Activities for terminally ill children, 26
Acute care facility, 13–14
  neonatal, 128. *See also* Neonatal Hospice Program
  See also Hospitalization of terminally ill children
Acute grief response, 253
Adult hospice care vs. pediatric hospice care, 7–10, 43
Alcoholics Anonymous (AA), 243
Amanda the Panda, 179–194
  Camp Amanda, 186–192
  Camp-A-Panda, 192–194
American Cancer Society, 71
Anger in grieving child, 208
Anticipating death
  neonatal, 140–142
  rehospitalization, 83
Anticipatory grief, 226–227
Art therapy, 18, 155–177. *See also* Expressive therapy
Autopsies, 83, 134, 141

Bach, S. R., 162
Bedrooms of inpatient units, 26
Bereaved Families of Ontario, 213*n.*
Bereavement, 101, 123, 219–220
  See also Grieving children; Grieving parents; Grieving staff; Mourning
Bluebond-Langner, M., 210, 211
Borkman, T., 256
Bowlby, J., 221

Cain, A. C., 214
Camp Amanda, 186–192
  funding, 193–194
Camp-A-Panda, 192–194
  funding, 193
Cancer, children with
  Camp-A-Panda, 192–194
  Candlelighters, 196, 238, 243–244, 249–251, 254–256, 258, 260
  home care for, 31–41, 65–86
Candlelighters, 196, 238, 243–244, 249–251, 254–256, 258
  newsletter, 260
Cardiac arrest, handling of, at home, 77
Caregivers
  Helen House, 111
  in home care programs, 68, 70
  needs of, 48–49
  in pediatric hospices, 9–10
  for respite care, 93–94, 96, 97–98
  see also Hospice caregivers; Hospital staff; Nursing services
Caregivers' stress, 261–276
  behavioral symptoms, 265

Caregivers' stress (*continued*)
being in relationships, importance of, 275–276
clinical experiences, 269–271
emotional, 264–265
grief, 264–265. *See also* Grieving staff
identification problems, 264
individual responses, 268–269
management of, 271–273
manifestations of, 265–266
mutual support for, 267–268
in neonatal deaths, 144–145
overinvolvement, 264
physical symptoms, 265
powerlessness, 264
preventive measures, 266–269
relationships, strains in, 266
role-related, 263–264
situational, 262–263
spiritual or value-related responses, 265–266
staff selection and, 266–267
staff supervision, 267
staff training and education, 267
suggested approaches to caring, 273–276
witnessing suffering, 264
Caring, definition of, 273
Certificate of Need, 23
Children
bereaved, *see* Grieving children
disabled, *see* Disabled children
dying, *see* Terminally ill children
as patients, distinctive elements of, 7–8
The Children's Hospital, Denver
Neonatal Hospice Program, 127–146. *See also* Neonatal Hospice Program
Childrens Hospital of Los Angeles (CHLA) home care program, 65–86
conclusion of services, 83–85
Crippled Childrens Services (CCS), 67
designing, 67–71
implementation of, 71–82
length of stay, 65
management of, 77–82
participants in, 65
preparation of program, 66–67
Chronically ill children, hospice care for, 114. *See also* Terminally ill children
Church groups and home care programs, 71
Clay, R. M., 112
Claypool, J., 259
Codden, P., 254
Collaboration model for care of the terminally ill, 50–59, 57 (fig.)
applying, 56, 58
assumptions of, 50–51
goals of, 52–53
intervention, 53–56
major components of, 52 (tab.)
recipients of, 53
values in, 51–52
Comfort of child at home, 76, 79, 124
Communication with life-threatened child
"open," 209–210
"protective," 209
Community response to death and dying, 241–242. *See also* Self-help groups
Community support and funding of respite care programs, 102
The Compassionate Friends (TCF), 137, 196, 238, 243–249, 252–258
newsletter, 260
policy statement, 254
Component development in pediatric hospice program, 23–27
Components of care, 10–11
Cooper, F., 244–247
Coordination of services
home care coordinator, *see* Home care coordinator
home care programs, 37–38
in hospitalization of terminally ill children, 52, 55–56
Cunningham, S., 43

Davidson, G. W., 227
Day/night care, 11, 12, 14
Death
  anticipating, 83–84, 140–142
  of children, response to, *see* Grieving parents
  children's impression of, 198–199. *See also* Expressive therapy; Grieving children
  denial of, 208
  finality of, cognitive problems with, 201–202
  at home, 83. *See also* Home care programs
  of parents, *see* Grieving children
  talking about, with children, 171, 174, 183, 186, 189–190
Denial
  of death, 208
  of terminal illness, 47
Dependent hospice model, 21
  formal organization, 23
Depression among terminally ill children, 161
Dimensions of care, 10–15
  child at home, 11–13
  child in health care facility, 13–14
  family after child's death, 14–15
Disabled children
  hospice care for, 114–115
  inpatient facilities for, 27
  respite care for, 89–90
Disorganization, definition of, 222
Disorientation, definition of, 222
Drama therapy, 18
Drawings, *see* Expressive therapy

Edmarc, 88–105. *See also* Respite care programs
Education
  of caregivers for terminally ill children, 52–53, 54–55, 131–132, 267
  in home care programs, 39
  in hospice objectives, 45
Emergencies, handling unplanned, at home, 76–77
Erikson, E., 215
Experiential knowledge, definition of, 256
Expressive therapy, 48, 155–177
  Ann, case example, 162–163, 163 (fig.)
  art therapy, 156, 157
  Billy and Carrie, case example, 165, 167
  components of, 156
  environment of, 159–160
  with grieving child, 167–176
  at home, 159
  at hospital, 159–160
  Jane, case example, 165, 166 (fig.)
  Jessica, case example, 171, 174–176, 175 (fig.), 176 (fig.)
  John, case example, 163–165, 164 (fig.)
  Kellie, case example, 169–171, 170 (fig.), 172 (fig.), 173 (fig.)
  levels of expression, 157
  premises of, 156
  with terminally ill child, 160–167
  therapeutic art process, 156–157
  understanding created expression, 157–159

Families of dying children, 120–124
  bereavement, *see* Grieving parents
  care provision by, 8
  distinctive elements of, 8–9
  follow-up services after death, 137–138, 142–144
  grief process, 14–15, 133–135, 137–144. *See also* Grieving parents
  helping others, 248–249. *See also* The Compassionate Friends
  home care, 11–13
  home care coordinator, conferring with, 73–74
  home care nurse dealing with needs of, 33–35, 81–82
  Home Care Project, Univ. of Minn., 32–35
  initial contact with home care team, 67–68

Families of dying children (*continued*)
needs of, 8–9, 33–35, 46–48, 81–82, 120–123. *See also* Home care programs; Respite care programs
in Neonatal Hospice Program, 133–135
nuclear, care problems of, 121
and respite care, 88, 90–93, 99–101
responsibilities of, 8
size, 8
Fears
of grieving children, 205–208
of terminally ill children, 161
Feasibility studies for pediatric hospice care, 19–22
Federal funds for respite care, 101–102
Fleming, S. J., 199
Formal organization of hospice program, 22–23
Frankl, V. E., 274
Freud, S., 199, 200
Funding
Camp Amanda and Camp-A-Panda, 193–194
Helen House, 109, 112
home care programs, 67, 71, 73
hospice programs, 22, 23
Neonatal Hospice Program, The Children's Hospital, Denver, 127*n.*
respite care programs, 101–104
Funeral arrangements, 83–84, 134, 141
Furman, E., 203, 204, 212

Grandparents, grieving parents and, 231–232
Grief
acute syndrome, 253
dynamics of, 221–222
features of, 219–220
see also Bereavement; Mourning
Grieving children (at death of sibling or parent), 155, 167–176, 186–187, 189–191, 195–196, 197–216
ability to express grief, 198–200
affective responses, 204–208
aggressiveness, 204
anger, 208
behavioral responses, 202–204
Camp Amanda, 186–192
cognitive responses, 201–202
communication during the dying process, effect of, 209–212
denial of death, 208
dependent behavior, 203–204
expressive therapy, 167–176. *See also* Expressive therapy
factors affecting outcome, 209–216
fear of abandonment and death, 205–208
fear of physicians, hospitals, and God, 208
identification with dead parent or sibling, 203
period of bereavement, 212–216
physiological responses, 201
remembering and longing, 203
searching for substitute parent, 203
Grieving parents, 14–15, 84–85, 101, 195–196, 219–239
abnormal grief, 223
adjustment, degree of, 234
anticipatory grief, 226–227
Candlelighters, 196, 238, 243–244, 249–251, 254–256, 258, 260
The Compassionate Friends, 137, 196, 238, 243–249, 252–258, 260
dynamics of grieving, 221–223
effect on daily functioning, 234–235
effect on employment, 235
effect on family friends, 231–232
effect on grandparents, 231–232
effect on marital relations, 229–230
effect on surviving siblings, 231. *See also* Siblings of dying children
guilt, 227
Home Care Project study of, 232–235
intensity of bereavement, period of, 232–234

model of parental grieving, 228–229, 228 (fig.)
mourning, 221–225. *See also* Mourning
neonatal deaths, 128, 133–135, 137–144
suggestions for helping, 236–238
Grieving staff, 144–145, 146, 264–265. *See also* Caregivers' stress
Grollman, E., 259
Guilt feelings
of dying children, 47–48
of grieving parents, 227
Gunther, F., 227

Handicapped children, *see* Disabled children
Harper, B. C., 266, 271–272
Hazzard, M. E., 50
Health professionals, *see* Caregivers
Helen House, Oxford, 62, 107–124
administration and finance, 112
aims of, 107–108
the building, 110
case histories, 116–120
children to be served, 113–116
emotional problems of children and their families, dealing with, 120–124
facilities and program, 110–112
founding of, 109
Helen, history of, 108–109
home care, 112
"hospice," definition of, 112–113
Joanne, history of, 119–120
liaison with other agencies and with families, 111
Mark, history of, 117–118
pattern of visits, 115
practical care of the child, 124
principles underlying care, 120–124
referrals, 115–116
Sammy, history of, 118–119
staff support, 112
Susanna, history of, 116–117
the team, 111
"terminal illness," definition of, 113
Helping groups, *see* Self-help groups
Hewett, J. H., 259
Hitchcock, V., 251
Home care coordinator
bringing child home, role in, 77–78
caregivers, securing, 68, 70
creation of position, 67
and implementation of program, 72 (tab.)
Home care nurse, 68, 70, 74–76
anticipating death, 83–84
and behavior problems of child, 80
community nurses, 66
consulting special expertise, 80–81
and daily activity pattern of child, 79–80
after death, visits, 84
first visit to home, 78
functions of, 33–36
and nutrition of child, 80
options and roles of, 74–76
parental needs, dealing with, 81
and physical comfort of child, 79
primary concerns of, 79–82
and psychological health of child, 79
qualifications of, 75
rewards and satisfactions of, 85
sibling needs, dealing with, 81
see also Nursing services
Home care programs, 11–13, 61–62, 65–86
administrative support for, 38
anticipating death, 83–84
bringing child home, 77–79
caregivers, selection of, 68, 70
caregivers' stress, *see* Caregivers' stress
Childrens Hospital of Los Angeles, 65–86
comfort of child as issue, 76, 79, 124
communication links with hospital, maintenance of, 78
conclusion of services, 83–85

Home care programs (*continued*)
coordination of services, 37–38, 67
coordination with hospital, 82
daily activity pattern of child, 79–80
after death, *see* Grieving parents
designing a, 67–71
emergencies, handling of, 76–77
family needs, dealing with, 81–82
funding of, 67, 71, 73
home care nurse, *see* Home care nurse
Home Care Project, Univ. of Minn., 31–41
and hospitalization, explaining alternatives between, 73–74
implementation, 71–77
institutionalization of, 37, 39
interdisciplinary hospice teams for, 68, 70
introducing, 71, 73–74
management, 77–82
medical support, degree of, 76–77
and nursing networks, 35–36
parental involvement, 38
preparing for a, 66–67
prerequisite conditions, 32
resistance to, 38
respite care, 90–96. *See also* Respite care
school teachers in, 71
sibling needs, dealing with, 81
special expertise needs, 80–81
for terminal cancer, 31–41
volunteers in, 71
Home Care Project, Univ. of Minn., 2, 31–41, 66
bereavement process study, 232–235
case study, 36–37
conferences with inpatient team, 82
institutionalization, 37–39
results of study, 32–36
Home health agencies, securing caregivers from, 66, 70
Hospice, definition of, 112–113
Hospice care
adult, *see* Adult hospice care
pediatric, *see* Pediatric hospice care
Hospice caregivers
coordination of care in hospital setting, 55–56
and education of hospital personnel in hospice practice, 54–55
in hospital setting, 52
see also Caregivers' stress
Hospice of Louisville, Kentucky, 2–3, 44–59
approach to improved care, 44–46
Hospice philosophy, collaboration model and, 49–56
Hospitalization of terminally ill children, 44–59
in anticipation of death, 83
collaboration model for improving care, 50–59
coordination with home care program, 82
coordination with hospice care, 55–56
home care vs., explaining alternatives to families, 73–74
interdisciplinary team approach, 49–50
needs of children and families, 46–48
needs of siblings, 48
needs of staff, 48–49
Hospital staff dealing with terminally ill children
education of, 52–53, 54–55
needs of, 48–49
needs of children and families, dealing with, 46–48
see also Caregivers' stress

Imara, M., 221, 273
Independent hospice model, 21
formal organization, 23
Infant Death Data Sheet, 134, 137, 149–151
Infant hospice programs, *see* Neonatal Hospice Program

Inpatient care, 13–14. *See also* Hospitalization of terminally ill children
Inpatient teams, conferences with home care teams, 82
Interdisciplinary team approach to terminal illness, 49–50
  for home care programs, 68, 70, 82
  Neonatal Hospice Program, 131–132, 145
International Work Group in Death, Dying and Bereavement
  assumptions, 50–51
  principles, 45–46, 52

Kaffman, M., 204
Kalish, R. A., 272
Karon, M., 210
Kollar, N., 264
Krell, R., 214, 215

LaGrand, L. E., 271
Lampl-deGroot, J., 200
Lay volunteers, *see* Volunteers
Legislative initiatives for home care programs, 39
Length of stay
  home care programs, 32, 65
  hospice programs, 7–8
  in program planning, 21
Lifton, R. J., 221–222
Lindemann, E., 253
Long-term home care program, St. Mary's Hospital for Children, 24 (tab.)

Mainstreaming, 89–90
  Edmarc, 89–90
  Helen House, 114–115
Manning, D., 238
Marital relations, effect of grieving on, 229–231
Martinson, I. M., 66, 212, 262
Maternal grieving, *see* Grieving parents
Media publicity for home care programs, 39
Medical support in home care programs, 31–32, 76–77
Miles, M. S., 227, 228
Miller, J. B. M., 199
Models for hospice care, 21–22
Moriarty, D. M., 199
Mourning, 199–200, 221–225
  abnormal grief, 223
  definition of, 199, 200, 221
  dynamics of grieving, 221–222
  goals of, 224–225
  tasks of, 223–224
  see also Grieving children; Grieving parents
Music therapy, 18

National Hospice Organization, 53
Neonatal care, hospice approach to, 62–63, 127–154
Neonatal Death Follow-up, 137, 152
Neonatal Hospice Program
  case studies, 138–142
  The Children's Hospital, Denver, 127–146
  decision-making process, 132–133
  effect of program on families, 138–144
  effect of program on staff, 144–145
  families, follow-up services for, 137–138, 142–144
  families, involvement of, 133–135
  the Family Room, 135–137
  Infant Death Data Sheet, 134, 137, 149–151
  life extension issues, 132–133
  Neonatal Death Follow-up, 137, 152
  Newborn Intensive Care Unit facilities, 130
  NICU floor plan, 135 (fig.)
  principles of, 129–130
  staff training and support, 131–132
Neonatal intensive care units (NICU), 127–128, 130, 135 (fig.)
  hospice principles, 128–129
Nouwen, H. J. M., 273
Nursing networks, 35–36

Nursing services
  for home care programs, 32–37, 66, 68, 70, 74–76
  Home Care Project, Univ. of Minn., 32–37
  options and roles for home care nurses, 74–76
  in pediatric hospice program, 16–17
  visiting nurse, 75
  see also Home care nurse

Occupational therapy, 18
Oehler, J., 141
Operational planning of hospice care, 22–23
Organ donations, 134, 135
Outpatient clinic care, 11, 12

Pain control in home care programs, 76
Palliative care, 6–7, 133
Parental fees, 103–104, 112. *See also* Funding
Parents
  death of, *see* Grieving children
  grieving, *see* Grieving parents
  see also Families of dying children
Parkes, C. M., 221
Pediatric home visit, suggested format for, 68, 69 (tab.)
Pediatric hospice care
  vs. adult, 43
  caregiver characteristics, 9–10
  after the child's death, 14–15, 84–85
  concept of, 5–6
  dimensions of care, 10–15
  distinctive elements of, 7–10
  Edmarc, 88–105. *See also* Respite care programs
  families of children, characteristics of, 8–9
  Helen House, 107–124
  home care, 11–13. *See also* Home care programs
  inpatient care, 13–14
  lack of, reasons for, 43–44
  and neonatal care, 127–146. *See also* Neonatal Hospice Program
  nursing services, 16–17
  physician services, 16
  program planning and development, 18–27
  and regulatory agencies, 10
  services to be provided, 15–18
  social work and counseling services, 17
  therapy services, 18. *See also* Expressive therapy
Pediatric nurses for home care programs, 68, 70. *See also* Home care nurses
Peppers, L. G., 259
Peterson, R., 238
Physical therapy, 18
Physician services in hospice program, 16
Piaget, J., 198
Planning and development of hospice program, 18–27
  detailed planning (component development), 23–27
  initial planning (feasibility), 19–22
  operational planning (formal organization), 22–23
Primary care nurse, 32–33. *See also* Home care nurse
Professional model of help vs. self-help groups, 256–258
Prognoses for terminally ill children, 21
Program planning, *see* Planning and development of hospice program
Publicity for home care programs, 39

Quality of care
  definition of, 52
  educating personnel in, 54–55
  for terminally ill children, 53, 55–56

Referrals, 22, 23
  Edmarc, 90–93
  Helen House, 115–116

Regulatory agencies and pediatric hospice care, 10
Rehospitalization in anticipation of death, 83
Reimbursement funding, *see* Funding
Reorganization, definition of, 222
Respiratory arrest at home, handling, 77
Respite care programs, 11, 12, 14, 62, 87–105
  Bereaved Parents Group, 101
  caregivers, 93–94, 96, 97–98
  case example, 94–95
  center-based, 96–99
  community support for, 102–103
  daily schedule, center-based, 98
  drop-in respite, 98–99
  Edmarc program, 87–105
  extended care program, 99
  facility equipment, center-based, 99
  families, needs of, 88
  families, referral, screening, and registration of, 90–93
  federal funds for, 101–102
  funding sources, 101–104
  Helen House, 107–108
  in-home, 90–96
  liability issues, 92, 96
  mainstreamed care, 89–90
  parent advisory board, 100
  parent fees, 103–104
  parent involvement, in center-based programs, 99–101
  parent support groups, 100
  referral system, 90–91
  registration process, 91–93
  screening process, 91
  siblings, care for, 93, 96–97
  staffing center-based care, 97–98
  state funds for, 101–102
  and the terminally ill child, 89
  volunteers in, 103

St. Christopher's Hospice, London, 113
St. Joseph's Hospice, London, 113
St. Mary's Hospital for Children, New York City, 2, 6, 19, 23, 24
  component development at, 26–27
  Palliative Care Center, 6–7
Saunders, C., 113
Schiff, H. S., 213, 215, 222, 260
School for home-bound children, 12–13
School teachers in home care programs, 71
Schwiebert, P., 141
Searching, definition of, 222
Self-help, definition of, 243
Self-help groups, 243–259
  professional intervention vs., 256–258
  support groups vs., 243
Selye, H., 261, 275
Separation anxiety, 89
Share, L., 209
Shneidman, E. S., 220
Shock and numbness, definition of, 221
Siblings of dying children, 122, 140–141
  bereavement, 212–215. *See also* Grieving children
  Camp Amanda, 186–192
  effect of parental grieving on, 231
  needs of, 48, 81
  respite care, 93, 96–97
Smith, A. A., 236
Social Adjustment Scale for bereaved parents, 213
Social work and counseling services in hospice care, 17. *See also* Caregivers' stress
Spinetta, J. J., 210–211
Staff
  Helen House, 111, 112
  Neonatal Hospice Program, 131–132
  respite care centers, 93–94, 96, 97–98
  see also Caregivers; Caregivers' stress; Hospital staff dealing with terminally ill children

State funds for respite care programs, 101–102
Stephens, S., 260
Stress, *see* Caregivers' stress; Grieving children; Grieving parents
Support groups vs. self-help groups, 243

Talking with children about death, 171, 174, 183, 186. *See also* Amanda the Panda; Expressive therapy
Terminal care, principles of, 45–46
Terminally ill, definition of, 113
Terminally ill children
  behavior problems of, 80
  Camp-A-Panda, 192–194
  community response to, 241–242
  daily activity pattern at home, 79–80
  initial contact with home care team, 67–68
  needs of, in hospital setting, 46–48
  nutrition of, at home, 80
  physical comfort of, at home, 76, 79, 124
  psychological health of, at home, 79
  and respite care, 89
  talking about dying with, 171, 174, 183, 186
Terminally ill parents, children's response to, *see* Grieving children
Therapy services in hospice program, 18. *See also* Expressive therapy
Title XX funds for respite care programs, 102
Toynbee, A., 220

United Way funding for respite care programs, 102

Vernick, J., 210
Visiting nurse, 75. *See also* Home care nurses
Volunteers
  for home care programs, 71
  in respite care programs, 103

Waechter, E. H., 85, 210
Williams, M., 276
Wilson, D. C., 211, 212
Withdrawal by terminally ill children, 161–162
Wolfenstein, M., 199–200
Worden, J. W., 200, 223

Yearning, definition of, 222